THE WASHINGTON MANUAL®

General Internal Medicine Consult

Third Edition

THE WASHINGTON MANUAL®

General Internal Medicine Consult
Third Edition

Editor

Thomas M. Ciesielski, MD

Instructor in Medicine
Division of Medical Education
Washington University School of Medicine
St. Louis, Missouri

Series Editor

Thomas M. De Fer, MD

Professor of Medicine
Division of Medical Education
Washington University School of Medicine
St. Louis, Missouri

Wolters Kluwer

Philadelphia · Baltimore · New York · London
Buenos Aires · Hong Kong · Sydney · Tokyo

Executive Editor: Rebecca Gaertner
Senior Product Development Editor: Kristina Oberle
Senior Production Project Manager: Alicia Jackson
Design Coordinator: Teresa Mallon
Senior Manufacturing Coordinator: Beth Welsh
Editorial Coordinator: Katie Sharp
Prepress Vendor: SPi Global

3rd edition

Copyright © 2017 by Department of Medicine, Washington University School of Medicine

Copyright © 2009, 2003 by Department of Medicine, Washington University School of Medicine
All rights reserved. This book is protected by copyright. No part of this book may be reproduced or transmitted in any form or by any means, including as photocopies or scanned-in or other electronic copies, or utilized by any information storage and retrieval system without written permission from the copyright owner, except for brief quotations embodied in critical articles and reviews. Materials appearing in this book prepared by individuals as part of their official duties as U.S. government employees are not covered by the above-mentioned copyright. To request permission, please contact Wolters Kluwer at Two Commerce Square, 2001 Market Street, Philadelphia, PA 19103, via email at permissions@lww.com, or via our website at lww.com (products and services).

9 8 7 6 5 4 3 2 1

Printed in China

Library of Congress Cataloging-in-Publication Data
Names: Ciesielski, Thomas, editor.
Title: The Washington manual general internal medicine consult / editor, Thomas Ciesielski.
Other titles: General internal medicine consult
Description: Third edition. | Philadelphia : Wolters Kluwer, [2017] | Includes bibliographical references and index.
Identifiers: LCCN 2016039528 | ISBN 9781496346322
Subjects: | MESH: Internal Medicine—methods | Handbooks
Classification: LCC RC55 | NLM WB 39 | DDC 616—dc23 LC record available at https://lccn.loc.gov/2016039528

This work is provided "as is," and the publisher disclaims any and all warranties, express or implied, including any warranties as to accuracy, comprehensiveness, or currency of the content of this work.

This work is no substitute for individual patient assessment based upon healthcare professionals' examination of each patient and consideration of, among other things, age, weight, gender, current or prior medical conditions, medication history, laboratory data and other factors unique to the patient. The publisher does not provide medical advice or guidance and this work is merely a reference tool. Healthcare professionals, and not the publisher, are solely responsible for the use of this work including all medical judgments and for any resulting diagnosis and treatments.

Given continuous, rapid advances in medical science and health information, independent professional verification of medical diagnoses, indications, appropriate pharmaceutical selections and dosages, and treatment options should be made and healthcare professionals should consult a variety of sources. When prescribing medication, healthcare professionals are advised to consult the product information sheet (the manufacturer's package insert) accompanying each drug to verify, among other things, conditions of use, warnings and side effects and identify any changes in dosage schedule or contraindications, particularly if the medication to be administered is new, infrequently used or has a narrow therapeutic range. To the maximum extent permitted under applicable law, no responsibility is assumed by the publisher for any injury and/or damage to persons or property, as a matter of products liability, negligence law or otherwise, or from any reference to or use by any person of this work.

LWW.com

To my family—Helen, Jack, and Charlotte—for your support during this process, and to Dr. Paula Ford Ciesielski and the late Dr. Peter Ford, for being my first mentors and teaching me that at the center of everything is the patient.

Contributors

Surachai Amornsawadwattana, MD
Fellow
Division of Gastroenterology
Washington University School of Medicine
St. Louis, Missouri

Anna Arroyo-Plasencia, MD
Assistant Professor of Medicine
Division of Hospital Medicine
Washington University School of Medicine
St. Louis, Missouri

Rachel H. Bardowell, MD
Assistant Professor of Medicine
Division of Hospital Medicine
Washington University School of Medicine
St. Louis, Missouri

Natalie C. Battle, MD
Instructor in Medicine
Division of Hospital Medicine
Washington University School of Medicine
St. Louis, Missouri

Melvin Blanchard, MD
Professor of Medicine
Division of Medical Education
Washington University School of Medicine
St. Louis, Missouri

Merilda O. Blanco-Guzman, MD
Fellow
Division of Infectious Diseases
Washington University School of Medicine
St. Louis, Missouri

Jaimie E. Bolda, MD
Resident
Division of Medical Education
Washington University School of Medicine
St. Louis, Missouri

Indra Bole, MD
Resident
Division of Medical Education
Washington University School of Medicine
St. Louis, Missouri

Steven H. Borson, MD
Resident
Division of Medical Education
Washington University School of Medicine
St. Louis, Missouri

Kelly M. Carlson, MD
Instructor in Medicine
Division of Hospital Medicine
Washington University School of Medicine
St. Louis, Missouri

Courtney D. Chrisler, MD
Instructor in Medicine
Division of Infectious Diseases
Washington University School of Medicine
St. Louis, Missouri

Thomas M. Ciesielski, MD
Instructor in Medicine
Division of Medical Education
Washington University School of Medicine
St. Louis, Missouri

Geoffrey Cislo, MD
Assistant Professor of Medicine
Division of Medical Education
Washington University School of Medicine
St. Louis, Missouri

William E. Clutter, MD
Associate Professor of Medicine
Division of Medical Education
Washington University School of Medicine
St. Louis, Missouri

John J. Cras, MD
Assistant Professor of Medicine
Division of Hospital Medicine
Washington University School of Medicine
St. Louis, Missouri

Stacy Dai, MD
Resident
Division of Medical Education
Washington University School of Medicine
St. Louis, Missouri

Thomas M. De Fer, MD
Professor of Medicine
Division of Medical Education
Washington University School of Medicine
St. Louis, Missouri

Melissa DeFoe, MD
Resident
Division of Medical Education
Washington University School of Medicine
St. Louis, Missouri

Erik R. Dubberke, MD
Associate Professor of Medicine
Division of Infectious Diseases
Washington University School of Medicine
St. Louis, Missouri

Gerome V. Escota, MD
Assistant Professor of Medicine
Division of Infectious Diseases
Washington University School of Medicine
St. Louis, Missouri

M. Phillip Fejleh, MD
Resident
Division of Medical Education
Washington University School of Medicine
St. Louis, Missouri

Emily Fondahn, MD
Assistant Professor of Medicine
Division of Medical Education
Washington University School of Medicine
St. Louis, Missouri

James Matthew Freer, MD
Assistant Professor of Medicine
Division of Hospital Medicine
Washington University School of Medicine
St. Louis, Missouri

Mark A. Gdowski, MD
Instructor in Medicine
Division of Medical Education
Washington University School of Medicine
St. Louis, Missouri

Anuradha Godishala, MD
Instructor in Medicine
Division of Hospital Medicine
Washington University School of Medicine
St. Louis, Missouri

Scott R. Goldsmith, MD
Resident
Division of Medical Education
Washington University School of Medicine
St. Louis, Missouri

Walter B. Gribben, MD
Instructor in Medicine
Division of Hospital Medicine
Washington University School of Medicine
St. Louis, Missouri

Patrick M. Grierson, MD, PhD
Resident
Division of Medical Education
Washington University School of Medicine
St. Louis, Missouri

Stephen Hasak, MD
Resident
Division of Medical Education
Washington University School of Medicine
St. Louis, Missouri

Kevin Hsueh, MD
Instructor in Medicine
Division of Infectious Diseases
Washington University School of Medicine
St. Louis, Missouri

Brett W. Jagger, MD
Fellow
Division of Infectious Diseases
Washington University School of Medicine
St. Louis, Missouri

Sushma Jonna, MD
Resident
Division of Medical Education
Washington University School of Medicine
St. Louis, Missouri

Caroline H. Kahle, MD
Assistant Professor of Medicine
Division of Hospital Medicine
Washington University School of Medicine
St. Louis, Missouri

Asrar Khan, MD
Resident
Division of Medical Education
Washington University School of Medicine
St. Louis, Missouri

Yevgeniy Khariton, MD
Resident
Division of Medical Education
Washington University School of Medicine
St. Louis, Missouri

Gina N. LaRossa, MD
Assistant Professor of Medicine
Division of Hospital Medicine
Washington University School of Medicine
St. Louis, Missouri

Eileen M. Lee, MD
Assistant Professor of Medicine
Division of Hospital Medicine
Washington University School of Medicine
St. Louis, Missouri

Lauren S. Levine, MD
Resident
Division of Medical Education
Washington University School of Medicine
St. Louis, Missouri

Stephen Y. Liang, MD
Assistant Professor of Medicine
Division of Infectious Diseases
Washington University School of Medicine
St. Louis, Missouri

Chien-Jung Lin, MD
Resident
Division of Medical Education
Washington University School of Medicine
St. Louis, Missouri

Michael Y. Lin, MD
Associate Professor of Medicine
Division of Hospital Medicine
Washington University School of Medicine
St. Louis, Missouri

David B. Liss, MD
Fellow
Division of Emergency Medicine
Washington University School of Medicine
St. Louis, Missouri

Adam Littich, MD
Instructor in Medicine
Division of Hospital Medicine
Washington University School of Medicine
St. Louis, Missouri

Robert J. Mahoney, MD
Associate Professor of Medicine
Division of Hospital Medicine
Washington University School of Medicine
St. Louis, Missouri

George Mansour, MD
Instructor in Medicine
Division of Hospital Medicine
Washington University School of Medicine
St. Louis, Missouri

Caline S. Mattar, MD
Fellow
Division of Infectious Diseases
Washington University School of Medicine
St. Louis, Missouri

Rachel K. McDonald, MD
Fellow
Division of Pulmonary Medicine
Washington University School of Medicine
St. Louis, Missouri

Cheryl R. McDonough, MD
Instructor in Medicine
Division of Hospital Medicine
Washington University School of Medicine
St. Louis, Missouri

Adam V. Meyer, MD
Assistant Professor of Medicine
Division of Hospital Medicine
Washington University School of Medicine
St. Louis, Missouri

Jennifer M. Monroy, MD
Assistant Professor of Medicine
Division of Immunology
Washington University School of Medicine
St. Louis, Missouri

Contributors | ix

Monalisa Mullick, MD
Assistant Professor of Medicine
Division of Hospital Medicine
Washington University School of Medicine
St. Louis, Missouri

Lemuel R. Non, MD
Fellow
Division of Infectious Diseases
Washington University School of Medicine
St. Louis, Missouri

Devin C. Odom, MD
Instructor in Medicine
Division of Hospital Medicine
Washington University School of Medicine
St. Louis, Missouri

Anupam S. Pande, MD
Fellow
Division of Infectious Diseases
Washington University School of Medicine
St. Louis, Missouri

Shadi Parsaei, MD
Instructor in Medicine
Division of Infectious Diseases
Washington University School of Medicine
St. Louis, Missouri

Vaiibhav Patel, MD
Resident
Division of Medical Education
Washington University School of Medicine
St. Louis, Missouri

Ashish Rastogi, MD
Resident
Division of Medical Education
Washington University School of Medicine
St. Louis, Missouri

Erin L. Reigh, MD
Fellow
Division of Allergy and Immunology
Washington University School of Medicine
St. Louis, Missouri

Hilary E. L. Reno, MD
Assistant Professor of Medicine
Division of Infectious Diseases
Washington University School of Medicine
St. Louis, Missouri

Lois F. Richard, MD
Assistant Professor of Medicine
Division of Hospital Medicine
Washington University School of Medicine
St. Louis, Missouri

Myra L. Rubio, MD
Associate Professor of Medicine
Division of Hospital Medicine
Washington University School of Medicine
St. Louis, Missouri

Joshua M. Saef, MD
Resident
Division of Medical Education
Washington University School of Medicine
St. Louis, Missouri

Maanasi Samant, MD
Resident
Division of Medical Education
Washington University School of Medicine
St. Louis, Missouri

Yeshika Sharma, MD
Resident
Division of Medical Education
Washington University School of Medicine
St. Louis, Missouri

Mosmi Surati, MD
Instructor in Medicine
Division of Hospital Medicine
Washington University School of Medicine
St. Louis, Missouri

Happy D. Thakkar, MD
Resident
Division of Medical Education
Washington University School of Medicine
St. Louis, Missouri

Mark S. Thoelke, MD
Associate Professor of Medicine
Division of Hospital Medicine
Washington University School of Medicine
St. Louis, Missouri

Megan E. Wren, MD
Associate Professor of Medicine
Division of Medical Education
Washington University School of Medicine
St. Louis, Missouri

Chairman's Note

Medical knowledge is increasing at an exponential rate, and physicians are being bombarded with new information at a pace that many find overwhelming. *The Washington Manual®* Subspecialty Consult Series was developed in this context for interns, residents, medical students, and other practitioners in need of readily accessible practical clinical information. This manual, therefore, provides an important resource in an era of information overload.

I would like to acknowledge the authors and editors who have contributed to this book, in particular, the manual's editor, Thomas M. Ciesielski, MD, and series editor, Thomas M. De Fer, MD. I'd also like to recognize Melvin Blanchard, MD, Chief of the Division of Medical Education in the Department of Medicine at Washington University, for his guidance and advice.

The efforts and outstanding skill of the lead authors are evident in the quality of the final product. I am confident that this series, including the *General Internal Medicine Consult*, will meet its desired goal of providing practical knowledge that can be directly applied to improving patient care.

Victoria Fraser, MD
Adolphus Busch Professor of Medicine
Chairman of Medicine
Washington University School of Medicine
St. Louis, Missouri

Preface

I am pleased to release this third edition of *The Washington Manual® General Internal Medicine Consult*. This manual is intended to be primarily used by residents who are called on to perform inpatient consults, for medical students working on an inpatient medicine service, and for specialists seeking information on the management of general medicine issues. The overall structure has been maintained from the last edition; however, each area has been updated, and a chapter on venous thromboembolic disease has been added.

This manual is not an in-depth review of hospital medicine. It is not possible to address the breadth of problems faced by today's hospitalist providers in a manual of this size. The content area was chosen based largely on the common general internal medicine consults requested at Barnes-Jewish Hospital and the Washington University School of Medicine. This approach allows me to focus the content within the provided space. It is a balance to provide adequate information in a readable clinical text of manageable size. Hopefully, this balance has been achieved.

This manual is part of series of subspecialty manuals published by Washington University and Lippincott Williams & Wilkins. The chapters are authored by residents, fellows, and faculty at Washington University School of Medicine. Some material contained herein is partially adapted from chapters from our other manuals and publications.

The medical management of many common problems remains an ongoing area of debate and discussion. This is what allows our profession to be progressive, dynamic, and exciting. This also means that not every physician will agree on management in even the most common clinical encounters. The guidelines proposed here are either those followed by our own clinical services or the most accepted approaches to management based on available evidence. On topics of great debate, we have chosen to present the appropriate clinical evidence and, when available, official guidelines advocated by major medical organizations. Clinicians, however, must decide which evaluations and interventions are most appropriate.

I have many people I would like to thank for the creation of this manual. First, my department chair, Dr. Victoria Fraser, has been an incredible role model in patient care, leadership, research, and education. My division chief, Dr. Melvin Blanchard, has been instrumental to my success and career development. Dr. Tom De Fer offered exceptional mentorship throughout this process. I would also like to offer my thanks to all the contributing authors and editors for their hard work and dedication. Katie Sharp has also been a wonderful resource.

T. M. C.

Contents

Contributors **vi**
Chairman's Note **x**
Preface **xi**

General Consultative Principles **1**
Caroline H. Kahle and Gina N. LaRossa

PART I. GENERAL ISSUES

1. Approach to Perioperative Care **7**
   Adam V. Meyer and Rachel H. Bardowell

2. Approach to Edema **29**
   Yevgeniy Khariton and Lois F. Richard

PART II. CARDIOVASCULAR

3. Approach to the Patient with Chest Pain **37**
   Anuradha Godishala

4. Acute Coronary Syndromes **44**
   Adam Littich

5. Approach to the Patient with Syncope **60**
   James Matthew Freer

6. Management of Heart Failure **68**
   Mark A. Gdowski

7. Atrial Fibrillation **80**
   Kelly M. Carlson

8. Anticoagulation and Surgery **90**
   Happy D. Thakkar and Mark S. Thoelke

PART III. PULMONARY

9. Dyspnea **99**
   Rachel H. Bardowell and Adam V. Meyer

10. Chronic Obstructive Lung Disease **103**
    Maanasi Samant and Thomas M. Ciesielski

11. Asthma **109**
    Jaimie E. Bolda and Walter B. Gribben

12. Solitary Pulmonary Nodule **119**
    Rachel K. McDonald and Thomas M. Ciesielski

PART IV. GASTROENTEROLOGY

13. Approach to Nausea and Vomiting **127**
    Cheryl R. McDonough

14. Approach to Gastrointestinal Bleeding **134**
    Cheryl R. McDonough

15. Approach to Abdominal Pain **143**
    Surachai Amornsawadwattana

16. Approach to Abnormal Liver Enzymes **150**
    James Matthew Freer

PART V. NEPHROLOGY

17. Approach to Acute Kidney Injury **159**
    Joshua M. Saef and Melvin Blanchard

18. Approach to Hyperkalemia and Hypokalemia **166**
    Stacy Dai and Melvin Blanchard

19. Approach to Hyponatremia and Hypernatremia **174**
    Asrar Khan and John J. Cras

20. Approach to the Patient with Hematuria **184**
    Melissa DeFoe and Melvin Blanchard

PART VI. INFECTIOUS DISEASE

21. Pneumonia **191**
    Indra Bole and Mark S. Thoelke

22. Urinary Tract Infections **196**
    Caline S. Mattar and Stephen Y. Liang

23. Cellulitis 200
    Brett W. Jagger and Myra L. Rubio

24. Osteomyelitis 204
    Kevin Hsueh

25. Approach to the Patient with Fever 209
    Anupam S. Pande and Stephen Y. Liang

26. Bacteremia 217
    Shadi Parsaei

27. Intravascular Catheter Infections 224
    Lemuel R. Non and Gerome V. Escota

28. Endocarditis 228
    Courtney D. Chrisler

29. Meningitis 237
    Steven H. Borson and Hilary E. L. Reno

PART VII. NEUROLOGY

30. Approach to Altered Mental Status 245
    Vaiibhav Patel and Thomas M. De Fer

31. Approach to the Patient with Vertigo 252
    Yeshika Sharma and Robert J. Mahoney

32. Approach to the Carotid Bruit 257
    Chien-Jung Lin and Megan E. Wren

PART VIII. HEMATOLOGY

33. Approach to Anemia 265
    Devin C. Odom

34. Thrombocytopenia 272
    Scott R. Goldsmith and George Mansour

35. Approach to a Prolonged Prothrombin Time/Partial Thromboplastin Time 279
    Patrick M. Grierson and Natalie C. Battle

36. Venous Thromboembolism 283
    Ashish Rastogi and Emily Fondahn

PART IX. ONCOLOGY

37. Pain Control in the Cancer Patient 297
    Eileen M. Lee

38. Neutropenic Fever 306
    Merilda O. Blanco-Guzman and Erik R. Dubberke

PART X. ENDOCRINOLOGY

39. Inpatient Diabetes Management 313
    Sushma Jonna and Michael Y. Lin

40. Thyroid Diseases 319
    Monalisa Mullick

41. Adrenal Insufficiency 329
    M. Phillip Fejleh and Mark S. Thoelke

42. Approach to the Adrenal Incidentaloma 333
    Lauren S. Levine and William E. Clutter

PART XI. RHEUMATOLOGY

43. Approach to the Patient with Positive Antinuclear Antibodies 339
    Adam Littich

44. Approach to Low Back Pain 346
    Mosmi Surati

PART XII. ALLERGY AND IMMUNOLOGY

45. Anaphylaxis 357
    Erin L. Reigh and Jennifer M. Monroy

46. Drug Reactions 360
    Jennifer M. Monroy

PART XIII. TOXICOLOGY

47. Alcohol Withdrawal 367
    Stephen Hasak and Geoffrey Cislo

48. General Toxicology and Opioid Intoxication and Withdrawal 374
    David B. Liss and Anna Arroyo-Plasencia

Index 381

General Consultative Principles

Caroline H. Kahle and Gina N. LaRossa

INTRODUCTION

Medical consultation is, fundamentally, the provision of internal medicine expertise to patients who are currently under the care of physicians not trained in internal medicine. While seemingly straightforward, the rendering of this service can at times be cumbersome and politically difficult. Common problems include disagreements regarding the relative importance of the medical issues compared to the problem for which the patient is being treated by the specialist, poor communication between the referring and consulting physicians, and lack of comfort in addressing the medical illness in the setting of a concurrent "nonmedical" problem. Overcoming these barriers and improving patient care is the duty of the medical consultant. Goldman et al.[1] suggested guiding principles for effective medical consultation in their "Ten Commandments." These concepts form the basis of the suggested approach to consultation that follows.

GENERAL PRINCIPLES

Determine the Question Being Asked

This is the first and most important task in providing any consultative service. Although the issue may seem obvious, disagreement may occur between the referring and consulting physicians regarding the clinical question. Direct communication between the services is essential if this is to be successfully avoided. Although it may be common practice, orders requesting consultations placed in the chart (and subsequently called by a secretary) should not be the sole initial communication between referring and consulting services. Ideally, the requesting service will call directly. If not, it is the duty of the consultant to contact the referring physician to discuss the clinical scenario and resulting question.

Not uncommonly, the clinical question is initially somewhat vague, and this is frequently a source of frustration for medical consultants. It must be remembered, however, that the precise problem may not be clear to the physician requesting the consult. Indeed, this may be the very reason a consult is being requested. Again, direct communication between the physicians involved is essential to resolve these difficulties. A series of diplomatic questions by the consultant will likely be useful in discerning the problem:

- What is the problem for which the patient is seeing you and what is the current status of that problem?
- What is the patient's medical history and are any of those problems out of control?
- Is the patient having a new problem?
- What are your major concerns and is there a problem on which we should focus?
- How can we best serve you?

On occasion, the requesting service will be unable to articulate a precise question even with the above prompting. Accepting that the physician and patient are in need of your expertise in this scenario is important to avoid frustration. An initial thoughtful evaluation of the patient usually reveals where the internist can be of assistance and where subsequent efforts should be focused.

Periodically, it will be clear after the introductory conversation with the referring physician that the clinical problem is beyond the scope of practice of a general medical consultant. For example, if a patient appears to be suffering an ST segment elevation myocardial infarction, there is no value to delaying the needed cardiology consultation by first reviewing the case. Under these circumstances, assistance in arranging timely consultation by the needed subspecialist is appropriate. More common, however, is the situation where the need and benefit of a general medical consult is unclear. One should err on the side of caution and evaluate the patient in this circumstance. This is much more likely to result in the appropriate decisions being made.

Establish Urgency

Although all consults should be seen in a timely fashion, some are clearly more urgent than others. This is of particular importance with regard to off-hours consultation requests. Emergent consults should, of course, be seen emergently without regard to time of day. Some, however, can clearly be deferred until regular hours. Discussion of the patient's clinical status with the requesting service is typically the best way to determine the proper approach. Appropriate triage can still be difficult, particularly when the referring service is unfamiliar with the management of the problem for which the consult is being requested. Under these circumstances, evaluating the patient is usually necessary. Regardless, the referring physician should be made aware of the time frame within which the consultation can be expected.

There will at times be consults that are of relative urgency based on nonclinical issues, such as surgical scheduling. While these consults cannot always be provided in a truly urgent fashion, the consultation should be completed as soon as feasible. Bear in mind that it is the patient who suffers most if a surgery is canceled or a discharge delayed because a medical consultation is still pending.

Look for Yourself

The recommendations of a medical consult should result from a thorough evaluation of the patient by the consultant. It is the responsibility of the medical consultant to independently gather and review the relevant clinical information. An independent history and physical examination should be performed, and relevant records and laboratory data should be reviewed from primary sources.

Although this may be time consuming, important information that was previously unrecognized can frequently be obtained. Never rely on the findings of others, which may lead to false assumptions and inappropriate recommendations.

Be as Brief as Appropriate

Overly long consult notes with long-winded recommendations will be difficult for the referring service to interpret. This will inevitably lead to poor implementation of the recommendations buried within the consultation. A succinct history and physical examination with a concise differential diagnosis and clearly marked recommendations will be easier for the requesting physician to follow.

Be Specific

Although brevity is important, so is clarity in the recommendations for management. Be certain that the medical problem being addressed is clearly stated and the management recommended exact. It should not be assumed that the referring physician will be familiar with drug choices and dosing, for example. Specific medications and dosing should be delineated (e.g., "start carvedilol 3.125 mg po bid" instead of "start β-blocker"). Similarly, specifics regarding recommended laboratory testing should be provided.

Provide Contingency Plans

It is the nature of medicine that initial management strategies will not always be successful and that recommended testing will lead to abnormal results. Unless one wishes to be called with every issue (or worse still, find that they have not been addressed until the patient is seen again), these situations should be anticipated and recommendations for their management provided. Of course, adhering to the tenet of brevity, not every eventuality can be addressed. Focus on those that are most likely and leave contact information in case questions arise.

Honor Thy Turf

As generalists, medical consultants frequently feel an obligation to address all of a patient's issues. In the role of consultant, however, it is most important to address the question asked, frequently leaving other, less important issues to be resolved later. Of course, should an urgent issue unrelated to the consultation question be discovered, it is appropriate to address it. Deciding what is and what is not important to address, particularly with medical–legal concerns omnipresent, is part of the art of being a consultant. Good communication with the primary service and arranging appropriate follow-up for unaddressed issues will typically resolve these dilemmas.

A related issue is determining the extent of the consultant's role in the care of the patient. For example, should the consultant write orders? Who will review laboratory results expected during off hours? Determining the expectations of the referring service is paramount to resolving these questions. Poor patient care and serious liability issues can occur should these questions be left unanswered. Again, there is no substitute for good communication between physicians.

Teach with Tact

Commonly, services will request medical consultations for uncomplicated medical issues. It must be remembered that physicians requesting medical consultations are not trained in internal medicine. Therefore, what are seen as straightforward medical issues by the consultant likely do not seem so clear cut to the requesting service. If they were comfortable managing the issue, there would not have been a consult! In these situations, the medical consultant should share his or her expertise gracefully. Condescension is never appropriate.

Follow-up

Most medical consultations will require at least one, if not several, follow-up visits. In many cases, the diagnosis will remain in question or the results of recommended therapies will have to be assessed. Moreover, adherence to recommendations is improved when follow-up visits are made. Should there be issues with compliance by the primary service, these should be resolved by direct discussion. Typically, there are well-founded reasons for recommendations not being followed, but this may also stem from a simple oversight. Both are best addressed via a simple conversation rather than chart notes. At teaching hospitals, attending to attending conversations may be necessary to resolve conflicts. Disparaging remarks should never be placed in the chart.

Communication, Communication, Communication

There is little else as important as communication between physicians who are caring for the same patient. Many questions can be answered and problems avoided if physicians merely speak directly to each other. Many institutions have a cultural bias against calling or paging other physicians. It is the belief of the authors that this is not in the best interests of patient care and should be overcome. Recommendations for management, particularly if viewed as critical, should be communicated directly to the requesting physician. One should not assume that a consult note will be read in a timely fashion. As has been suggested many times throughout this chapter, there is no substitute for direct personal communication.

CONCLUSION

Adherence to the above principles will assist in successful completion of the medical consultation. Not addressed, however, is the last issue raised as a barrier to effective medical consultation in the introductory paragraph to this chapter: the consultant's lack of comfort in addressing medical issues while the patient is being treated for another illness. The authors of this manual hope that the chapters that follow will allow readers to overcome this obstacle as they seek to improve patient care in the role of medical consultant.

REFERENCE

1. Goldman L, Lee T, Rudd P. Ten commandments for effective consultations. *Arch Intern Med* 1983;143:1753.

General Issues

Approach to Perioperative Care

Adam V. Meyer and Rachel H. Bardowell

INTRODUCTION

- The main focus of the preoperative evaluation is to identify those patients at increased risk for perioperative morbidity and mortality.
- The role of the medical consultant is to risk-stratify patients, determine the need for further evaluation, prescribe possible interventions, and optimize chronic medical conditions to mitigate risk.
- Preoperative consultations often focus on cardiac risk, but it is essential to remember that poor outcomes can result from significant disease in other organ systems. Evaluation of the entire patient is necessary to provide optimal perioperative care.

Preoperative Cardiac Evaluation

GENERAL PRINCIPLES

Epidemiology

- Of the 200 million surgeries performed worldwide each year, 1 million patients will die in the 30-day postoperative period.[1] Depending on the definition of cardiac complication, type of noncardiac surgery performed, and population studied, cardiac complication rates can be as high as 5%.[2]
- Of those who have a perioperative myocardial infarction (MI), the risk of in-hospital mortality is estimated to be 10–15%.[3]

Pathophysiology

- Autopsy data suggest that fatal perioperative MIs occur via the same mechanisms as nonperioperative MIs.[4]
- Type 1 (plaque rupture) and type 2 MIs (oxygen supply–demand mismatch) have both been documented.
- The distribution between type 1 and type 2 MIs in the perioperative period is not entirely clear; however, one angiographic study found evidence of plaque rupture (type 1) in up to 50% of patients undergoing noncardiac surgery.[5]
- Oxygen supply–demand mismatch physiology is frequently associated with tachycardia in the perioperative period.[6] Hypotension and anemia can also contribute to this.

DIAGNOSIS

Clinical Presentation

History

The focus of the history is to identify factors and comorbid conditions that will affect perioperative risk. Various risk stratification models have been developed, but in general, each focuses on the identification of known cardiovascular disease or one of its risk factors. Eliciting signs or symptoms of active cardiac disease is of particular importance.

- **Evidence of active cardiac conditions:**
  - Unstable angina or acute coronary syndrome
  - Recent MI (within 60 days if no coronary intervention)
  - Symptoms of decompensated congestive heart failure (CHF)
  - Significant arrhythmias (does *not* include chronic, rate-controlled atrial fibrillation)
  - Severe valvular disease
- **Other significant risk factors:**
  - Preexisting, stable coronary artery disease (CAD)
  - Stable CHF
  - Diabetes mellitus
  - Prior cerebrovascular accident (CVA) or transient ischemic attack (TIA)
  - Renal insufficiency (creatinine >1.5 or 2, depending on risk calculator)
  - Intra-abdominal, intrathoracic, or vascular surgery

Physical Examination
A complete physical exam is essential. Specific attention should be paid to:

- Vital signs, particularly blood pressure (BP) and evidence of **hypertension**.
  - Systolic blood pressure (SBP) <180 and diastolic blood pressure (DBP) <110 mm Hg are generally considered acceptable with no significant increase in cardiac risk.
  - It may be reasonable to delay surgery for SBP >180 or DBP >110 if it is a new diagnosis of hypertension or there is evidence of end organ damage.[7]
- Murmurs suggestive of **significant valvular lesions**, particularly aortic stenosis (AS). Symptomatic stenotic lesions such as mitral stenosis and AS are thought to be associated with the greatest risk.
- **Aortic stenosis** (AS).
  - **Symptomatic** severe AS (valve area <1.0 cm^2 or mean gradient ≥40 mm Hg) is associated with increased perioperative MI and 30-day mortality.[8,9]
  - The perioperative risk for **asymptomatic**, moderate, and severe AS appears to be less, and no further intervention is required prior to elective low- and elevated-risk surgery.[9,10]
- **Mitral stenosis.**
  - Percutaneous balloon commissurotomy should be performed prior to elective surgery for patients with severe mitral stenosis who meet standard criteria for intervention.[9]
  - Elevated risk of noncardiac surgery can likely be performed on patients with **asymptomatic** severe mitral stenosis who don't meet criteria for percutaneous intervention.[9]
- Symptomatic mitral regurgitation and aortic regurgitation are generally tolerated perioperatively and can be managed medically.
- For all significant valvular lesions, the need for **endocarditis prophylaxis** should be considered.
- Evidence of CHF (elevated jugular venous pulse [JVP], crackles, S3, etc.).

Diagnostic Testing

12-Lead ECG
- Routine preoperative ECG testing is not indicated in asymptomatic patients prior to low-risk surgery.
- The 2014 American College of Cardiology/American Heart Association (ACC/AHA) guidelines make the following recommendations:
  - It is reasonable to obtain a preoperative ECG in patients with known CAD, cardiac risk factors, or structural heart disease undergoing a surgery with elevated risk.[9]
  - Asymptomatic patients undergoing a surgery with elevated risk may benefit from a preoperative baseline ECG, but studies are conflicting on the utility of this.[9,11]

Imaging
- In general, the indications for echocardiographic evaluation in the preoperative setting are no different than in the nonoperative setting. **An echocardiogram is not routinely necessary**.
- New murmurs found on physical exam suggestive of significant underlying valvular disease should be evaluated by an echocardiogram.
- An assessment of left ventricular (LV) function should be considered when there is clinical concern for undiagnosed or worsening CHF, or any new dyspnea of unknown origin.[9]

Diagnostic Testing
Stress testing should be guided by an assessment of preoperative risk as detailed below (see section on Risk Stratification). Routine stress evaluation of all patients undergoing surgery is not warranted and, in general, not indicated for low-risk noncardiac surgery.

- **Exercise testing**:
  - Patients must be able to walk on a treadmill and exercise to 85% of their predicted maximal heart rate.
  - Baseline ECG must be interpretable. The presence of a left bundle-branch block should prompt pharmacologic stress testing instead.
  - Exercise ECG stress testing (no imaging):
    - Although it is not as frequently pursued, this test can still be useful.
    - Baseline ECG should have no abnormalities that preclude interpretation of the test (e.g., LV strain, ST segment depressions >1 mm).
- **Exercise stress testing with imaging** (echo or nuclear perfusion):
  - Neither imaging modality is clearly superior to the other for purposes of risk stratification.
  - Patient comorbidities (e.g., obesity impeding echo windows) and additional questions to be answered (e.g., valvular disease making an echo more useful) should be considered in selecting the modality.
- **Pharmacologic stress testing**:
  - Vasodilator nuclear perfusion imaging and dobutamine echocardiography are the generally available options.
  - Neither is clearly superior to the other for risk stratification.
  - Consideration must be given to patient comorbidities that make utilization of a modality's pharmacologic agent undesirable (e.g., supraventricular arrhythmias with dobutamine and bronchospasm with adenosine).

Risk Stratification

The ACC/AHA published revised guidelines for perioperative cardiac evaluation and management in 2014, and these are described in Figure 1-1.[9]

Step 1: Establish the Urgency of Surgery

- Emergency surgery (within 6 hours) warrants no further testing.
- As time allows, evaluate preoperatively, and suggest management strategies.
- It is important to note that many surgeries, though not absolutely emergent, are urgent (within 6–24 hours) and are unlikely to allow for a time-consuming evaluation.

Step 2: Assess for Active Cardiac Conditions

- As defined above (see section on History):
  - Acute coronary syndrome (ST-segment-elevation MI [STEMI], non–ST-segment-elevation MI [NSTEMI], unstable angina, recent MI)

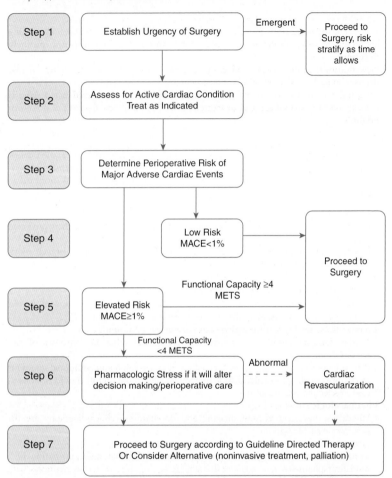

FIGURE 1-1 Algorithm for preoperative cardiac evaluation for noncardiac surgery. MACE, major adverse cardiac event; MET, metabolic equivalent. (Adapted from Fleisher LA, Fleischmann KE, Auerbach AD, et al. 2014 ACC/AHA guideline on perioperative cardiovascular evaluation and management of patients undergoing noncardiac surgery: a report of the American College of Cardiology/American Heart Association Task Force on practice guidelines. *J Am Coll Cardiol* 2014;64:e77–137.)

- Decompensated heart failure
- Unstable arrhythmias
- Severe valvular disease
- Delaying surgery to allow for further management of these conditions is recommended.

Step 3: Determine Perioperative Risk of Major Adverse Cardiac Events

- It is important to determine the risks of major adverse cardiac events (MACE) in the perioperative period.

- The clinical risk factors are adapted from the **Revised Cardiac Risk Index** (RCRI)[12–14]:
  - Ischemic heart disease
  - History of TIA or CVA
  - History of CHF
  - Renal insufficiency (serum creatinine ≥ 2.0)
  - Diabetes mellitus requiring insulin
  - Surgical risk—defined as intraperitoneal, intrathoracic, or suprainguinal vascular surgery
- Patients with **one or no clinical risk factors** are at low risk (<0.9%) and may proceed to surgery without further testing.
- Patients with **two or more clinical risk factors** are at an elevated risk of adverse cardiac events, particularly with vascular surgery. The risks and benefits of further cardiac testing should be considered.
- The RCRI may not effectively predict risk associated with vascular surgery.[14]
- The American College of Surgeons (ACS) National Surgical Quality Improvement Program (NSQIP) risk calculators may better determine cardiac risk associated with vascular surgery; however, the surgical risk calculator has >20 risk inputs, which may be cumbersome or not available (http://riskcalculator.facs.org/RiskCalculator/, last accessed 9/7/16).[15,16]

Step 4: Patients at Low Risk

- Low-risk surgery is defined as a procedure with combined patient and procedural risk <1% MACE.
- Patients can generally undergo low-risk procedures without further evaluation.

Step 5: Evaluation of Patients at Elevated Risk

- Elevated risk surgery is defined as a procedure with combined patient and procedural risk >1% MACE.
- The 2014 AHA/ACC perioperative guidelines have combined previously labeled intermediate- and high-risk procedures into this category due to similar management recommendations.
- Assess the patient's functional capacity.
  - Patients with good functional capacity ≥ 4 metabolic equivalents of task (MET) are unlikely to suffer serious cardiovascular complications and can proceed to surgery.[9]
  - Poor functional capacity (<4 METs) is associated with an increased risk of perioperative cardiac events.[17]
  - Functional capacity can be reliably estimated by patient self-report of daily activities.[18,19]
  - Table 1-1 highlights METs for certain activities.

Step 6: Evaluation of Patients at Elevated Risk with Poor or Unknown Functional Capacity

- It is important to develop a plan for patients at elevated risk, MACE > 1%, and poor (<4 METs) or an unknown functional capacity.

TABLE 1-1 METABOLIC EQUIVALENTS (METs) FOR CERTAIN ACTIVITIES

METs	Representative Activities
≥ 4	Walking at 4 mph on level ground, climbing stairs, climbing hills, riding a bicycle at 8 mph, golfing, bowling, throwing a baseball/football, carrying 25 pounds (groceries from the store to the car), scrubbing the floor, raking leaves, mowing the lawn
>7	Jogging at 5 mph on level ground, carrying a 60-pound object

- Pharmacologic stress testing may be indicated if the additional diagnostic information will affect management decisions.
- Any plan for preoperative revascularization should take into account the limitations discussed below.

Step 7: Proceeding to Surgery in Patients at Elevated Risk

- Many patients with elevated perioperative risk will proceed to surgery without pharmacologic stress testing.
- Guideline-directed medical therapy (GDMT) should be followed in all patients regardless of testing.
- Alternative therapies such as noninvasive treatments or palliation should be considered in patients at greatest risk of a cardiac complication.

TREATMENT

Revascularization

The best available data on preoperative revascularization come from the CARP trial—a prospective study of patients scheduled to undergo vascular surgery.[20]

- All patients studied had angiographically proven significant CAD.
- Patients were randomized to revascularization (coronary artery bypass grafting [CABG] in 41% and percutaneous coronary intervention [PCI] in 59%) versus no revascularization.
- Notable exclusions from the study population were patients found to have significant left main disease, severe LV dysfunction, severe AS, and the presence of severe coexisting illnesses.
- There was no difference between the groups in the occurrence of MI or death at 30 days or in mortality with long-term follow-up.
- **Based on these results, routine coronary revascularization as a method of decreasing perioperative cardiac risk is not recommended**. It is important to identify those high-risk subsets who may obtain a survival benefit from revascularization independent of their need for noncardiac surgery in accordance with GDMT.
- Additional considerations in patients **who have undergone PCI preoperatively** apply:
  - If a **bare metal stent** is utilized, elective noncardiac surgery should not be done in the first 30 days following PCI.[21,22] This is thought to be largely due to increased risk of in-stent restenosis.
  - Elective noncardiac surgery should be delayed 12 months after placement of **drug-eluting stents (DES)**, especially if dual antiplatelet therapy cannot be discontinued perioperatively.[9,21,23] Consideration of surgery 6 months post DES is reasonable in certain circumstances after discussion with the patient's cardiologist.[24]
  - For angioplasty alone, a 2-week delay is recommended.[9]

Medical Therapy

- **β-Blockers**
  - Initial interest into the cardioprotective benefit of β-blockers in the perioperative setting was based on relatively small studies that showed favorable cardiac risk and mortality benefit.
  - However, several notable subsequent studies failed to demonstrate clear benefit in patients with diabetes undergoing noncardiac surgeries and in vascular surgery populations.[25–27]
  - Most recently, the large POISE trial (8351 patients) demonstrated an increase in total mortality and strokes in the treatment group (perioperative metoprolol) despite a decrease in cardiac events.[28]

- The current ACC/AHA recommendations for perioperative β-blockade are as follows[9]:
  - β-blockers should be continued perioperatively for patients already on chronic β-blocker therapy (class 1).
  - It may be reasonable to begin perioperative β-blockers in patients with intermediate- or high-risk ischemia noted on stress test (IIb), patients with three or more RCRI risk factors (IIb), and patients with long-term indication for β-blocker therapy (IIb).
- If initiating therapy, β-blockers should be started >1 day prior to and **not on the day of surgery**.
- Attention should be paid to the presence of any contraindications to β-blocker use.
- **α2-Agonists**: Based on the POISE-2 trial, there is no indication for starting α-2 agonists perioperatively for noncardiac surgery. α-2 Agonists showed no reduction in risk of nonfatal MI or death, but there was an increase in nonfatal cardiac arrest and hypotension.[29]
- **Statins**: Current studies suggest a likely benefit to the perioperative use of statins.
  - Reduced in-hospital mortality associated with statin use was demonstrated in a retrospective cohort study of patients undergoing a variety of major noncardiac surgeries.[30]
  - A retrospective cohort evaluating statins in noncardiac nonvascular surgery showed reduction in the 30-day mortality in the treatment group.[31]
  - Current recommendations:
    - Statins should be continued perioperatively in patients on chronic statin therapy.
    - Patients undergoing vascular surgery may benefit from starting a statin perioperatively.[9,32,33]
    - Statin therapy may be started perioperatively in patients undergoing elevated-risk surgeries if indicated in guideline-directed therapy.[9]
- **Aspirin**
  - Traditionally, aspirin is withheld for ~1 week prior to invasive procedures to minimize bleeding risk.
  - However, some evidence suggests that withdrawal of aspirin in patients with stents may be associated with an increased risk of cardiac events.[34]
  - The POISE-2 trial demonstrated no cardiac or mortality benefit in starting aspirin perioperatively, but did identify an increased risk of major bleeding in the treatment arm.[35]
  - Recommendations
    - In general, it is not recommended to initiate or continue aspirin to prevent cardiac events in patients with no history of cardiac stenting undergoing noncardiac non-carotid surgery. However, it can be considered if the risk of myocardial ischemia is greater than bleeding risk.[9]
    - Any decision regarding change in antiplatelet therapy for patient with recent PCI (<30 days BMS, <365 days DES) should be made in coordination with the patient's cardiologist and surgeons based on risk of bleeding and in-stent thrombosis.[9]

FOLLOW-UP

The current ACC/AHA guidelines recommend:[9]

- Obtaining **ECG** on patients with clinical signs or symptoms of myocardial ischemia or arrhythmia.
- **Troponin measurements** are recommended only for patients with clinical signs or symptoms of MI.
- There is no indication to perform surveillance in the absence of signs or symptoms of myocardial ischemia.

Perioperative Hypertension

GENERAL PRINCIPLES

Severe hypertension (BP > 180/110 mm Hg) preoperatively often results in wider fluctuations in intraoperative BP and has been associated with an increased rate of perioperative cardiac events.[36] Specific concerns regarding chronic antihypertensive agents:

- Discontinuing chronic **β-blocker** therapy can lead to tachycardia.
- Abrupt cessation of **clonidine** may result in rebound hypertension, sometimes severe.
- **Angiotensin-converting enzyme (ACE) inhibitors** and **angiotensin II-receptor blockers** are associated with higher risk of intraoperative hypotension, but do not appear to have a negative outcome on mortality or cardiac event outcomes.[37]

TREATMENT

- Hypertension in the postoperative period is a common problem with multiple possible causes.
- All **remediable causes of hypertension**, such as pain, agitation, hypercarbia, hypoxia, hypervolemia, and bladder distention, should be excluded or treated.
- Review the patient's home medication list, and resume any medications discontinued preoperatively, as clinically indicated.
- Parenteral or oral antihypertensive medications are available based on the patient's clinical status. Transdermal clonidine is also an option, but the onset of action is delayed.

Preoperative Pulmonary Evaluation

GENERAL PRINCIPLES

Epidemiology

Clinically significant postoperative **pulmonary complications are at least as common as cardiac complications**, and the occurrence of one increases the risk of the other.[38] Pulmonary complications increase length of stay.[39] These complications include[40]

- Pneumonia
- Respiratory failure
- Atelectasis
- Exacerbation of underlying chronic lung disease

Etiology

As with cardiovascular complications, both patient and surgery-specific risk factors combine to produce the level of risk. These are reviewed in detail in a 2006 guideline from the American College of Physicians.[41]

Risk Factors

- Patient risk factors
  - **Age:** Even if healthy or with good functional status, risk increases starting at age 50.[42]
  - **Smoking**: Especially those with >40 pack-year history.[43]
  - **Chronic obstructive pulmonary disease** (COPD).[40] However, **there is no identified degree of COPD that is an absolute contraindication to surgery**.
  - **Obstructive sleep apnea**, especially in patients who are noncompliant with their continuous positive airway pressure (CPAP) therapy. Perioperative CPAP may be a management strategy to reduce this risk.[44]

- **Pulmonary hypertension**, when combined with a history of pulmonary embolism, worse New York Heart Association (NYHA) class, or evidence of right ventricular hypertrophy, is associated with increased morbidity and mortality in patients undergoing longer periods (>3 hours) of general anesthesia.[45]
- Congestive heart failure.[41]
- **General health status**: patients with functional dependence or higher American Society of Anesthesiologists class (ASA class >2).[42,46]
- **Asthma** that is compensated does not appear to be a significant risk factor.[47]
- **Obesity** does not appear to be a significant risk factor.[42]
- Procedure-related risk factors:
  - **Surgical site** is generally considered the greatest determinant of risk, increasing with proximity to the diaphragm.[40,42] Repair of abdominal aortic aneurysms appears to pose the greatest surgical risk.[48]
  - **Emergent surgery**.[41]
  - **Duration of surgery**: >2–3 hours.[49]
  - **Type of anesthesia:** Data are conflicting but neuraxial anesthesia may be less risky than general anesthesia.[50]

DIAGNOSIS

Clinical Presentation

History

The preoperative pulmonary evaluation should focus on evaluating the presence and severity of patient-dependent risk factors, as detailed above. Particular attention should be paid to determining whether the patient is functioning at their baseline or whether there has been any recent deterioration, such as increased dyspnea or cough with sputum production. Though exacerbations of chronic conditions or acute infections are not an absolute contraindication to surgery, it may be prudent to postpone an elective procedure in such cases. If there is consideration of undiagnosed sleep apnea, a screening questionnaire (e.g., Berlin Questionnaire, STOP-BANG) can be administered.[44]

Physical Examination

Attention should be paid to evidence of chronic lung disease or heart failure such as the presence of adventitious lung sounds, decreased breath sounds, or prolonged expiration. Persistent coughing after a voluntary cough as well as a maximum laryngeal height of <4 cm have been associated with pulmonary complications.[43]

Diagnostic Testing

Laboratories
- **Arterial blood gas:**
  - Preoperative arterial blood gas (ABG) is unlikely to add to the estimate of preoperative pulmonary risk beyond other clinically derived variables and should not be part of the routine preoperative evaluation.[40]
  - An ABG should be obtained when otherwise clinically necessary.
- **Serum albumin**:
  - A decreased serum albumin level (defined variably but generally <3.5 mg/dL) is a potent predictor of pulmonary risk.[42]
  - Supplemental nutrition (enteral or parenteral) **does not** appear to decrease risk.[51]

Imaging
- Preoperative chest radiography should not be used routinely in the preoperative pulmonary evaluation but **may be considered in patients undergoing higher-risk procedures who are over the age of 50 with known cardiopulmonary disease**.[41]

- Increased abnormalities are noted with advancing age. However, many findings deemed abnormal are chronic and do not affect management.[52]

Diagnostic Procedures
- The value of preoperative pulmonary function tests (PFTs) is unclear and controversial outside of lung resection surgery and should **not** be part of the routine preoperative pulmonary evaluation.[41]
- Although PFTs can clearly be used to define lung disease, in the setting of nonpulmonary surgery, there is concern that they add little beyond what can be gathered clinically.[53]
- PFTs could be considered in patients whose baseline cannot be clinically determined and may benefit from aggressive preoperative management.

Estimating Risk
- There are few tools for estimating perioperative pulmonary complications unlike cardiac risk stratification.
- In general, patients are deemed to be at an elevated risk for complications if they are undergoing high-risk procedures and have one or more of the identified patient-dependent risk factors.
- Risk indexes for predicting postoperative respiratory failure and pneumonia have been developed.[48,54] These risk indices were validated on patients who were receiving care through the VA hospital system and were nearly all men.
- The ARISCAT Risk Index stratifies patients as low, intermediate, and high risk of pulmonary complications using a weighted point score of seven risk factors.[55]

TREATMENT

- **Modifiable patient-related risk factors:**
  - Smoking cessation has been shown to decrease postoperative pulmonary complications if patients stop smoking at least 8 weeks before surgery. Previous concerns about a paradoxical increase in complications have not been proven.[56]
  - COPD therapy should be optimized. Symptoms should be aggressively managed preoperatively.
    - A preoperative course of **steroids** is reasonable for symptomatic patients already receiving **maximal bronchodilator therapy** who are not at their best personal baseline as determined by history and examination.
    - Patients with recent sputum changes may benefit from a preoperative course of **antibiotics**.
- **Modifiable procedure-related risk factors:**
  - Consideration of alternative procedures with the lowest possible pulmonary risk should be undertaken for high-risk patients. Laparoscopic procedures cause less disruption of lung function postoperatively.[57] Whether this translates to fewer clinically relevant complications is not clear.[51]
  - Although the choice of anesthesia is the province of the anesthesiologist, use of neuraxial/regional anesthetic methods should be considered where possible, especially in high-risk patients.
- **Postoperative interventions:**
  - Lung expansion maneuvers, such as incentive spirometry or deep breathing exercises, should be employed.
  - CPAP should be used routinely in patients with known sleep apnea. These patients should also be monitored with continuous pulse oximetry.[44]
    - CPAP or other noninvasive positive pressure ventilation (NPPV) devices may reduce the need for endotracheal ventilation in patients with acute respiratory failure following upper abdominal surgery.[58]

- Because of the potential complications of its use, patients being treated with NPPV should be monitored closely in the postanesthesia care unit (PACU), intensive care unit (ICU), or surgical observation unit.
  - Adequate analgesia is essential to prevent splinting, but oversedation must be carefully avoided. When appropriate, NSAIDs, acetaminophen, and regional analgesia should be considered. Postoperative epidural analgesia has been shown to reduce the incidence of pulmonary complications.[40]
  - A strategy of selective nasogastric tube placement rather than routine use has also been shown to decrease the risk of pulmonary complications.[51]
  - Prophylaxis for deep venous thrombosis (DVT) should be considered.

Transfusion Issues in Surgery

GENERAL PRINCIPLES

The transfusion of blood products is associated with substantial risks, including transmission of blood-borne infections, transfusion reactions, transfusion-related acute lung injury (TRALI), and possibly immunomodulatory effects. The threshold at which a red blood cell transfusion should be administered is unclear.

- A study of ICU patients suggested that the historical transfusion threshold of hemoglobin of 10 g/dL was too liberal, as patients treated with a more restrictive strategy (transfusion threshold of 7 g/dL) had outcomes that were at least equivalent and in some cases better.[59]
- More recently, The FOCUS trial showed no mortality difference between a restrictive (Hg < 8 g/dL) and liberal (Hg < 10 g/dL) transfusion threshold in high-risk (known or have risk factors for cardiovascular disease) patients after hip surgery.[60]

DIAGNOSIS

- Preoperative anemia is present in 5–35% of patients depending on the definition of anemia and type of surgery studied.[61]
- A history of anemia, hematologic disease, or bleeding diathesis should be noted on history or review of medical records.
- Any clinical signs of anemia (e.g., pallor) or coagulopathy (e.g., petechiae) should prompt further evaluation.
- For low-risk procedures, there is no evidence that routine testing of asymptomatic individuals increases safety.[62]
- For higher-risk procedures, particularly those with higher bleeding risk, a baseline complete blood count (CBC) and coagulation profile are typically obtained. Further testing should be performed as indicated.

TREATMENT

It is generally agreed that **transfusion is not required when the hemoglobin exceeds 10 g/dL**. Likewise, it is generally agreed that **a hemoglobin <7 g/dL necessitates transfusion**. For patients with hemoglobin between 7 and 10 g/dL:

- In stable patients, transfusion may be considered at hemoglobin 7–8 g/dL.
- In stable patients with cardiovascular disease, a transfusion threshold of 8 g/dL should be utilized.
- In patients with signs or symptoms of active cardiac ischemia, transfusions may be indicated to achieve a hemoglobin of 8–10 g/dL.

- Measures to reduce the need for allogeneic blood should be utilized where feasible.
  - Preoperative **autologous blood donation** should be considered for elective procedures where the anticipated need for transfusion is high.
  - **Preoperative erythropoietin** is generally not indicated but can be considered in patients with a decreased hemoglobin concentration; however, its use has been associated with increased risk for DVT.[63]
  - **Intraoperative measures** include normovolemic hemodilution for surgeries with high expected blood loss. Intraoperative blood salvage and autotransfusion and positional blood pooling are other options.
- Patients with **sickle cell anemia** require transfusion to a hemoglobin of 10 g/dL preoperatively to decrease the incidence of complications.[64]

Surgery in the Patient with Liver Disease

GENERAL PRINCIPLES

Patients with cirrhosis (with or without portal hypertension) suffer an increased risk of morbid outcomes when undergoing surgery such as increased in-hospital mortality and hospital length of stay.[65] The myriad systemic effects of liver dysfunction result in an increased frequency of other complications as well, such as bleeding, sepsis, encephalopathy, and renal failure.[66] Patients at risk must be identified and medically optimized prior to surgery to reduce postoperative complications.

Classification
- The best validated measure of perioperative risk in patients with cirrhosis is the Child-Pugh score, reflecting increased risk of perioperative morbidity and mortality with greater degrees of hepatic dysfunction, though recent evidence suggests the Model for End-stage Liver Disease (MELD) score can also be used.[67]
- Child-Pugh class C and MELD score >15 are considered contraindications to elective surgeries. A patient with a MELD score of 10–15 can undergo elective or semiurgent procedures with caution.

DIAGNOSIS

Clinical Presentation
As part of the preoperative history and physical exam, evidence of liver disease should be sought.

- Historical details include alcohol or drug abuse and prior blood transfusion.
- Physical examination evidence of liver dysfunction may be obvious, such as icterus and abdominal distension with ascites, but other abnormalities, such as spider angiomata, palmar erythema, and testicular atrophy in men, may be more subtle.
- Other indicators of risk for liver disease may be noted in the preoperative evaluation (e.g., family history of hemochromatosis).

Laboratories
Routine laboratory screening for hepatic dysfunction in patients presenting for surgery who are without clinically suspected or known liver disease is **not** recommended.[68] Patients with known or suspected liver disease should undergo evaluation of liver and kidney functions, including serum electrolytes, hepatic enzymes, bilirubin, albumin, coagulation studies, and creatinine.

TREATMENT

- Patients with **acute viral or alcoholic hepatitis** tolerate surgery poorly, and **delaying surgery until recovery** is recommended.
- Patients with **chronic hepatitis** without evidence of hepatic decompensation generally tolerate surgery well. Based on the high perioperative mortality rates in patients with **advanced cirrhosis**, nonoperative alternatives should be strongly considered. For patients who do require surgery, steps should be taken to optimize the preoperative status.
  - **Coagulopathy** is common in patients with liver disease.
    - Vitamin K is conventionally given if the international normalized ratio (INR) is elevated. The coagulopathy is likely to be refractory to this measure as the abnormality is secondary to hepatic dysfunction and not a nutritional deficiency. Fresh frozen plasma and cryoprecipitate may be required.
    - Administration of blood products may increase the patient's risk of volume overload or lung injury but won't necessarily improve bleeding risk.[69]
  - **Thrombocytopenia** is a common occurrence and should generally be corrected if severe. The general recommendation for most surgical procedures is a minimum platelet count of 50,000.
  - **Electrolyte abnormalities** should be addressed to reduce the risk of cardiac arrhythmias and encephalopathy.
  - Changes in **renal function** should be noted and addressed.
  - Careful attention should be paid to **volume status**. Many patients with liver disease develop hypervolemic **hyponatremia,** and restriction of free water may be required in certain cases for management. This can be complicated in the perioperative setting by NPO status, recent diuretic use, administration of IV fluids, etc.
  - **Ascites** may influence respiratory mechanics and increase the risk of abdominal wound dehiscence or herniation and so should be aggressively managed.
    - If time permits and the patient also has lower extremity edema, **diuretic therapy** should be instituted.
    - **Paracentesis** should be considered preoperatively if diuretics are ineffective or if time constraints prevent their use. Ascites may also be completely drained during surgery.
    - Preoperative placement of transjugular intrahepatic portosystemic shunt (**TIPS**) before elective abdominal surgeries has not been shown to reduce intraoperative blood loss, postoperative complications, or to improve cumulative survival.[70]
  - **Encephalopathy** should be investigated and treated.
    - **Lactulose** titrated to two to four soft bowel movements per day should be started in patients with encephalopathy. Rifaximin may also be considered, especially if the patient has had frequent episodes.
    - **Sedatives and other narcotics** can precipitate or worsen encephalopathy. They should be used cautiously, and dose reductions should be considered.

Management of Perioperative Diabetes

GENERAL PRINCIPLES

- Hospitalized patients with diabetes and hyperglycemia are at increased risk for poor outcomes.[71,72]
- Poor preoperative and postoperative glucose control is associated with an increased risk of postoperative infections.[73,74]

- While the benefits of glucose control in the perioperative period are not disputed, there are conflicting data on optimal target glucose levels.[75]
  ○ A single institutional study found a morbidity and mortality benefit of strict glucose control (<110 mg/dL) in surgical intensive care patients.[76]
  ○ A subsequent randomized, multicenter trial showed increased mortality among mixed surgical and medical intensive care patients with strict glucose control (81–108 mg/dL) versus "standard" glucose control (<180 mg/dL).[77] Of note, there was a substantial increased risk for severe hypoglycemia in the strict glucose control group.
- Diabetics are at increased risk for cardiovascular disease, and appropriate risk stratification for cardiac complications of surgery is vital to the perioperative evaluation of these patients.

Classification

Establishing the etiology of hyperglycemia has important implications for subsequent patient care.

- **Stress hyperglycemia** can occur in the perioperative setting because of the body's response to surgery with the release of counterregulatory hormones and cytokines that impede glucose metabolism. These patients need adequate glucose control during the perioperative period but are unlikely to require such treatment later.
- Type 2 diabetes is generally underdiagnosed, and the notation of perioperative hyperglycemia may be the first indication of its presence.
- It is also essential to distinguish between type 1 and type 2 diabetes mellitus.
  ○ **Type 1 diabetics** will require a continuous supply of insulin to prevent ketoacidosis—regardless of glucose level and oral intake.
  ○ The insulin requirement, if any, of **type 2 diabetics** during the perioperative period, will vary.

DIAGNOSIS

Laboratory Studies

Most patients should have a **hemoglobin A1c** obtained. This can assist in differentiating perioperative stress hyperglycemia from undiagnosed diabetes. Knowledge of recent glycemic control in known diabetics is also helpful in determining what therapy is required. Evaluating **renal function** is also recommended, given the increased prevalence of renal disease in diabetics. Cardiovascular risk stratification may require other evaluations (see section on Preoperative Cardiac Evaluation).

TREATMENT

Elective surgery in patients with uncontrolled diabetes mellitus should preferably be scheduled after acceptable glycemic control has been achieved. If possible, the operation should be scheduled for early morning to minimize prolonged fasting. Frequent monitoring of blood glucose levels is required in all situations.

- **Type 1 diabetes:**
  ○ Some form of basal insulin is required at all times.
  ○ On the evening prior to surgery, the regularly scheduled basal insulin should be continued. If taken in the morning, it is still recommended to give the regularly scheduled basal insulin without dose adjustment.[78] However, dose reduction may be considered if the patient has a history of hypoglycemic events.

- **Glucose infusions** (e.g., D5-containing fluids) can be administered to avoid hypoglycemia while the patient is NPO and until tolerance of oral intake postoperatively is established.
- For complex procedures and procedures requiring a prolonged NPO status, a **continuous insulin infusion** will likely be necessary.
- **Caution should be exercised with the use of subcutaneous insulin** in the intraoperative and critical care settings, as alterations in tissue perfusion may result in variable absorption.
- **Type 2 diabetes**: Treatment of type 2 diabetics varies according to their preoperative requirements and the complexity of the planned procedure. Consideration should be given to the efficacy of the patients' current regimen. If they are not well controlled at baseline, then an escalation in therapy may be required.
  - **Diet-controlled type 2 diabetes**: This can generally be managed without insulin therapy. Glucose values should be checked regularly, and elevated levels (>180 mg/dL) can be treated with intermittent doses of short-acting insulin.
  - **Type 2 diabetes managed with oral therapy:**
    - **Short-acting sulfonylureas** and **other oral agents** should be withheld on the operative day.
    - **Metformin** and **long-acting sulfonylureas** (e.g., chlorpropamide) should be withheld 1 day before planned surgical procedures. Metformin is generally held for 48 hours postoperatively. Renal function should be normal prior to resuming treatment. Other oral agents can be resumed when patients are tolerating their preprocedure diet.
    - Most patients can be managed without an insulin infusion.
    - Glucose values should be checked regularly, and elevated levels (>180 mg/dL) can be treated with intermittent doses of short-acting insulin.
  - **Type 2 diabetes managed with insulin:**
    - If it is anticipated that the patient will be able to eat postoperatively, basal insulin is still given on the morning of surgery.
    - If given as long-acting insulin (e.g., glargine insulin) and the patient usually takes the dose in the morning, 50–100% of the usual dose can be given.[78]
    - If the patient utilizes intermediate-acting insulin (e.g., neutral protamine hagedorn [NPH]), one-half to two-thirds of the usual morning dose is given to avoid periprocedural hyperglycemia.
    - Dextrose-containing IV fluids may be required to avoid hypoglycemia.
    - Patients undergoing major procedures will typically require an insulin drip perioperatively.
    - Glucose and potassium will need to be administered concomitantly to avoid hypoglycemia and hypokalemia, respectively. The **presence of renal dysfunction** may, however, contraindicate the use of potassium.
    - The usual insulin treatment can be resumed once oral intake is established postoperatively.
- **Target glucose levels**: There are no generally agreed-upon target glucose levels applicable to the entire postsurgical population.
  - In a general medical–surgical population, recurring glucose values >200 mg/dL were associated with a poor outcome.[71]
  - Pending further research, the current American Associate of Clinical Endocrinologists clinical practice guidelines recommend[79]
    - A premeal glucose <140 mg/dL and random blood glucose <180 mg/dL in general medical and surgical inpatients.
    - For patients in the ICU, a target glucose range of 140–180 mg/dL is recommended.

Perioperative Management of Corticosteroids

GENERAL PRINCIPLES

Surgery is a potent activator of the hypothalamic–pituitary axis (HPA). Patients with adrenal insufficiency may lack the ability to respond appropriately to surgical stress. Further, patients receiving corticosteroids as medical therapy for indications other than adrenal dysfunction may develop adrenal insufficiency. How to best identify and treat these patients has undergone considerable change since the case reports of postoperative crises in the 1950s.

Pathophysiology

The subtype of adrenal insufficiency has implications on management.

- **Tertiary adrenal insufficiency** due to exogenous corticosteroid administration is the most common adrenal problem encountered. These patients should have intact mineralocorticoid function and therefore require only glucocorticoid supplementation.[80]
- **Secondary adrenal insufficiency** should not result in mineralocorticoid deficiency. The possibility of deficits in other hormones due to pituitary disease should be considered.
- **Primary adrenal insufficiency** requires replacement of both mineralocorticoids and glucocorticoids.
- The dose and duration of exogenous corticosteroids required to produce clinically significant tertiary adrenal insufficiency are highly variable, but general principles can be outlined.[81]
  - Daily therapy with **≤5 mg prednisone** (or its equivalent), **alternate-day corticosteroid therapy**, and **any dose given for <3 weeks** should not result in clinically significant adrenal suppression.
  - Patients receiving **>20 mg/d of prednisone (or equivalent) for >3 weeks** and patients who are clinically **cushingoid in appearance** can be expected to have **significant suppression of adrenal responsiveness**.
  - The function of the HPA **cannot be readily predicted** in **patients receiving doses of prednisone 5–20 mg for >3 weeks**.

DIAGNOSIS

Clinical Presentation

History
- The dose and duration of prior corticosteroid therapy should be clarified.
- The coexistence of diseases that suggest the possibility of primary adrenal insufficiency should be sought (e.g., autoimmune thyroid disease, malignant tumors that metastasize to the adrenal glands such as lung cancer, etc.).

Physical Examination
Physical exam findings suggestive of adrenal hypofunction, such as hyperpigmentation, should be noted. As above, inspection for features of a cushingoid appearance should be performed.

Diagnostic Testing

- For patients in whom clinical prediction of adrenal function is difficult, a **cosyntropin stimulation test** can be performed. A cortisol level >18, 30 minutes after administration of cosyntropin, confirms a normal functioning HPA. Administration of perioperative stress-dose steroids should be considered in patients with a level <18.

- **Electrolyte abnormalities** should be evaluated in patients with primary adrenal insufficiency. Patients with other forms of adrenal insufficiency are unlikely to manifest the classic hyperkalemia and hyponatremia due to intact mineralocorticoid function.

TREATMENT

- **Patients expected to have an intact adrenal function** (as outlined above) should take their regularly scheduled dose of corticosteroid.[82] No further treatment is required.
- **Patients with known or expected adrenal insufficiency** should be treated with perioperative glucocorticoids.
- In **patients whose HPA status is uncertain** and there is inadequate time to perform a cosyntropin stimulation test, corticosteroids can be administered preoperatively with dosing determined by the expected amount of surgical stress.
- There is currently no uniform recommendation on the specific dose of corticosteroid to give perioperatively.[83,84] Please refer to Chapter 41, Adrenal Insufficiency, for further management recommendations.
- Additional **mineralocorticoid supplementation** for patients with primary adrenal insufficiency may or may not be necessary, depending on the dose and mineralocorticoid potency of the corticosteroid given.

Perioperative Care of Chronic Kidney Disease and End-Stage Renal Disease

GENERAL PRINCIPLES

Chronic kidney disease (CKD) is an independent risk factor for **perioperative cardiac complications**, so many patients with renal disease will need appropriate cardiac risk stratification. **Patients with end-stage renal disease (ESRD)** have a substantial mortality risk when undergoing surgery.[85,86]

TREATMENT

- **Volume status**: Every effort should be made to **achieve euvolemia** preoperatively so as to reduce the incidence of volume-related complications intra- and postoperatively.[87] Although this typically entails removing volume, some patients will be hypovolemic and thus require hydration.
  - Patients with CKD not receiving hemodialysis may require treatment with loop diuretics.
  - Patients being treated with **hemodialysis** should undergo dialysis preoperatively.
    - This is commonly performed on the day prior to surgery.
    - Hemodialysis can be performed on the day of surgery as well. The possibility that transient electrolyte abnormalities and hemodynamic changes postdialysis can occur should be considered.
- **Electrolyte abnormalities**
  - **Hyperkalemia** in the preoperative setting should be treated, particularly as tissue breakdown associated with surgery may elevate the potassium level further postoperatively.
    - For patients on dialysis, preoperative dialysis should be utilized.
    - For patients with CKD not undergoing dialysis, alternative methods of potassium excretion will be necessary.

- **Loop diuretics** can be utilized, particularly if the patient is also hypervolemic.
- **Sodium polystyrene sulfonate (SPS) resins** can also be utilized. The possibility that intestinal necrosis with SPS resins occurs more frequently in the perioperative setting has been suggested.[88]
  - **Metabolic acidosis**: Although chronic metabolic acidosis has not been associated with elevated perioperative risk, some local anesthetics have reduced efficacy in acidotic patients. Preoperative metabolic acidosis should be corrected with sodium bicarbonate infusions or dialysis.
- **Bleeding diathesis: Platelet dysfunction** has long been associated with uremia.
  - Preoperative bleeding time does not predict postoperative bleeding and is not recommended.[89]
  - Patients who evidence perioperative bleeding should, however, be treated.
    - **Dialysis** for patients with ESRD will improve platelet function.
    - **Desmopressin** (0.3 µg/kg IV or intranasally) can be utilized.
    - **Cryoprecipitate** is also an additional option.
    - In patients with coexisting anemia, **red blood cell transfusions** can improve uremic bleeding.
  - For patients **with a history of prior uremic bleeding**, preoperative desmopressin or **conjugated estrogens** (0.6 mg/kg/d IV or PO for 5 days) should be considered.
  - **Heparin** given with dialysis can increase bleeding risk. **Heparin-free dialysis** should be discussed with the patient's nephrologist when surgery is planned.

Perioperative Care of Acute Renal Failure

GENERAL PRINCIPLES

Acute kidney injury (AKI) can occur in the surgical population for various reasons.[90] Patients with **CKD** are at increased risk of AKI. The approach to AKI in the perioperative setting is not substantially different from that in the nonoperative setting. However, certain additional factors have to be considered in evaluating the cause in the perioperative setting:

- **Intraoperative hemodynamic changes**, particularly hypotension, should be considered. A careful review of the operative record is advised.
- Certain procedures can have an adverse effect on renal function (e.g., aortic clamping). Therefore, careful attention to the details of the procedure is necessary.
- The possibility that bleeding is responsible for a prerenal state deserves special attention.

REFERENCES

1. Weiser TG, Regenbogen SE, Thompson KD, et al. An estimation of the global volume of surgery: a modelling strategy based on available data. *Lancet* 2008;372:139–44.
2. van Waes JA, Nathoe HM, de Graaff JC, et al. Myocardial injury after noncardiac surgery and its association with short-term mortality. *Circulation* 2013;127:2264–71.
3. Adesanya AO, de Lemos JA, Greilich NB, et al. Management of perioperative myocardial infarction in noncardiac surgical patients. *Chest* 2006;130:584–96.
4. Dawood MM, Gutpa DK, Southern J, et al. Pathology of fatal perioperative myocardial infarction: implications regarding pathophysiology and prevention. *Int J Cardiol* 1996;57:37–44.
5. Gualandro DM, Campos CA, Calderaro D, et al. Coronary plaque rupture in patients with myocardial infarction after noncardiac surgery: frequent and dangerous. *Atherosclerosis* 2012;222:191–5.

6. Landesberg G, Beattie WS, Mosseri M, et al. Perioperative myocardial infarction. *Circulation* 2009;119:2936–44.
7. Howell SJ, Sear JW, Foex P. Hypertension, hypertensive heart disease and perioperative cardiac risk. *Br J Anaesth* 2004;92:570–83.
8. Agarwal S, Rajamanickam A, Bajaj NS, et al. Impact of aortic stenosis on postoperative outcomes after noncardiac surgeries. *Circ Cardiovasc Qual Outcomes* 2013;6:193–200.
9. Fleisher LA, Fleischmann KE, Auerbach AD, et al. 2014 ACC/AHA guideline on perioperative cardiovascular evaluation and management of patients undergoing noncardiac surgery: a report of the American College of Cardiology/American Heart Association Task Force on practice guidelines. *J Am Coll Cardiol* 2014;64:e77–137.
10. Calleja AM, Dommaraju S, Gaddam R, et al. Cardiac risk in patients aged >75 years with asymptomatic, severe aortic stenosis undergoing noncardiac surgery. *Am J Cardiol* 2010;105:1159–63.
11. van Klei WA, Bryson GL, Yang H, et al. The value of routine preoperative electrocardiography in predicting myocardial infarction after noncardiac surgery. *Ann Surg* 2007;246:165–70.
12. Lee TH, Marcantonio ER, Mangione CM, et al. Derivation and prospective validation of a simple index for prediction of cardiac risk of major noncardiac surgery. *Circulation* 1999;100:1043–9.
13. Devereaux PJ, Goldman L, Cook DJ, et al. Perioperative cardiac events in patients undergoing noncardiac surgery: a review of the magnitude of the problem, the pathophysiology of the events and methods to estimate and communicate risk. *CMAJ* 2005;173:627–34.
14. Ford MK, Beattie WS, Wijeysundera DN. Systematic review: prediction of perioperative cardiac complications and mortality by the revised cardiac risk index. *Ann Intern Med* 2010;152:26–35.
15. Gupta PK, Gupta H, Sundaram A, et al. Development and validation of a risk calculator for prediction of cardiac risk after surgery. *Circulation* 2011;124:381–7.
16. Cohen ME, Ko CY, Bilimoria KY, et al. Optimizing ACS NSQIP modeling for evaluation of surgical quality and risk: patient risk adjustment, procedure mix adjustment, shrinkage adjustment, and surgical focus. *J Am Coll Surg* 2013;217:336–46, e1.
17. Reilly DF, McNeely MJ, Doerner D, et al. Self-reported exercise tolerance and the risk of serious perioperative complications. *Arch Intern Med* 1999;159:2185–92.
18. Hlatky MA, Boineau RE, Higginbotham MB, et al. A brief self-administered questionnaire to determine functional capacity (the Duke Activity Status Index). *Am J Cardiol* 1989;64:651–4.
19. Myers J, Bader D, Madhavan R, et al. Validation of a specific activity questionnaire to estimate exercise tolerance in patients referred for exercise testing. *Am Heart J* 2001;142:1041–6.
20. McFalls EO, Ward HB, Moritz TE, et al. Coronary-artery revascularization before elective major vascular surgery. *N Engl J Med* 2004;351:2795–804.
21. Kaluza GL, Joseph J, Lee JR, et al. Catastrophic outcomes of noncardiac surgery soon after coronary stenting. *J Am Coll Cardiol* 2000;35:1288–94.
22. Wilson SH, Fasseas P, Orford JL, et al. Clinical outcome of patients undergoing non-cardiac surgery in the two months following coronary stenting. *J Am Coll Cardiol* 2003;42:234–40.
23. Berger PB, Kleiman NS, Pencina MJ, et al. Frequency of major noncardiac surgery and subsequent adverse events in the year after drug-eluting stent placement results from the EVENT (Evaluation of Drug-Eluting Stents and Ischemic Events) Registry. *JACC Cardiovasc Interv* 2010;3:920–7.
24. Holcomb CN, Graham LA, Richman JS, et al. The incremental risk of noncardiac surgery on adverse cardiac events following coronary stenting. *J Am Coll Cardiol* 2014;64:2730–9.
25. Yang H, Raymer K, Butler R, et al. The effects of perioperative beta-blockade: results of the Metoprolol after Vascular Surgery (MaVS) study, a randomized controlled trial. *Am Heart J* 2006;152:983–90.
26. Brady AR, Gibbs JS, Greenhalgh RM, et al. Perioperative beta-blockade (POBBLE) for patients undergoing infrarenal vascular surgery: results of a randomized double-blind controlled trial. *J Vasc Surg* 2005;41:602–9.
27. Juul AB, Wetterslev J, Gluud C, et al. Effect of perioperative beta blockade in patients with diabetes undergoing major non-cardiac surgery: randomised placebo controlled, blinded multicentre trial. *BMJ* 2006;332:1482.
28. Group PS, Devereaux PJ, Yang H, et al. Effects of extended-release metoprolol succinate in patients undergoing non-cardiac surgery (POISE trial): a randomised controlled trial. *Lancet* 2008;371:1839–47.
29. Devereaux PJ, Sessler DI, Leslie K, et al. Clonidine in patients undergoing noncardiac surgery. *N Engl J Med* 2014;370:1504–13.

30. Lindenauer PK, Pekow P, Wang K, et al. Lipid-lowering therapy and in-hospital mortality following major noncardiac surgery. *JAMA* 2004;291:2092–9.
31. Raju MG, Pachika A, Punnam SR, et al. Statin therapy in the reduction of cardiovascular events in patients undergoing intermediate-risk noncardiac, nonvascular surgery. *Clin Cardiol* 2013;36:456–61.
32. Durazzo AE, Machado FS, Ikeoka DT, et al. Reduction in cardiovascular events after vascular surgery with atorvastatin: a randomized trial. *J Vasc Surg* 2004;39:967–75.
33. Desai H, Aronow WS, Ahn C, et al. Incidence of perioperative myocardial infarction and of 2-year mortality in 577 elderly patients undergoing noncardiac vascular surgery treated with and without statins. *Arch Gerontol Geriatr* 2010;51:149–51.
34. Ferrari E, Benhamou M, Cerboni P, et al. Coronary syndromes following aspirin withdrawal: a special risk for late stent thrombosis. *J Am Coll Cardiol* 2005;45:456–9.
35. Devereaux PJ, Mrkobrada M, Sessler DI, et al. Aspirin in patients undergoing noncardiac surgery. *N Engl J Med* 2014;370:1494–503.
36. Hollenberg M, Mangano DT, Browner WS, et al. Predictors of postoperative myocardial ischemia in patients undergoing noncardiac surgery. The Study of Perioperative Ischemia Research Group. *JAMA* 1992;268:205–9.
37. Rosenman DJ, McDonald FS, Ebbert JO, et al. Clinical consequences of withholding versus administering renin-angiotensin-aldosterone system antagonists in the preoperative period. *J Hosp Med* 2008;3:319–25.
38. Fleischmann KE, Goldman L, Young B, et al. Association between cardiac and noncardiac complications in patients undergoing noncardiac surgery: outcomes and effects on length of stay. *Am J Med* 2003;115:515–20.
39. Lawrence VA, Hilsenbeck SG, Mulrow CD, et al. Incidence and hospital stay for cardiac and pulmonary complications after abdominal surgery. *J Gen Intern Med* 1995;10:671–8.
40. Smetana GW. Preoperative pulmonary evaluation. *N Engl J Med* 1999;340:937–44.
41. Qaseem A, Snow V, Fitterman N, et al. Risk assessment for and strategies to reduce perioperative pulmonary complications for patients undergoing noncardiothoracic surgery: a guideline from the American College of Physicians. *Ann Intern Med* 2006;144:575–80.
42. Smetana GW, Lawrence VA, Cornell JE, et al. Preoperative pulmonary risk stratification for noncardiothoracic surgery: systematic review for the American College of Physicians. *Ann Intern Med* 2006;144:581–95.
43. McAlister FA, Khan NA, Straus SE, et al. Accuracy of the preoperative assessment in predicting pulmonary risk after nonthoracic surgery. *Am J Respir Crit Care Med* 2003;167:741–4.
44. Vasu TS, Grewal R, Doghramji K. Obstructive sleep apnea syndrome and perioperative complications: a systematic review of the literature. *J Clin Sleep Med* 2012;8:199–207.
45. Ramakrishna G, Sprung J, Ravi BS, et al. Impact of pulmonary hypertension on the outcomes of noncardiac surgery: predictors of perioperative morbidity and mortality. *J Am Coll Cardiol* 2005;45:1691–9.
46. Hall JC, Tarala RA, Hall JL, et al. A multivariate analysis of the risk of pulmonary complications after laparotomy. *Chest* 1991;99:923–7.
47. Woods BD, Sladen RN. Perioperative considerations for the patient with asthma and bronchospasm. *Br J Anaesth* 2009;103(Suppl 1):i57–65.
48. Arozullah AM, Daley J, Henderson WG, et al. Multifactorial risk index for predicting postoperative respiratory failure in men after major noncardiac surgery. The National Veterans Administration Surgical Quality Improvement Program. *Ann Surg* 2000;232:242–53.
49. Kroenke K, Lawrence VA, Theroux JF, et al. Operative risk in patients with severe obstructive pulmonary disease. *Arch Intern Med* 1992;152:967–71.
50. Rodgers A, Walker N, Schug S, et al. Reduction of postoperative mortality and morbidity with epidural or spinal anaesthesia: results from overview of randomised trials. *BMJ* 2000;321:1493.
51. Lawrence VA, Cornell JE, Smetana GW, et al. Strategies to reduce postoperative pulmonary complications after noncardiothoracic surgery: systematic review for the American College of Physicians. *Ann Intern Med* 2006;144:596–608.
52. Joo HS, Wong J, Naik VN, et al. The value of screening preoperative chest x-rays: a systematic review. *Can J Anaesth* 2005;52:568–74.
53. De Nino LA, Lawrence VA, Averyt EC, et al. Preoperative spirometry and laparotomy: blowing away dollars. *Chest* 1997;111:1536–41.

54. Arozullah AM, Khuri SF, Henderson WG, et al. Development and validation of a multifactorial risk index for predicting postoperative pneumonia after major noncardiac surgery. *Ann Intern Med* 2001;135:847–57.
55. Canet J, Gallart L, Gomar C, et al. Prediction of postoperative pulmonary complications in a population-based surgical cohort. *Anesthesiology* 2010;113:1338–50.
56. Barrera R, Shi W, Amar D, et al. Smoking and timing of cessation: impact on pulmonary complications after thoracotomy. *Chest* 2005;127:1977–83.
57. Bablekos GD, Michaelides SA, Analitis A, et al. Effects of laparoscopic cholecystectomy on lung function: a systematic review. *World J Gastroenterol* 2014;20:17603–17.
58. Faria DA, da Silva EM, Atallah AN, et al. Noninvasive positive pressure ventilation for acute respiratory failure following upper abdominal surgery. *Cochrane Database Syst Rev* 2015;(10):CD009134.
59. Hebert PC, Wells G, Blajchman MA, et al. A multicenter, randomized, controlled clinical trial of transfusion requirements in critical care. Transfusion Requirements in Critical Care Investigators, Canadian Critical Care Trials Group. *N Engl J Med* 1999;340:409–17.
60. Carson JL, Terrin ML, Noveck H, et al. Liberal or restrictive transfusion in high-risk patients after hip surgery. *N Engl J Med* 2011;365:2453–62.
61. Musallam KM, Tamim HM, Richards T, et al. Preoperative anaemia and postoperative outcomes in non-cardiac surgery: a retrospective cohort study. *Lancet* 2011;378:1396–407.
62. Benarroch-Gampel J, Sheffield KM, Duncan CB, et al. Preoperative laboratory testing in patients undergoing elective, low-risk ambulatory surgery. *Ann Surg* 2012;256:518–28.
63. Goodnough LT, Monk TG, Andriole GL. Erythropoietin therapy. *N Engl J Med* 1997;336: 933–8.
64. Howard J, Malfroy M, Llewelyn C, et al. The Transfusion Alternatives Preoperatively in Sickle Cell Disease (TAPS) study: a randomised, controlled, multicentre clinical trial. *Lancet* 2013;381:930–8.
65. Csikesz NG, Nguyen LN, Tseng JF, et al. Nationwide volume and mortality after elective surgery in cirrhotic patients. *J Am Coll Surg* 2009;208:96–103.
66. Wiklund RA. Preoperative preparation of patients with advanced liver disease. *Crit Care Med* 2004;32(Suppl):S106–15.
67. O'Leary JG, Friedman LS. Predicting surgical risk in patients with cirrhosis: from art to science. *Gastroenterology* 2007;132:1609–11.
68. Rizvon MK, Chou CL. Surgery in the patient with liver disease. *Med Clin North Am* 2003;87: 211–27.
69. Rai R, Nagral S, Nagral A. Surgery in a patient with liver disease. *J Clin Exp Hepatol* 2012;2: 238–46.
70. Vinet E, Perreault P, Bouchard L, et al. Transjugular intrahepatic portosystemic shunt before abdominal surgery in cirrhotic patients: a retrospective, comparative study. *Can J Gastroenterol* 2006;20:401–4.
71. Umpierrez GE, Isaacs SD, Bazargan N, et al. Hyperglycemia: an independent marker of in-hospital mortality in patients with undiagnosed diabetes. *J Clin Endocrinol Metab* 2002;87:978–82.
72. Frisch A, Chandra P, Smiley D, et al. Prevalence and clinical outcome of hyperglycemia in the perioperative period in noncardiac surgery. *Diabetes Care* 2010;33:1783–8.
73. King JT Jr, Goulet JL, Perkal MF, et al.Glycemic control and infections in patients with diabetes undergoing noncardiac surgery. *Ann Surg* 2011;253:158–65.
74. Dronge AS, Perkal MF, Kancir S, et al. Long-term glycemic control and postoperative infectious complications. *Arch Surg* 2006;141:375–80.
75. Buchleitner AM, Martinez-Alonso M, Hernandez M, et al. Perioperative glycaemic control for diabetic patients undergoing surgery. *Cochrane Database Syst Rev* 2012;(9):CD007315.
76. van den Berghe G, Wouters P, Weekers F, et al. Intensive insulin therapy in critically ill patients. *N Engl J Med* 2001;345:1359–67.
77. Finfer S, Chittock DR, Su SY, et al. Intensive versus conventional glucose control in critically ill patients. *N Engl J Med* 2009;360:1283–97.
78. Clement S, Braithwaite SS, Magee MF, et al. Management of diabetes and hyperglycemia in hospitals. *Diabetes Care* 2004;27:553–91.
79. Handelsman Y, Bloomgarden ZT, Grunberger G, et al. American association of clinical endocrinologists and American college of endocrinology—clinical practice guidelines for developing a diabetes mellitus comprehensive care plan—2015. *Endocr Pract* 2015;21(Suppl 1):1–87.

80. Cooper MS, Stewart PM. Corticosteroid insufficiency in acutely ill patients. *N Engl J Med* 2003;348:727–34.
81. Schiff RL, Welsh GA. Perioperative evaluation and management of the patient with endocrine dysfunction. *Med Clin North Am* 2003;87:175–92.
82. Yong SL, Marik P, Esposito M, et al. Supplemental perioperative steroids for surgical patients with adrenal insufficiency. *Cochrane Database Syst Rev* 2009;(4):CD005367.
83. Coursin DB, Wood KE. Corticosteroid supplementation for adrenal insufficiency. *JAMA* 2002;287:236–40.
84. Jung C, Inder WJ. Management of adrenal insufficiency during the stress of medical illness and surgery. *Med J Aust* 2008;188:409–13.
85. Kellerman PS. Perioperative care of the renal patient. *Arch Intern Med* 1994;154:1674–88.
86. Schneider CR, Cobb W, Patel S, et al. Elective surgery in patients with end stage renal disease: what's the risk? *Am Surg* 2009;75:790–3.
87. Joseph AJ, Cohn SL. Perioperative care of the patient with renal failure. *Med Clin North Am* 2003;87:193–210.
88. Gerstman BB, Kirkman R, Platt R. Intestinal necrosis associated with postoperative orally administered sodium polystyrene sulfonate in sorbitol. *Am J Kidney Dis* 1992;20:159–61.
89. Lind SE. The bleeding time does not predict surgical bleeding. *Blood* 1991;77:2547–52.
90. Kheterpal S, Tremper KK, Englesbe MJ, et al. Predictors of postoperative acute renal failure after noncardiac surgery in patients with previously normal renal function. *Anesthesiology* 2007;107:892–902.

Approach to Edema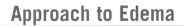

Yevgeniy Khariton and Lois F. Richard

GENERAL PRINCIPLES

- Edema refers to an excess of fluid that has accumulated in skin and subcutaneous tissue.
- Edema is the result of an increase in net filtration of fluid from the vascular bed, which is dependent on the following changes to existing Starling forces:
  - Increased vascular hydrostatic pressure
  - Decreased oncotic pressure (low protein state)
  - Increased vascular permeability (inflammatory response)[1]
- Other factors include compensatory retention of sodium and water by the kidney, efficiency of venous and lymphatic flow, and regulation of capillary flow by the precapillary sphincter.[2]
- Although more common in the lower extremities, edema can also occur in the upper extremities, torso, and genitalia.
- Edema is characterized as local, regional, or generalized. Localized edema is often associated with a focal process (e.g., lymphatic obstruction, insect bite), while generalized or peripheral edema is often associated with a systemic process, such as congestive heart failure (CHF).

DIAGNOSIS

Clinical Presentation

History
- If the edema is localized, ask about:
  - Chronicity and progression of symptoms
  - Presence of pain (localized obstruction and congenital forms are typically painless)
  - Previous injury or insect bites
  - Prior surgery
  - Risk factors for deep venous thrombosis (DVT), which include prolonged immobilization, recent surgery, malignancy, pregnancy
- If edema is bilateral lower extremity or generalized, ask about:
  - Congestive heart failure
  - Diet
  - Toxic exposures (chemicals, insect bites)
  - Smoking history, alcohol, and illicit substance use
  - Chronic liver disease
  - Renal failure
  - Endocrinopathies (i.e., infiltrative disorders, thyroid disorders)
- If acute-onset edema, ask about:
  - Symptoms of or history of anaphylaxis
  - New medication or chemical exposures (i.e., nonsteroidal anti-inflammatory drugs (NSAIDs), steroids, calcium channel blockers, sex hormones)
  - Major changes in weight (i.e., malignancy, cirrhosis, CHF)

- Chest discomfort or shortness of breath (i.e., pulmonary embolism [PE], heart failure, valvular disorders)
- Paroxysmal nocturnal dyspnea and/or orthopnea (i.e., heart failure)
- Syncope/presyncope (i.e., PE, heart failure, valvular disorders)
- Changes in urine output (i.e., hepatic, renal, cardiac disorders)
- Abdominal swelling (i.e., CHF, cirrhotic liver disease)
- History of smoking and history of procoagulable conditions (i.e., DVT/PE)
- History of injection drug use (i.e., screening for hepatitis exposure, emboli, infection)[3]

Physical Examination
- **Vital signs**
  - A trend of hemodynamic measurements, blood pressure in particular, is often useful in distinguishing between acute and chronic conditions.
  - Relative hypotension is a feature consistent with cirrhotic liver disease due to the predominance of local and systemic vasodilators; it is notable in cardiogenic shock due to impaired contractility and inotropy.
  - Pronounced hypertension is often characteristic of a chronic hypertensive state as well as primary renal disease.
- **Acuity and distribution of edema**
  - Examine the skin for signs of chronicity, such as brawny skin changes, hemosiderosis, lymphostatic verrucosis (dark, wart-like projections), or venous stasis ulcers.
  - Rapid onset of severe edema may result in pain and erythema mimicking cellulitis.
  - Angioedema is typically rapid onset (within minutes to hours) and is frequently localized to the lips, head, or neck.
  - Periorbital edema occurring acutely or chronically in the setting of bilateral upper extremity edema may suggest superior vena cava obstruction (malignancy) or may simply reflect an isolated protein-losing nephropathy.
- It is important to differentiate **pitting edema from nonpitting edema**.
  - **Pitting edema** is traditionally graded using the pit recovery time (PRT) on a scale of 1–4: a finger is pressed to the select area for approximately 5–10 seconds, after which a delayed return to original skin depth every 30 seconds is assigned an additional point.[4]
  - **Nonpitting edema**
    - Lipedema: a chronic disorder of adipose tissue and lymphatic dysfunction, frequently affecting lower extremities and sparing the feet.[5]
    - Myxedema: deposition of protein and mucopolysaccharides in the dermis, which bind water and cause boggy edema, most commonly seen in the pretibial region and associated with severe hypothyroidism.[6]
- In the patient with suspected or known heart failure, document the following:
  - Jugulovenous distention (JVD)
  - Hepatojugular reflux
  - S3/S4 gallop
  - Cardiac murmurs (new or old)
- In the patient with suspected or known chronic liver disease, document the following:
  - Ascites
  - Spider angiomata
  - Palmar erythema
  - Parotid enlargement
  - Caput medusa
  - Hemorrhoids
  - Asterixis or generalized delirium
- JVD will be abnormally elevated in right-sided heart failure and normal in portal hypertension.
- In patients with localized peripheral edema, especially if unilateral, the presence of an underlying DVT may exhibit warmth, tenderness, or a palpable venous cord.

- A torn medial gastrocnemius head may have a palpable mass, purpura from tendon or fascial bleeding, or a depression with tenderness in the midcalf area.
- A ruptured Baker cyst typically exhibits a tender popliteal fossa.[2,4]

Differential Diagnosis
- Common causes of localized edema[4]
  - Venous obstruction/insufficiency (DVT)
  - Lymphatic obstruction
  - Local trauma (ruptured Baker cyst, insect bites, burns) or postsurgical
  - Angioedema (hereditary, acquired, medication induced)
  - Radiation-induced injury
  - Rheumatic disease
  - Localized malignancy
  - Soft tissue infection (cellulitis)
  - Crystalline arthropathies (gout)
- Common causes of generalized edema or bilateral edema[4]
  - Venous obstruction (inferior vena caval obstruction, valvular incompetency)
  - Chronic kidney disease (CKD) (i.e., glomerulonephropathy)
  - Chronic hepatic insufficiency (portal hypertension)
  - Heart failure (right-sided insufficiency due to cor pulmonale, left-sided heart failure, or primary valvular disease)
  - Excessive intravenous fluids or sodium-rich products
  - Localized malignancy or fibrosis
  - Low protein state (nephrotic-range proteinuria, cirrhosis, protein–calorie malnutrition, and protein-losing enteropathy)
  - Angioedema (hereditary, acquired, medication-induced, i.e., angiotensin-converting enzyme [ACE] inhibitors, NSAIDs)
  - Medications (calcium channel blockers, vasodilators, steroids, sex hormones, NSAIDs, cyclooxygenase [COX]-2 inhibitors)
  - Pregnancy and premenstrual period

Diagnostic Testing

Laboratories
- Blood and urine evaluation should be guided by history and exam and should rule out systemic disease. Initial evaluation commonly includes the following:
  - Creatinine and electrolytes (renal function and electrolyte stability)
  - Total serum protein and albumin (liver dysfunction, malnutrition)
  - Hepatic function panel (synthetic hepatic activity vs. extrinsic injury)
  - Thyroid-stimulating hormone (TSH) to evaluate for myxedema
  - Brain naturetic peptide (BNP), a nonspecific marker of volume overload
  - Urinalysis (proteinuria and glomerulonephropathy)
- In select patients, consider the following:
  - 24-hour urine protein collection and lipid panel (nephrotic syndrome)
  - Serum and urine electrophoresis (infiltrative paraproteinemia, amyloidosis)

Imaging
Imaging should be guided by results of the history, physical, and lab evaluation and should be used to evaluate for specific causes of edema.

- Doppler ultrasound of extremities (DVT, ruptured Baker cyst)
- Renal ultrasound (acute renal failure, nephrotic syndrome)
- Liver ultrasound with Doppler images (Budd-Chiari syndrome, portal hypertension, ascites)

- Transthoracic echocardiogram (heart failure, valvular abnormalities)
- CXR (heart failure, acute or chronic)
- CT abdomen/pelvis (retroperitoneal fibrosis or obstructing masses)

TREATMENT

- Treatment should be directed at the underlying disorder.
- Address the following questions to ensure appropriate management:
- When must edema be treated?
  - Pulmonary edema is **urgently** addressed with IV diuretics, often accompanied by nitrate therapies, for preload reduction and symptomatic relief.
  - Marked peripheral edema due to advanced renal failure and CHF may become uncomfortable and warrant nonurgent fluid removal.
  - Rapid fluid shifts induced by volume removal in patients with cirrhosis have the capacity to cause delirium as well as precipitate hepatorenal syndrome.
- What are the clinical consequences of fluid removal?
  - The clinical implications of vascular underfilling translate to relative tissue malperfusion and compensatory renal retention to restore venous return to the heart.
  - The consequences of fluid removal entail a loss of effective circulating volume, which has the potential to reduce cardiac output and systemic blood flow; nevertheless, most patients experience a therapeutic benefit from the appropriate use of diuretics despite these transient reductions.
  - Excess caution must be used in patients with severe cardiac insufficiency or those recently treated with high-dose diuretics.
  - Interstitial edema secondary to DVT and lymphatic insufficiency should not be addressed with volume removal but rather managed with an emphasis on compression stockings and elastic wraps.
  - The practitioner should be mindful that there are select cases where an acceptable level of edema must be tolerated at the cost of preserving organ homeostasis.
- How rapidly should edema fluid be removed?
  - Cumulative mobilization of excess fluid is dependent on the underlying condition as well as the influence of diuretic resistance.
  - In patients with a clinical presentation of decompensated heart failure, the mobilization of plasma fluid may be rapid and effective.
  - A more cautious approach may be useful in localized edema (i.e., ascites) where accelerated diuresis may result in poor therapeutic outcomes.[2]

Medications

- Loop diuretics, namely furosemide, are the medications of choice.
- Loop diuretics (e.g., furosemide, bumetanide, torsemide) excrete 20–25% of nephron sodium.
- Second-line agents include thiazide-type diuretics (hydrochlorothiazide), which are responsible for about 3–5% of the filtered sodium load at the distal tubule and have limited efficacy due to compensatory resorption at the cortical collecting duct.
- Potassium-sparing diuretics (e.g., aldactone, triamterene, amiloride) have the smallest capacity to induce effective natriuresis and have the largest therapeutic role in the treatment of cirrhosis and ascites in concert with loop diuretics.
- Diuretic-mediated treatment strategies are often limited by the practice of high-sodium diets as well as time limitations in diuretic activity (i.e., loop diuretics given as a bolus have a duration of action of 6 hours).
- Several sequential strategies, in order of preference, to augment appropriate diuretic response are as follows:

- Implement a low-sodium diet (<2 g daily).
- Increase the dose of loop diuretic until ceiling dose is achieved.
- Increase the frequency of loop diuretic administration or consider continuous IV infusion.
- Add a thiazide diuretic (IV or PO) to the regimen.[2]
* Due to the rapidity in which a compensatory state is achieved (2–3 weeks), both chronic diuretic doses and dietary restrictions should be encouraged.
* When administering intravenous diuretic therapy, monitor for the following:
  - Hypotension in naive patients
  - Electrolyte depletion and secondary cardiac arrhythmias
* The use of ultrafiltration as a strategy for volume removal, in the context of diuretic unresponsiveness, is seldom implemented and will not be discussed in this chapter.

Other Nonpharmacologic Therapies

Other nonpharmacologic therapies include compression stockings, elastic wraps, elevation of the affected extremity, and low-sodium diets.[2]

REFERENCES

1. Hall JE, Guyton A. *Medical Physiology*. 11th ed. Philadelphia: Elsevier Saunders, 2006.
2. Rose B, Post T. *Clinical Physiology of Acid-Base and Electrolyte Disorders*. New York: McGraw-Hill Education, 2001.
3. Stern SC, Cifu AS, Altkorn D. *Symptom to Diagnosis: An Evidence-Based Guide*. 3rd ed. New York: McGraw-Hill, 2014.
4. Kasper DL, Faucy AS, Hauser SL, et al. *Harrison's Principles of Internal Medicine*. 19th ed. McGraw-Hill, 2015.
5. Herbst KL. Rare adipose disorders (RADs) masquerading as obesity. *Acta Pharmacol Sin* 2012;33:155–72.
6. Fatourechi V. Pretibial myxedema: pathophysiology and treatment options. *Am J Clin Dermatol* 2005;6:295–309.

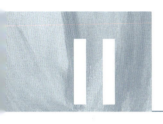

Cardiovascular

Approach to the Patient with Chest Pain

3

Anuradha Godishala

GENERAL PRINCIPLES

- Chest pain is one of the most common reasons for emergency department (ED) visits and hospital admission. Of the 8–10 million visits to the ED annually for chest pain, >1 million result in hospitalization for an acute coronary syndrome (ACS).[1-4]
- Prompt and accurate evaluation of chest pain has immense implications for patient morbidity and mortality. Chest pain due to **myocardial infarction (MI), pulmonary embolism (PE), aortic dissection, or pneumothorax** may result in sudden death.
- Given the broad differential diagnosis of chest pain (Table 3-1), the immediate goal should be to exclude the four life-threatening causes bolded above.
- The initial diagnostic approach includes a focused history and physical exam, as well as emergent ECG, optimally completed within 10 minutes of presentation.
- Results of the initial assessment guide further diagnostic tests and therapeutic interventions.
- High-risk patients (including those who appear ill, have abnormal vital signs, or possess risk factors for coronary disease) need immediate IV access and cardiac monitoring.

DIAGNOSIS

Clinical Presentation

History
- Establish the location, quality, and severity of chest discomfort, onset and duration of symptoms, aggravating and alleviating factors, and any associated symptoms.
- It is important to note that patients with underlying coronary ischemia often deny chest pain per se, but instead use terms such as sharp, crushing, tearing, squeezing, or pressure to describe their symptoms.
- With this information, patients can be assigned to one of three categories (Table 3-2):
  ○ Typical (definite) angina
  ○ Atypical (possible or probable) angina
  ○ Nonanginal symptoms. However, typical features may be lacking in ACSs (e.g., precipitating or relieving factors)
- Estimate the probability of coronary disease based on age, sex, prior history of angina, MI, or cardiac arrest, history of percutaneous coronary intervention (PCI) or coronary artery bypass graft, coronary artery disease documented by angiography, results of previous cardiac testing, and cardiac risk factors.
- Pertinent cardiac risk factors to elicit in the history include hypertension, hypercholesterolemia, peripheral or cerebrovascular disease, diabetes, smoking, and family history of coronary heart disease (CHD). Notably, diabetes is considered a CHD equivalent; the risk of cardiac events in diabetic patients is similar to that of patients with a prior MI.[5]
- Other diagnoses that should not be missed include the following:
  ○ **Pulmonary embolism**: Chest pain onset usually coincides with shortness of breath; may be pleuritic, accompanied by cough, or associated with palpitations, dizziness, or light-headedness. Assess for predisposing factors including recent surgery, immobilization, malignancy, or hypercoagulability. Validated risk scores such as the Wells criteria can also be used to estimate the risk of PE.

TABLE 3-1 DIFFERENTIAL DIAGNOSIS OF CHEST PAIN

Cardiac
- Coronary artery disease (angina pectoris, unstable angina, myocardial infarction, coronary vasospasm)
- Pericarditis
- Aortic stenosis
- Hypertrophic cardiomyopathy

Vascular
- Aortic dissection
- Pulmonary embolism
- Pulmonary hypertension

Pulmonary
- Pneumothorax or tension pneumothorax
- Pneumonitis, pleuritis (e.g., connective tissue disease or TB), or tracheobronchitis
- Pulmonary neoplasm

Gastrointestinal
- Gastroesophageal reflux disease, esophagitis
- Diffuse esophageal spasm, mucosal tear, rupture, or infection (e.g., esophageal candidiasis)
- Peptic ulcer disease
- Biliary colic or cholecystitis
- Pancreatitis

Musculoskeletal and neurologic
- Muscle strain (especially intercostal, interscalene, pectoralis)
- Costochondritis
- Subacromial bursitis
- Cervical spine disease with referred pain
- Herpes zoster

Psychiatric
- Emotional, anxiety related, panic disorder

TB, tuberculosis

- ○ **Aortic dissection**: Classically presents with severe, tearing pain radiating to the back.
- ○ **Pneumothorax**: Typically presents with sudden, sharp pleuritic chest pain and dyspnea.
- ○ **Pericarditis**: Pain typically worse with recumbency, relieved by sitting upright or leaning forward. Fever and persistent chest pain may be additional clues.
- The history should also include questions aimed at assessing the risk of antiplatelet and anticoagulant therapy, such as known bleeding diathesis, prior gastrointestinal or intracranial bleeding, recent surgery, as well as relevant over-the-counter and prescribed medications.

TABLE 3-2 HISTORICAL FEATURES ASSOCIATED WITH ANGINA

Clinical Feature	Typical Angina	Atypical Angina	Nonanginal Symptoms
Location	Substernal ± radiation to neck, arm, shoulder	Epigastric, right sided; to back, teeth, or ear	Radiation to lower abdomen or legs
Quality	Pressure, tightness, squeezing, heaviness	Burning, cramping, gas	Stabbing, sharp
Time course	Builds over 5–10 min (sometimes sudden in myocardial infarction)	Duration >30 min without other signs of ACS	Lasts only seconds
Aggravating factors	Exercise, stress, cold weather	Occurs at rest (although myocardial infarction, unstable angina, and Prinzmetal angina may occur at rest)	Deep breathing, change in position
Alleviating factors	Rest, nitroglycerin	Belching, antacids	
Associated symptoms	Dyspnea, diaphoresis, nausea and vomiting		

Physical Examination

An abbreviated exam, including vital signs and oxygen saturation, jugular venous pulsation, lungs, heart, chest wall, abdomen, extremities, and pulses, may suggest a cause of chest pain (Table 3-3). However, physical exam lacks sensitivity and specificity for reaching a diagnosis.

Diagnostic Testing

Laboratories

Lab markers of myocardial injury, such as troponin and CK-MB assays, are sensitive and specific indications of cardiac muscle necrosis. See Chapter 4 (Acute Coronary Syndromes) for further details.

Electrocardiography
- A 12-lead ECG provides the most important initial data. The ECG is valuable for both risk stratification and diagnosis of ACS. Approximately 80% of patients with acute MI have abnormalities on their ECG, of which half are diagnostic.[6] Table 3-4 lists the significance of common ECG abnormalities.
- Obtain ECG within 10 minutes of presentation; repeat if pain recurs or persists, or with any change in symptoms.
- Assume that all abnormalities are new unless proven otherwise. Obtain old ECGs.

TABLE 3-3 FEATURES FROM PHYSICAL EXAM SUGGESTING A SPECIFIC CAUSE

Physical Finding	Diagnoses to Consider
S3, S4, or mitral regurgitation murmur during pain	Myocardial ischemia
Friction rub or pericardial knock	Pericarditis
Tachycardia, tachypnea, hypotension, hypoxemia	Pulmonary embolism, myocardial infarction with cardiogenic shock
Loud P2 with fixed split of S2	Pulmonary hypertension, pulmonary embolism
Pleural friction rub	Pneumonia, pulmonary embolism
Aortic insufficiency murmur, asymmetric pulses or blood pressures	Aortic dissection
Unilateral decreased breath sounds and tympany	Pneumothorax
Chest wall tenderness and worse with movement	Musculoskeletal causes
Vesicular rash, dermatomal distribution	Herpes zoster

Imaging
- Although rarely diagnostic, **chest radiography** can help rule out less common causes of chest pain as well as complications of MI. It is more useful if comparison films are available.
  - Findings on CXR that may point to a pulmonary cause of chest pain include a focal infiltrate (pneumonia), interstitial or airspace opacity (pulmonary edema), unilateral radiolucency (pneumothorax) or radiodensity (effusion), or wedge-shaped density (PE with infarction).
  - CXR findings that may suggest a cardiovascular etiology of chest pain: cardiomegaly (pericardial effusion or MI complicated by left ventricular failure or free-wall rupture), mediastinal widening, or abnormal aorta (aortic dissection).
  - Other causes seen on CXR: pneumomediastinum (esophageal rupture), rib fracture, or dislocation.
- **Echocardiography** can show segmental myocardial dysfunction but cannot distinguish between acute MI, ischemia, and prior infarction. The absence of regional wall motion abnormalities does not rule out MI; however, an echocardiogram can help when other data are equivocal.

Disease-Specific Confirmatory Testing
- **Suspected myocardial ischemia.** Once acute MI has been excluded by serial ECGs and cardiac enzymes, patients with unstable angina should undergo further testing to identify anatomic abnormalities or inducible ischemia.
  - Patients with a thrombolysis in myocardial infarction (TIMI) risk score >4 (see Chapter 4) derive greater benefit from early coronary angiography when compared with lower-risk patients.
  - Others should have a functional ischemic evaluation, such as an exercise or pharmacologic stress test.

TABLE 3-4 SIGNIFICANT ECG FINDINGS IN CHEST PAIN

ECG Finding	Likely Diagnosis	Differential Diagnosis
≥1 mm ST-segment elevation in at least two contiguous leads	Acute MI	Coronary vasospasm Pericarditis Early repolarization Left ventricular aneurysm
≥1 mm ST-segment depression	Myocardial ischemia or infarction	Normal variant LVH with strain Digitalis toxicity Electrolyte abnormalities
T-wave inversions in at least two contiguous leads	Myocardial ischemia or infarction	Normal variant CNS disease Hypertrophic obstructive cardiomyopathy
Q waves ≥1 mm and 0.04 s in two contiguous leads	MI, age undetermined	Dilated cardiomyopathy LVH, hypertrophic obstructive cardiomyopathy, COPD Pulmonary embolism
Tall R waves ± T-wave inversions in V1/V2, right axis deviation, new right bundle branch block	Pulmonary embolism	Pulmonary hypertension

CNS, central nervous system; COPD, chronic obstructive pulmonary disease; LVH, left ventricular hypertrophy; MI, myocardial infarction.

- Recently cardiac CT has emerged as an alternative noninvasive imaging modality for the evaluation of patients suspected to have ACS. However, the role of cardiac CT angiography in risk stratification has not yet been clearly defined.
- The American College of Cardiology/American Heart Association guidelines recommend cardiac catheterization for patients with the following:
  - Prior revascularization
  - Congestive heart failure (left ventricular ejection fraction < 50%)
  - Ventricular arrhythmias
  - Persistent or recurrent angina
  - Noninvasive study indicating high risk
- Either an early invasive or early conservative strategy may be undertaken.[7]
- **Pericarditis/Pericardial Effusion**
  - ST-segment elevation is often present in acute pericarditis, leading to an erroneous diagnosis of ST-segment elevation myocardial infarction (STEMI). However, the classic ECG changes of pericarditis are diffuse, concave upward ST-segment elevations, and concurrent PR-segment depressions.
  - Pericarditis may also be associated with pericardial effusion. Pericardial effusions may result from myriad causes, although the most common etiology is idiopathic.

- An echocardiogram can reveal the presence of fluid in the pericardial sac as well as signs of hemodynamic compromise or cardiac tamponade.
- Adjunctive laboratory markers that are sometimes elevated in pericarditis include the erythrocyte sedimentation rate and C-reactive protein.
- **Pulmonary Embolism**
  - The Wells criteria combined with a D-dimer assay and imaging study can efficiently and reliably diagnose PE in most patients.[8]
  - A ventilation/perfusion (V/Q) scan and CT pulmonary angiogram (CTA) are both appropriate diagnostic tests.
  - The gold standard, pulmonary angiography, should be reserved for cases in which less invasive studies are equivocal.
  - For high suspicion, empiric anticoagulation is usually recommended and should not be delayed until testing is complete.
  - In patients who have a documented PE and concomitant hypoxia and/or hypotension that is refractory to supportive therapy, the use of thrombolytics may be considered.
- **Aortic Dissection**
  - Transesophageal echocardiography (TEE), CT with contrast (using a dissection protocol), magnetic resonance imaging (MRI), and aortography can show details of aortic anatomy.
  - If dissection is a possibility, one of these should be performed before initiating anticoagulation in suspected MI or PE.
  - In addition, an ECG should be performed immediately to look for signs of myocardial ischemia, particularly in the inferior leads (II, III, aVF), which would be suggestive of a dissection extending into the right coronary cusp.
  - Patients who have an underlying connective tissue disorder such as Marfan syndrome should be evaluated with a high degree of suspicion for aortic dissection.
- **Esophageal Disease**
  - Upper endoscopy is useful for visualizing structural lesions of the esophagus and stomach, including reflux esophagitis and peptic ulcer disease.
  - Twenty-four-hour esophageal pH monitoring can document acid reflux.
  - Contrast radiography of the upper gastrointestinal tract (e.g., barium swallow) in combination with esophageal manometry can diagnose motility disorders such as diffuse esophageal spasm, which can be mistaken for angina.

TREATMENT

- Patients who are thought to be experiencing an ACS should chew a 325-mg aspirin tablet. In the absence of contraindications, oxygen, β-blockers, nitrates, and analgesics (e.g., morphine) should also be considered.
- In patients with ACS who have been ruled out for other life-threatening causes of chest pain, appropriate antiplatelet and anticoagulant therapy should be administered.
- Patients with STEMI or new left bundle branch block (LBBB) generally proceed directly to cardiac catheterization. The national goal for administration of fibrinolytics (door-to-needle time) is within 30 minutes of ED arrival, and door-to-balloon time is within 90 minutes.

REFERENCES

1. Cannon CP. Acute coronary syndromes: risk stratification and initial management. *Cardiol Clin* 2005;23:401–9.
2. Pope JH, Selker HP. Acute coronary syndromes in the emergency department: diagnostic characteristics, tests, and challenges. *Cardiol Clin* 2005;23:423–51.

3. Owens PL, Barrett ML, Gibson TB, et al. Emergency department care in the United States: a profile of national data sources. *Ann Emerg Med* 2010;56:150–65.
4. Mozaffarian D, Benjamin EJ, Go AS, et al. Heart disease and stroke statistics—2015 Update: a report from the American Heart Association. *Circulation* 2015;131:e29–e322.
5. Haffner SM, Lehto S, Rönnemaa T, et al. Mortality from coronary heart disease in subjects with type 2 diabetes and in nondiabetic subjects with and without prior myocardial infarction. *N Engl J Med* 1998;339:229–34.
6. Lee T, Goldman L. Evaluation of the patient with acute chest pain. *N Engl J Med* 2000;342:1187–95.
7. Scanlon PJ, Faxon DP, Audet A, et al. ACC/AHA Guidelines for Coronary Angiography. A report of the American College of Cardiology/American Heart Association Task Force on practice guidelines (Committee on Coronary Angiography). Developed in collaboration with the Society for Cardiac Angiography and Interventions. *J Am Coll Cardiol* 1999;33:1756–824.
8. Perrier A, Roy PM, Aujesky D, et al. Diagnosing pulmonary embolism in outpatients with clinical assessment, D-Dimer measurement, venous ultrasound, and helical computed tomography: A multicenter management study. *Am J Med* 2004;116:291–9.

Acute Coronary Syndromes 4

Adam Littich

GENERAL PRINCIPLES

- Coronary artery disease (CAD) is the leading cause of death in the United States in both men and women and accounts for a large portion of US health care expenditure.[1] Encouragingly, the death rate attributable to CAD has been declining.[1]
- In the United States, of the more than 12 million Americans with a diagnosis of CAD, more than 50% have had a history of myocardial infarction (MI).[1]
- Annually, more than 1 million Americans suffer a coronary event.[1]
- The spectrum of CAD ranges from silent disease to chronic angina to acute coronary syndromes (ACS) to sudden cardiac death (SCD).
- ACS can be classified into three distinct syndromes: unstable angina (UA), non–ST-segment elevation myocardial infarction (NSTEMI), and ST-segment elevation myocardial infarction (STEMI). The underlying pathologic and histologic changes are different in each of these syndromes.
  - Patients with STEMI usually have significant myocardial necrosis, often with transmural involvement and associated electrocardiographic (ECG) changes of ST-segment elevation in contiguous leads.
  - Patients with NSTEMI have less significant myocardial necrosis, but without the resultant ST-segment elevation.[2]
  - Patients with UA do not demonstrate any ECG changes or enzymatic evidence of myocardial necrosis.[2] For classification purposes, UA and NSTEMI are often grouped together because of significant overlap in their pathogenesis and treatment.
- ACS includes a variety of etiologies, often culminating in acute myocardial ischemia.
  - In most cases, ACS results from atherosclerosis-mediated plaque rupture and subsequent thrombosis, which is now termed a **type I MI**.[2]
  - Systemic inflammatory mediators play a large role in the genesis of plaque rupture, initiating a sequence of platelet aggregation, fibrin deposition, and vasoconstriction that eventually occludes the artery.
  - However, it is important to note that not all ACS is caused by plaque rupture. The term **type II MI** has come into use to account for other causes including vasospasm (idiopathic and cocaine induced), supply–demand mismatch, systemic hypotension, severe hypertension, anemia, hypoxia, tachy-/bradyarrhythmias, vasculitis, and less commonly, extension of an aortic dissection.[2]

DIAGNOSIS

Clinical Presentation

History

Rapid recognition is the key to outcome: a targeted history, physical, and 12-lead ECG should be completed prehospital by emergency medical technicians or within 10 minutes of presentation to an emergency department.[3] The **most critical part of the evaluation is the ECG**, focusing on prompt recognition of ST-segment elevation, in which case the patient should be immediately assessed for thrombolysis or percutaneous revascularization.[4]

- Often, patients with **typical angina** complain of crushing discomfort described as substernal or left sided, with or without radiation to the left arm, neck, shoulder, back, or jaw. Onset is usually during exertion, but may be at rest. Pain lasting only seconds, pleuritic pain, or pain localizable with one finger is unlikely to be of cardiac origin. Ischemic chest discomfort is often accompanied by dyspnea, diaphoresis, nausea, vomiting, palpitations, and an overwhelming sense of doom.
- ACS may also occur with atypical chest discomfort or none at all, particularly in the following patients: postoperative, elderly, women, or diabetics. In fact, depending on cohort studied, up to 25% of MIs are initially unrecognized because of silent or atypical symptoms.[5]
- In addition, clinical history should attempt to identify similarities to previous symptoms, especially in patients who have had a prior MI. UA and MI are usually differentiated from stable angina by lack of relief with rest and/or nitroglycerin (NTG) as well as prolonged discomfort lasting >20 minutes.
- Focused past medical, family, and social histories should determine if the patient has a history of CAD, aspirin use, hypertension, hypercholesterolemia, diabetes mellitus, smoking, and family history of CAD; these are useful in calculating the thrombolysis in myocardial infarction (TIMI) score—see Table 4-1.[6]

Physical Examination

The goals of the physical exam are as follows:

- **Determine hemodynamic stability**: Assess for cardiogenic shock with pulse rate and blood pressure measurement (both arms if dissection is suspected). Assess for hypoxia with pulse oximetry. The presence of an S3 gallop, jugular venous distention, and pulmonary rales is suggestive of concomitant heart failure.

TABLE 4-1 TIMI RISK SCORE

Number of Risk Factors[a]	Rates of All-Cause Mortality, Myocardial Infarction, and Severe Recurrent Ischemia Prompting Urgent Revascularization Through 14 d After Randomization (%)
0–1	4.7
2	8.3
3	13.2
4	19.9
5	26.2
6–7	40.9

[a]Risk factors (1 point each) = age ≥ 65 y, ≥3 risk factors for CAD (family history of CAD, hypertension, hypercholesterolemia, diabetes, current smoker), known CAD (≥50% stenosis), ST deviation > 0.5 mm, severe angina (≥2 anginal episodes/24 h), ASA use in past 7 d, and elevated cardiac biomarkers.

Adapted from Antman, EM, Cohen, M, Bernink PJ, et al. The TIMI risk score for unstable angina/non-ST elevation MI: a method for prognostication and therapeutic decision making. *JAMA* 2000;284(7):835–42, Ref.[6]

- **Detect mechanical complications of MI** such as papillary muscle dysfunction, free wall rupture, and ventricular septal defect. The presence of a new systolic murmur and a paradoxical S2 is suggestive of mitral valve dysfunction as a result of myocardial ischemia.
- **Detect the presence of other areas of atherosclerotic burden**: Careful examination of the carotid, femoral, and distal pulses should be undertaken to assess for the presence of peripheral vascular disease, which can also help guide arterial cannulation when urgent cardiac catheterization is planned.
- **Evaluate for other possible etiologies of chest discomfort**: Especially, evaluate for the ability to reproduce chest pain on palpation.

Differential Diagnosis

For a detailed discussion on the differential diagnosis of chest pain, see Chapter 3.

Diagnostic Testing

The diagnosis of the spectrum of ACS can be made by the presence of some combination of the following criteria:

- Prolonged chest discomfort or anginal equivalent
- ECG changes consistent with ischemia or infarction
- Elevated cardiac enzymes

Laboratories

- Troponin I (or newer assays of troponin T) has the highest sensitivity and specificity for myocardial ischemia.[3]
  - Troponin I often increases 2–12 hours after the onset of symptoms[7] and peaks at 24–48 hours before returning to baseline up to 14 days later.[3]
  - Because of the possible lag of the troponin peak, it is recommended to check troponin at presentation as well as 2–6 hours after the symptom onset in all patients.[3]
  - Those with ECG changes or intermediate to high clinical risk may have additional serial troponin measurement every 6 hours, until the possible lag of 12 hours has passed.[3] This is termed ACS rule-out.
  - Note that there are many causes of mildly elevated troponin: cardiac injury not related to ischemia (e.g., contusion, myocarditis, etc.), decreased renal clearance, stroke, pulmonary embolism, or heart failure. Thus, history and ECG remain centrally important to assessing the significance of troponin. Troponin measurement should be reserved for patients suspected of having ACS.
- Other cardiac enzymes such as creatine kinase, creatine kinase-MB (CK-MB), and myoglobin are no longer recommended.[3] See Table 4-2 for time courses of the

TABLE 4-2 CARDIAC ENZYMES WITH TIMING AND SPECIFICITY

Cardiac Enzyme	Time to Positive (h)	Time to Peak (h)	Time to Normal	Specificity
Troponin I/T	2–12	24–48	7–14 d	Very high
CK-MB	4–6	18–24	72 h	High (95%)
Myoglobin	1–4	—	—	Intermediate

CK-MB, creatine kinase-MB.

various cardiac enzymes. CK-MB may be falsely positive with myopathy or other muscle injury.
- Myoglobin, though present as early as 1 hour, is not specific for cardiac muscle.

Electrocardiography
- **ECG should be completed within 10 minutes of arrival.**[3] Always obtain old ECGs for comparison if possible. Consider serial ECG every 15–30 minutes in those with ongoing symptoms.[3]
- Definitive ECG diagnosis of STEMI requires ≥1 mm of ST-segment elevation in at least two contiguous leads.[4]
- **New left bundle-branch block (LBBB)** with ACS symptoms is managed like STEMI (suggests proximal occlusion of the left anterior descending coronary artery). Ischemia can still be identified in patients with known old LBBB.[4]
- ST depression ≥5 mm or T-wave inversion of ≥2 mm are diagnostic of NSTEMI.[3]
- Distribution of ischemic changes is helpful in determining the location of the occluded vessel, assessing prognosis, and predicting complications.
- Consider posterior (V_7–V_9) or right-sided (V_3R–V_6R) leads if the initial ECG negative and strong clinical suspicion persists.[3]

Diagnostic Procedures
Consider appropriate stress testing in low- and intermediate-risk patients (discussed below) who have negative troponins and ECG.[8–10] It is also reasonable to substitute resting CT coronary angiography in the same population, provided the patient does not have known CAD.[11,12]

- Patients with TIMI score of 0–1 (Table 4-1) with negative ECG along with negative troponin at presentation and 2 hours had a negative predictive value of >99% for a major cardiac event; these patients can be discharged safely without stress testing.[13–15]
- For appropriate patients (see below), stress testing can be performed either in the emergency department or in an observation unit. Prompt discharge can also be considered for those who have negative stress testing[9] or negative CT coronary angiography.[11]
- Admit all patients with continuing anginal symptoms, significant ECG changes, significantly elevated troponin (with evidence of rise or fall), positive stress test, or positive CT coronary angiography.
  - Patients with persistent symptoms or hemodynamic instability should be admitted to a coronary care unit with continuous rhythm monitoring, high nurse–patient ratio, frequent assessment, and quick access to defibrillation.
  - Patients who are symptom free should be admitted to the hospital floor with continuous rhythm monitoring.

TREATMENT OF UA/NSTEMI

Treatment goals include controlling ischemia by increasing myocardial oxygen delivery and reducing demand, providing antiplatelet and anticoagulation therapy, revascularizing when appropriate, risk stratifying and finally, preventing future events through risk factor modification.

Medications
Anti-Ischemic Therapy
The goal of anti-ischemic therapy involves measures to improve the balance of myocardial oxygen supply and demand. Nonpharmacologic measures include bed rest and supplemental O_2. Traditionally, oxygen was administered to all patients with ACS regardless of respiratory status. However, based on recent evidence, it is recommended to use supplemental oxygen only in patients with true hypoxemia.[16]

- **Nitroglycerin (NTG)** works as a venous, coronary, and systemic arterial vasodilator. It reduces preload and afterload, resulting in lower myocardial oxygen demand, and dilates coronary arteries to improve myocardial oxygen supply.
  - Use of NTG is based more on pathophysiologic rationale and historical observation rather than high-level evidence.[3]
  - Start with a 0.4-mg sublingual tablet or NTG spray, monitoring for hypotension. If ischemic symptoms are not completely relieved, repeat q5 minutes until three doses are given.
  - Provide IV NTG if symptoms persist after three doses of immediate-release NTG. Also consider IV NTG for those with heart failure or persistent hypotension. Initiate IV NTG at 10 mcg/min and increase by 10 mcg/min q3–5 minutes until symptoms resolve or BP falls.
  - Use with caution when SBP ≤ 110 mm Hg or has fallen by ≥25%. Remember that readministration of sublingual NTG will deliver much more NTG (400 mcg) in a short time than increasing the IV drip rate.
  - Therefore, if recurrent ischemia develops, administer sublingual NTG before increasing the drip.
  - Once a patient has been symptom free for 12–24 hours, change to topical or long-acting oral nitrates or consider discontinuation. If there are no recurrent ischemic symptoms, initiate a daily nitrate-free interval to prevent nitrate tolerance.
  - Nitrates are contraindicated if sildenafil or other phosphodiesterase inhibitors were used in the previous 24 hours.
  - Be cautious in administration to patients with right ventricular infarction, as this can precipitate cardiogenic shock.
- **Morphine Sulfate**: Its primary function is to reduce preload via venodilation and reduce heart rate and systolic blood pressure (SBP) via decreased central sympathetic outflow. Both these effects serve to improve the supply of oxygen to ischemic myocardial tissue. In addition, morphine sulfate also has potent **analgesic** and anxiolytic properties.
  - Give 1–5 mg IV for symptoms refractory to three doses of immediate-release NTG.
  - Repeat dosing q5–30 minutes if necessary. It should be noted, however, that excessive use of morphine is not recommended for persistent chest pain, as it can mask the symptoms of coronary ischemia, often delaying urgent revascularization.
  - It can also cause hypotension and respiratory depression. Its use, therefore, has been downgraded to a class IIb recommendation in the most recent American College of Cardiology/American Heart Association (ACC/AHA) guidelines.[3]
  - No randomized controlled trial has been performed, but one large observational study suggested possible harm.[17] This may be due to selection bias as patients who receive morphine often have persistent symptoms despite appropriate anti-ischemic therapy and thus may be acutely ill.
- **β-Blockers** inhibit $β_1$ receptors and therefore reduce the cardiac rate and contractility and reduce myocardial oxygen demand. Also, diastole is prolonged, thus improving coronary perfusion and myocardial oxygen supply.
  - Meta-analysis data suggest that β-blockers in UA/NSTEMI reduce the progression to acute myocardial infarction (AMI) by 18%; however, no mortality benefit has been demonstrated in the reperfusion era.[18]
  - In the 45,000-patient Chinese COMMIT study, which mainly investigated STEMI patients, the composite of death, reinfarction, or cardiac arrest was not reduced with the use of early intravenous then oral β-blockade.[19]
  - There is no clear evidence that any specific β-blocker is superior. Choice is usually based on clinician familiarity. Commonly used agents in acute ischemia include metoprolol, atenolol, or esmolol. If there is concern about the tolerability of β-blockers, use a short-acting agent such as metoprolol or ultra–short-acting esmolol.

- Typical dosing regimens are as follows:
  - **Metoprolol** tartrate: 25–50 mg PO q6–12 hours. Can consider a switch to long-acting metoprolol succinate or carvedilol at discharge, especially if there is evidence of concomitant heart failure.
  - **Atenolol**: 25–50 mg every 12 hours. Can switch to daily dosing at discharge or change to metoprolol succinate or carvedilol if heart failure.
  - **Esmolol**: Use if continuous IV administration is needed. Start with 50 mcg/kg/min IV, titrating up by 50 mcg/kg/min q10 minutes to a max of 300 mcg/kg/min, as heart rate and BP tolerate.
- Contraindications are as follows:
  - Signs of acute heart failure or those at risk of cardiogenic shock.
  - Bradycardia or heart block—avoid β-blockers if heart rate ≤50, PR interval >240 ms, or there is any type of second- or third-degree heart block.
  - Active bronchospastic lung disease—most patients with a history of chronic obstructive pulmonary disease (COPD) will still tolerate a cardioselective β-blocker at a low dose.
- **Calcium channel blockers (CCB)**: Meta-analyses have shown **no significant mortality benefit** for CCB in UA/NSTEMI[20]; use of nondihydropyridine CCB (e.g., diltiazem and verapamil) is limited primarily to symptomatic relief in those who have a contraindication to β-blockers,[3] though some studies showed decreased reinfarction occurrence.[21] There is **no role for immediate-release dihydropyridine CCB** (e.g., short-acting nifedipine) in ACS as studies have shown higher mortality.[22] In general, CCB are second-line agents whose use is limited to the following situations:
  - Refractory ischemia in patients already receiving nitrates and β-blockers
  - Patients with contraindications to β-blockers
  - Patients with variant or Prinzmetal angina from coronary vasospasm
  - CCB are contraindicated in severe left ventricular (LV) dysfunction, Wolff-Parkinson-White syndrome (CCB in IV form), or heart block.
- Inhibitors of the Renin–Angiotensin–Aldosterone System
  - **Angiotensin-converting enzyme (ACE) inhibitors** have been shown to decrease mortality in patients with ACS, especially those with concomitant LV dysfunction.[23]
  - **Angiotensin receptor blockers (ARB)** can be used as an alternative in patients who have ACE inhibitor intolerance.[24]
  - Start an ACE inhibitor or ARB in all patients with ACS and ejection fraction <40%, as well as those with hypertension, diabetes mellitus, or stable CKD.[3] Contraindications include acute renal failure or hypotension.
  - Aldosterone antagonists such as eplerenone have also been shown to improve mortality in patients with ACS who have concomitant LV dysfunction, heart failure, or diabetes.[25] This benefit likely exists for spironolactone as well, though not proven. Contraindications include renal dysfunction (creatinine > 2.5 mg/dL) or hyperkalemia (K^+ > 5.0 mEq/L). Therapeutic doses should first be reached for ACE/ARB and β-blockers.[3]
- **Statins**
  - High-intensity statin should be initiated or continued in all patients presenting with ACS, except for those with contraindication.[3]
  - High-intensity statin therapy reduced recurrent ischemic events,[26] mortality, and major adverse cardiovascular events.[27]
  - The mechanism is primarily mediated through reduction of low-density lipoprotein cholesterol (LDL-C), though there may be other anti-inflammatory or antithrombotic effects as well. Dosing is as follows:
    - Atorvastatin 40–80 mg daily
    - Rosuvastatin 20–40 mg daily

Antiplatelet Therapy
- **Aspirin (ASA)** is a cyclooxygenase (COX) inhibitor that prevents thromboxane A_2–mediated platelet aggregation and should be administered immediately to all patients with suspected ACS unless contraindicated as below.[3] It should be continued indefinitely.[3]
  - Multiple large studies have consistently demonstrated reduction in death or MI. Pooled data suggest a relative risk reduction of 19% for the combined end point of cardiovascular death, MI, or stroke and 31% relative risk reduction for MI alone.[28]
  - The initial dose (162–325 mg) should not be coated and may be chewed to speed absorption. Subsequent doses (81–325 mg PO daily) may be enteric coated.
  - Recent dose comparison studies found no difference in outcome after percutaneous intervention between high dose (300–325 mg) and low dose (75–100 mg) ASA,[29-31] but did show increased major bleeding with high dose.[30,31] Most recent guidelines give a class IIa recommendation to 81 mg dose for maintenance therapy, instead of traditional 325 mg.[3]
  - Contraindications include allergy, serious active bleeding, and severe uncontrolled hypertension (risk of intracranial hemorrhage).
- **$P2Y_{12}$ inhibitors** (including clopidogrel, ticagrelor, prasugrel) irreversibly inhibit the activation of $P2Y_{12}$, which subsequently blocks activation of downstream GP IIb/IIIa, ultimately inhibiting platelet aggregation. When combined with aspirin, the antiplatelet effect is synergistic. Clopidogrel or ticagrelor is indicated for all patients with ACS who are treated with either early invasive or ischemia-guided strategy.[3]
  - **Clopidogrel** is a prodrug, which requires CYP2C19 for activation; thus, the onset of action is slower. It is an irreversible inhibitor of $P2Y_{12}$. Some patients with low levels of CYP2C19 may not get the full platelet inhibitory effect.[32]
    - Clopidogrel added to aspirin in patients with UA/NSTEMI reduced cardiovascular death, MI, and stroke.[33] In addition, clopidogrel has been shown to be beneficial when used in patients with NSTEMI undergoing PCI.[34]
    - Give a loading dose of 300–600 mg PO followed by 75 mg PO daily. Loading dose of 600 mg is preferred in STEMI[4] and is also reasonable in patients being managed with early invasive approach.[29]
  - **Prasugrel** has more rapid onset than clopidogrel, though it also is a prodrug. It is a stronger $P2Y_{12}$ inhibitor than the other drugs and is irreversible.
    - Prasugrel, compared with clopidogrel, showed no difference in mortality, MI, stroke, or bleeding in patients with ACS on aspirin not undergoing PCI.[35]
    - When compared with clopidogrel in patients on aspirin undergoing PCI, prasugrel reduces risk of MI and stent thrombosis, but increases bleeding risk, with no overall difference in mortality.[36]
    - Prasugrel should not be used in patients with prior stroke or transient ischemic attack.[3,4,36]
    - Most recent 2014 AHA/ACC guidelines do not recommend using prasugrel as upfront therapy in patients with ACS/NSTEMI,[3] but it may be used in patients with STEMI.[4]
    - Give prasugrel 60 mg loading dose followed by 10 mg daily dose.[4]
  - **Ticagrelor** is a reversible $P2Y_{12}$ inhibitor with more rapid onset and shorter half-life. It is not a prodrug and is thus not dependent on the cytochrome P450 system.
    - Ticagrelor had lower rates of overall mortality and MI and similar rates of bleeding when compared to clopidogrel in patients with ACS on aspirin.[37]
    - Most recent 2014 AHA/ACC guidelines give preference to ticagrelor over clopidogrel, a class IIa recommendation.[3]
    - Give a 180-mg loading dose, then 90 mg twice daily. The shorter half-life and twice-daily dosing are a concern in patients prone to medication noncompliance.

- **Glycoprotein IIb/IIIa inhibitors** (tirofiban, eptifibatide, abciximab) block platelet aggregation by interfering with platelet binding to fibrinogen.
  - The PRISM-PLUS trial (tirofiban)[38] and PURSUIT trial (eptifibatide)[39] showed benefits of GP IIb/IIIa inhibitors in patients with ACS, with less death and MI, but with greater bleeding.
  - Eptifibatide and tirofiban are indicated in ACS patients with positive troponin when early invasive strategy is planned.[3] These two drugs may be started on initial management (class IIb recommendation).[3]
  - It is also reasonable to **defer** GP IIb/IIIa inhibition to the time of PCI, as the major studies of early administration versus administration at the time of PCI did not show convincing differences in UA/NSTEMI[40,41] or STEMI.[42,43]
  - Abciximab should be reserved for use at the time of PCI, as major studies were all designed in this manner,[44,45] and trials examining upstream use are lacking or demonstrate a negative outcome.[43]
  - In the GUSTO IV-ACS trial, there was no clinical benefit of abciximab in troponin-negative patients[46]; thus routine use of GP IIb/IIIa inhibitors is not recommended in this setting.
  - Dosing
    - Eptifibatide: loading 180 mcg/kg (max 22.6 mg) then 2 mcg/kg/min for 18–24 hours
    - Tirofiban: loading 25 mcg/kg then 0.15 mcg/kg/min for 18–24 hours. Renal adjustment recommended
    - Abciximab: loading 0.25 mg/kg then 0.125 mcg/kg/min for 12 hours

Anticoagulation Therapy
- In our practice, it is typical to use unfractionated heparin (UFH) in most patients with ACS. It is reasonable to use a low molecular weight heparin (LMWH) such as enoxaparin as an alternative, except in STEMI or in patients with creatinine clearance < 30. Given their ease of subcutaneous administration, enoxaparin and a factor Xa inhibitor, such as fondaparinux, are reasonable alternatives to UFH when an ischemia-guided approach (see below) is chosen, provided creatinine clearance is >30. Given its increased cost, need for continuous IV drip, and concern for increased acute stent thrombosis, we rarely use bivalirudin.
- Heparin agents are indirect thrombin inhibitors that complex with antithrombin to inactivate thrombin (aka factor IIa) and factor Xa, subsequently preventing coagulation. **Anticoagulation should be added to antiplatelet therapy in all patients with ACS.** Guidelines for ACS/NSTEMI do not specify a preference between UFH, LMWH, fondaparinux, or the bivalirudin,[3] while STEMI guidelines support either UFH or bivalirudin.[4]
- Studies showing benefit of heparins versus placebo were generally performed in the era prior to early revascularization and P2Y$_{12}$ inhibitors, such as clopidogrel. Nonetheless, a pooled analysis of smaller trials showed a significant 47% reduction in death or MI at 7 days with either UFH or LMWH versus placebo.[47]
- **Unfractionated heparin**: Dosage should be weight based. Start with an initial loading dose of 60 IU/kg (maximum 4000 IU) and an infusion rate of 12 IU/kg/h (maximum 1000 IU/h).[3] Adjust the dose based on institutional nomograms. Follow the complete blood count daily to monitor for heparin-induced thrombocytopenia. The optimal duration of therapy is not established, but in most trials, it was continued for 2–4 days.
- **Low molecular weight heparin** (LMWH) such as enoxaparin and dalteparin have a molecular weight one-third that of UFH and have less anti-IIa effect. Anti–factor Xa levels can be measured to monitor the antithrombotic effect of LMWH, though it is not required.

- Earlier trials comparing LMWH with UFH showed small benefits of LMWH in terms of death, MI, recurrent angina, or need for revascularization.[48-50] These trials mainly used an ischemia-guided approach.
- However, the best evidence probably comes from the SYNERGY trial, which compared UFH to enoxaparin in patients treated with dual antiplatelet therapy, most of whom underwent revascularization. No significant difference was found in death or MI, but there was a small increase in bleeding with LMWH.[51]
- LMWH is generally accepted to have similar efficacy, require less monitoring due to predictable anticoagulant effects, and induce less thrombocytopenia than does UFH. However, the level of anticoagulation is difficult to assess, and effects are harder to reverse. For this reason, we prefer UFH if early invasive approach (see below) is utilized. Based on the ATOLL study,[52] UFH is also preferred for STEMI.[4]
- Typical dosing of enoxaparin is 1 mg/kg SC q12 hours in patients up to 100 kg.[3] The renal dose adjustment (creatinine clearance < 30 mL/min) is 1 mg/kd SC q24 hours; obesity dosing is unclear.[3]

- **Direct thrombin inhibitors (DTIs)**: Hirudin was one of the earliest DTIs to be studied, but initial results were unconvincing, leading to the development of a synthetic DTI called **bivalirudin**. Bivalirudin should be reserved for patients planning to undergo PCI,[3,4] as it has not been studied outside of this indication.
  - Most trials of bivalirudin versus heparin are confounded by glycoprotein IIb/IIIa inhibitor use, overwhelmingly in the heparin group. Three studies compared bivalirudin alone versus heparin plus GP IIb/IIIa and showed no difference in death, MI, or urgent revascularization, but significantly less bleeding in the bivalirudin group.[53-55]
  - In the ACUITY trial, bivalirudin, with or without a GP IIb/IIIa inhibitor, was compared with heparin plus a GP IIb/IIIa inhibitor; the results showed bivalirudin alone to be noninferior to the control group in terms of death, MI, and unplanned revascularizations, with less bleeding.[56]
  - Bivalirudin plus GP IIb/IIIa inhibitor had similar findings, but with increased bleeding.[56]
  - A major caveat to bivalirudin usage is found in the HEAT-PPCI trial, which was a more direct comparison of bivalirudin to heparin, with similar rates of usage of GP IIb/IIIa inhibitors in both groups.[57] It showed an increase in the composite outcome in the bivalirudin group, seemingly driven mainly by a **large increase in acute stent thrombosis (within 24 hours)**, with 3.91 relative risk for bivalirudin (3.4% in bivalirudin, 0.9% in heparin).[57] A meta-analysis confirmed this finding with 3.86 relative risk of acute stent thrombosis in bivalirudin groups compared to heparin groups.[58]
  - Given the high cost of bivalirudin and recent concerns of increased acute stent thrombosis, **we use heparin in preference to bivalirudin**, though AHA/ACC guidelines (published before the HEAT-PPCI trial[57] or the 2014 meta-analysis)[58] consider them equivalent.[3,4]
  - However, it may be reasonable to use bivalirudin in patients at high risk for bleeding, given the apparent superior bleeding profile. When used in this setting, the loading dose should be at 0.10 mg/kg followed by 0.25 mg/kg/h.[3] Continue until PCI or a few hours after PCI.

- **Factor Xa inhibitors**: These drugs tend to inhibit downstream coagulation reactions, reducing the production of thrombin. The prototype, **fondaparinux**, is renally cleared, does not need to be monitored by laboratory testing, has a longer half-life, and behaves in a more predictable manner in terms of its pharmacokinetics. Fondaparinux was compared with LMWH in the OASIS-5 study, with the results demonstrating similar primary composite outcomes with less bleeding.[59] It should be noted, however, that there was an increased incidence of catheter-associated thrombus, which prompted the addition of UFH to the fondaparinux group. Based on this, if coronary angiography/PCI is planned, we use UFH. Fondaparinux may be used as alternative to LMWH or UFH in patients who have a high bleeding risk and are being managed noninvasively.[3] Dosing is 2.5 mg/kg SC q24 hours; avoid in patients with a creatinine clearance < 30.

Other Nonpharmacologic Therapies

There are two approaches to the treatment of UA/NSTEMI: the early invasive and ischemia-guided strategies.

- The early invasive approach involves cardiac catheterization with possible revascularization of the target lesion.
  - This approach more quickly identifies patients at very low risk (e.g., no significant CAD) and very high risk (e.g., left main or three-vessel CAD). It offers immediate revascularization of the culprit lesion and prevention of recurrent angina and ischemia.
  - Multiple meta-analyses suggest that the early invasive strategy is superior to the ischemia-guided approach, especially when examining long-term outcomes.[60–62] This is especially true for patients with high-risk features, with decreasing returns seen in low-risk patients, highlighting the importance of risk stratification (see below).
  - The latest update to the AHA/ACC guidelines recommends this early invasive strategy for patients with UA and any of the following **high-risk features**[3]:
    - Recurrent angina or ischemia at rest or low-level activity despite intensive medical therapy
    - Hemodynamic instability
    - Signs or symptoms of heart failure or new/worsening mitral regurgitation
    - Sustained ventricular tachycardia or fibrillation
    - Elevated cardiac markers with temporal change
    - New ST depression
    - LV ejection fraction $\leq 40\%$
    - PCI with stent in previous 6 months
    - Prior coronary artery bypass graft (CABG)
    - Elevated cardiac risk score (see below)
- The ischemia-guided approach involves cardiac catheterization and revascularization only for patients with refractory ischemia, hemodynamic instability, or a markedly abnormal noninvasive stress test.[3]
  - This approach may avoid risks and costs associated with unnecessary coronary angiography while achieving similar outcomes in low-risk patients.
  - An ischemia-guided approach is also recommended for patients with extensive comorbidities (e.g., hepatic failure, renal failure, respiratory failure, malignancy) where the risks of invasive approach outweigh the benefits.[3]
  - Consider an echocardiogram; if LV dysfunction is present, then angiography should be performed to rule out left-main or three-vessel coronary disease because CABG improves survival in this setting.[3]
- Often, risk calculation scores, such as the TIMI[6] or GRACE[63,64] scores, are helpful to facilitate the decision to pursue either the early invasive or ischemia-guided strategy.
  - The TIMI scoring system[6] is a well-validated instrument to predict cardiovascular risk (Table 4-1). Patients who have a TIMI risk score of ≥ 2 derive a greater benefit from the early invasive strategy.[3]
  - The GRACE score is another commonly used prospectively studied and validated scoring system, though it is significantly more complicated to calculate (Table 4-3).[63,64]
  - If the ischemia-guided strategy is chosen, a noninvasive stress test can establish the presence of myocardial ischemia and identify high-risk patients who would benefit from angiography. There are two groups of patients who may **not** require a noninvasive stress test:
    - Those at highest risk (patients with recurrent rest angina despite maximal therapy, severe LV dysfunction, hemodynamic instability, TIMI score ≥ 2) who will require angiography regardless of the results.[3]

TABLE 4-3 GRACE RISK SCORE

Killip Class	Points	Systolic Blood Pressure	Points
I (No CHF)	0	<80	58
II (Rales and/or JVD)	20	80–99	53
III (Pulmonary edema)	39	100–119	43
IV (Cardiogenic Shock)	39	120–139	34
		140–159	24
		160–199	10
		≥200	0

Heart Rate	Points	Age	Points
<50	0	<30	0
50–69	3	30–39	8
70–89	9	40–49	25
90–109	15	50–59	41
110–149	24	60–69	58
150–199	38	70–79	75
≥200	46	80–89	91
		≥90	100

Creatinine Level (mg/dL)	Points		
0–0.39	1	**Cardiac Arrest at Admission**	**Points**
0.40–0.79	4	Yes	39
0.8–1.19	7	**ST-Segment Deviation > 5 mm**	**Points**
1.2–1.59	10	Yes	39
1.6–1.99	13	**Elevated Cardiac Enzyme Levels**	**Points**
2.0–3.99	21	Yes	14
≥4.0	28		

Add all values.

Scores > 140 generally favorable to early invasive strategy within 24 h.

Scores 109–140 generally favorable to early invasive strategy 25–72 h.

CHF, congestive heart failure; JVD, jugulovenous distension

Adapted from Fox KA, Dabbous OH, Goldberg RJ, et al. Prediction of risk of death and myocardial infarction in the six months after presentation with acute coronary syndrome: prospective multinational observational study (GRACE). *BMJ* 2006;333:1091–4, Ref.[63]; Elbarouni B, Goodman SG, Yan RT, et al. Validation of the global registry of acute coronary event (GRACE) risk score for in-hospital mortality in patients with acute coronary syndrome in Canada. *Am Heart J* 2009;158(3):392–9, Ref.[64]

- Those at lowest risk (atypical symptoms without CAD risk factors) who would not be considered for angiography and revascularization regardless of the results because the risk of true disease is so low that angiography would not offer significant benefit. Patients with TIMI score of 0–1 with negative ECG along with serial negative troponins at presentation and 2 hours had a negative predictive value of >99% for a major cardiac event and can be discharged safely without stress testing.[13–15]
- Stress testing is discussed earlier as well as in Chapter 1.

TREATMENT OF STEMI

The initial goals in managing STEMI are as follows[4]:

- Rapid confirmation of diagnosis with ECG showing ST elevation or new LBBB, preferably by EMS (as described earlier)
- Assessment and implementation of possible reperfusion strategies, preferably PCI
- Administration of antithrombotic and antiplatelet therapy and other adjunctive medications
- Recognition and correction of hemodynamic abnormalities
- Control of ischemic pain

Medications

Once the diagnosis of STEMI has been established, consider the following adjunctive medications while evaluating for reperfusion (see earlier text for details): aspirin, a $P2Y_{12}$ inhibitor, GP IIb/IIIa inhibitor, heparin, β-blocker, ACE inhibitor or ARB, high-intensity statin, NTG, and morphine sulfate.[4]

Reperfusion

- **Percutaneous coronary intervention (PCI)**
  - Optimal time to PCI is 90 minutes from first medical contact.[4]
  - If the patient first arrives to a non–PCI-capable hospital, the recommended strategy is to transfer to a PCI-capable hospital, provided PCI can be performed within 120 minutes from first medical contact.[4]
  - If this is not possible, consider thrombolysis (see below).[4]
  - Some patients delay in seeking medical care after onset of symptoms[65]; however, it is still recommended to perform acute reperfusion within 12 hours of symptom onset in patients with ST-segment elevation or new LBBB.[4]
  - Patients with >12 hours but <24 hours of symptoms should still be considered for reperfusion if there is clinical or ECG evidence of ongoing ischemia.[4] PCI should be performed in all patients with STEMI complicated by acute severe heart failure or cardiogenic shock regardless of time from symptom onset; thrombolysis should not be performed in these patients.[4]
  - Emergent percutaneous coronary intervention
    - Emergent PCI has advantages of increased early efficacy in opening occluded arteries, lower rates of hemorrhagic stroke, and improved survival.
    - A systematic review of randomized clinical trials found that primary PCI versus thrombolysis reduced short-term mortality by 27% (number needed to treat [NNT] 43), nonfatal reinfarction by 65% (NNT 23), total stroke by 54% (NNT 93), and hemorrhagic stroke by 95% (NNT 93).[66] Given the lower stroke risk and higher efficacy, **PCI is the reperfusion method of choice** in hospitals with the capacity for emergent PCI and adequate experience.[4]

- If PCI is not available or if thrombolysis is contraindicated, transfer to a facility capable of emergent PCI should be considered as outlined above.[4]
- As a note of caution, data suggest only that 30% of transferred patients meet this goal of transfer for PCI within 120 minutes; the median time was 149 minutes.[67]
- **Thrombolysis**
  - Advantages of thrombolysis are widespread availability and fast administration.
  - The benefit of early thrombolytic therapy (within 12 hours of symptom onset) is well studied. Pooled data from the Fibrinolytic Therapy Trialists' Collaborative Group showed an 18% reduction in mortality.[68]
  - However, thrombolytics increase the risk of hemorrhage, including hemorrhagic stroke in 1%.[66] Predictive factors for stroke and intracranial hemorrhage include age ≥65 years, weight < 70 kg, and HTN on admission.
  - **Time: 30 minutes** from first medical contact.
  - **Agents**: Fibrin specific (tissue plasminogen activator [tPA], reteplase, anistreplase, tenecteplase) are preferred to nonfibrin specific (streptokinase).[4]
  - Perform thrombolysis only on STEMI patient who cannot be transferred for a PCI within 120 minutes.[4] Never perform thrombolysis in NSTEMI or UA.[3]
  - **Contraindications** should always be carefully considered (Table 4-4).
  - **Rescue PCI**: As 15–50% of patients do not achieve coronary artery patency with thrombolytics,[69] patients with ongoing symptoms and persistent ST-segment elevation after thrombolysis should be considered for emergent transfer for rescue PCI.[4] Even for successful thrombolysis, guidelines recommend PCI for all patients 3–24 hours after thrombolysis.[4]

TABLE 4-4 CONTRAINDICATIONS TO THROMBOLYSIS

Absolute contraindications

Active internal bleeding (not including menstruation)

Suspected aortic dissection

Major trauma or surgery within previous 2 wk

History of hemorrhagic stroke

Recent head trauma or known intracranial neoplasm

Hemorrhagic retinopathy

Relative contraindications

Uncontrolled HTN (BP > 180/110) or history of chronic, severe HTN

History of any stroke

Bleeding diathesis or use of anticoagulant medications

Prolonged, traumatic CPR

Active peptic ulcer disease

Pregnancy

BP, blood pressure; CPR, cardiopulmonary resuscitation; HTN, hypertension.

Adapted from O'Gara PT, Kushner FG, Ascheim DD, et al. 2013 ACCF/AHA guideline for the management of ST-elevation myocardial infarction: executive summary. *Circulation* 2013;127:529–55.

REFERENCES

1. Mozaffarian D, Benjamin EJ, Go AS, et al. Executive summary: heart disease and stroke statistics—2015 update: a report from the American Heart Association. *Circulation* 2015;131:434–41.
2. Thygesen K, Alpert JS, Jaffe AS, et al. ESC/ACCF/AHA/WHF expert consensus document: third universal definition of myocardial infarction. *Circulation* 2012;126:2020–35.
3. Amsterdam EA, Wenger NK, Brindis RG, et al. 2014 AHA/ACC guideline for the management of patients with non-ST-elevation acute coronary syndromes: executive summary. *Circulation* 2014;130:2354–94.
4. O'Gara PT, Kushner FG, Ascheim DD, et al. 2013 ACCF/AHA guideline for the management of ST-elevation myocardial infarction: executive summary. *Circulation* 2013;127:529–55.
5. Valensi P, Logis L, Cottin Y. Prevalence, incidence, predictive factors, and prognosis of silent myocardial infarction: a review of the literature. *Arch Cardiovasc Dis* 2011;104(3):178–88.
6. Antman EM, Cohen M, Bernink PJ, et al. The TIMI risk score for unstable angina/non-ST elevation MI: a method for prognostication and therapeutic decision making. *JAMA* 2000;284(7):835–42.
7. Reichlin T, Irfan A, Twerenbold R, et al. Utility of absolute and relative changes in cardiac troponin concentrations in the early diagnosis of acute myocardial infarction. *Circulation* 2011;124:136–45.
8. Farkouh ME, Smars PA, Reeder GS, et al. A clinical trial of a chest-pain observation unit for patients with unstable angina. *N Engl J Med* 1998;339:1882–8.
9. Amsterdam EA, Kirk JD, Diercks DB, et al. Immediate exercise testing to evaluate low-risk patients presenting to the emergency department with chest pain. *J Am Coll Cardiol* 2002;40(2):251–6.
10. Bholasingh R, Cornel JH, Kamp O, et al. Prognostic value of predischarge dobutamine stress echocardiography in chest pain patients with a negative cardiac troponin T. *J Am Coll Cardiol* 2003;41(4):596–602.
11. Litt HI, Gatsonis C, Synder B, et al. CT angiography for safe discharge of patients with possible acute coronary syndromes. *N Engl J Med* 2012;366(15):1393–403.
12. Hoffman U, Truong QA, Schoenfeld DA, et al. Coronary CT angiography versus standard evaluation in acute chest pain. *N Engl J Med* 2012;367(4):299–308.
13. Than M, Cullen L, Reid CM, et al. A 2-h diagnostic protocol to assess patients with chest pain symptoms in the Asia-Pacific region (ASPECT): a prospective observational validation study. *Lancet* 2011;377:1077–84.
14. Than M, Cullen L, Aldous S, et al. 2-Hour accelerated diagnostic protocol to assess patients with chest pain symptoms using contemporary troponins as the only biomarker. *J Am Coll Cardiol* 2012;59(23):2091–8.
15. Cullen L, Mueller C, Parsonage WA, et al. Validation of high-sensitivity troponin I in a 2-hour diagnostic strategy to assess 30-day outcomes in emergency department patients with possible acute coronary syndrome. *J Am Coll Cardiol* 2013;62(14):1242–9.
16. Stub D, Smith K, Bernard S, et al. Air versus oxygen in ST-segment-elevation myocardial infarction. *Circulation* 2015;131:2143–50.
17. Meine TJ, Roe MT, Chen AY, et al. Association of intravenous morphine use and outcomes in acute coronary syndromes: results from the CRUSADE quality improvement initiative. *Am Heart J* 2005;149(6):1043–9.
18. Bangalore S, Makani H, Radford M, et al. Clinical outcomes with β-blockers for myocardial infarction: a meta-analysis of randomized trials. *Am J Med* 2014;127:939–53.
19. Chen ZM, Pan HC, Chen YP, et al.; COMMIT collaborative group. Early intravenous then oral metoprolol in 45,852 patients with acute myocardial infarction: randomized placebo-controlled trial. *Lancet* 2005;366:1622–32.
20. Held PH, Yusuf S, Furberg CD. Calcium channel blockers in acute myocardial infarction and unstable angina: an overview. *BMJ* 1989;299:1187–92.
21. Gibson RS, Boden WE, Theroux P, et al. Diltiazem and reinfarction in patients with non-Q-wave myocardial infarction: results of a double-blind, randomized, multicenter trial. *N Engl J Med* 1986;315(7):423–9.
22. Furberg CD, Psaty BM, Meyer JV. Nifedipine: dose-related increase in mortality in patients with coronary heart disease. *Circulation* 1995;92(5):1326–31.
23. ACE inhibitor myocardial infarction collaborative group. Indications for ACE inhibitors in the early treatment of acute myocardial infarction: systematic overview of individual data from 100,000 patients in randomized trials. *Circulation* 1998;97(22):2202–12.

24. Pfeffer MA, McMurray JJ, Velazquez EJ, et al. Valsartan, captopril, or both in myocardial infarction complicated by heart failure, left ventricular dysfunction, or both. *N Engl J Med* 2003;349(20):1893–906.
25. Pitt B, Remme W, Zannad F, et al. Eplerenone, a selective aldosterone blocker, in patients with left ventricular dysfunction after myocardial infarction. *N Engl J Med* 2003;348(14):1309–21.
26. Schwartz GG, Olsson AG, Ezekowitz MD, et al. Effects of atorvastatin on early recurrent ischemic events in acute coronary syndromes: the MIRACL study: a randomized controlled trial. *JAMA* 2001;285(13):1711–8.
27. Cannon CP, Braunwald E, McCabe CH, et al. Intensive versus moderate lipid lowering with statins after acute coronary syndromes. *N Engl J Med* 2004;350(15):1495–504.
28. Baigent C, Blackwell L, Collins R, et al. Antithrombotic trialists' (ATT) collaboration: aspirin in the primary and secondary prevention of vascular disease: collaborative meta-analysis of individual participant data from randomized trials. *Lancet* 2009;3373:1849–60.
29. Mehta SR, Bassand JP, Chrolavicius S, et al. CURRENT-OASIS 7 investigators: dose comparisons of clopidogrel and aspirin in acute coronary syndromes. *N Engl J Med* 2010;363(10):930–42.
30. Jolly SS, Pogue J, Haladyn K, et al. Effects of aspirin dose on ischaemic events and bleeding after percutaneous coronary intervention: insights from the PCI-CURE study. *Eur Heart J* 2009;30(8):900–7.
31. Xian Y, Wang TY, McCoy LA, et al. Association of discharge aspirin dose with outcomes after acute myocardial infarction: insights from the treatment with ADP receptor inhibitors: longitudinal assessment of treatment patterns and events after acute coronary syndrome (TRANSLATE-ACS) study. *Circulation* 2015;132:174–81.
32. Giusti B, Gori AM, Marcucci R, et al. Relation of cytochrome P450 2C19 loss-of-function polymorphism to occurrence of drug-eluting coronary stent thrombosis. *Am J Cardiol* 2009; 103(6):806–11.
33. Yusuf S, Zhao F, Mehta SR, et al. Effects of clopidogrel in addition to aspirin in patients with acute coronary syndromes without ST-segment elevation. *N Engl J Med* 2001;345(7):494–502.
34. Mehta SR, Yusuf S, Peters RJ, et al. Effects of pretreatment with clopidogrel and aspirin followed by long-term therapy in patients undergoing percutaneous coronary intervention: the PCI-CURE study. *Lancet* 2001;358:527–33.
35. Roe MT, Armstrong PW, Fox KA, et al. Prasugrel versus clopidogrel for acute coronary syndromes without revascularization. *N Engl J Med* 2012;367(14);1297–309.
36. Wiviott, SD, Braunwald E, McCabe CH, et al. Prasugrel versus clopidogrel in patients with acute coronary syndromes. *N Engl J Med* 2007;357(20):2001–15.
37. Wallentin L, Becker RC, Budaj A, et al. Ticagrelor versus clopidogrel in patients with acute coronary syndromes. *N Engl J Med* 2009;361(11):1045–57.
38. The platelet receptor inhibition in ischemic syndrome management in patients limited by unstable signs and symptoms (PRISM-PLUS) study investigators. Inhibition of the platelet glycoprotein IIb/IIIa receptor with tirofiban in unstable angina and non-Q-wave myocardial infarction. *N Engl J Med* 1998;338(21):1488–97.
39. The PURSUIT trial investigators. Inhibition of platelet glycoprotein IIb/IIIa with eptifibatide in patients with acute coronary syndromes. *N Engl J Med* 1998;339(7):436–43.
40. Stone GW, Bertrand ME, Moses JW, et al. Routine upstream initiation vs deferred selective use of glycoprotein IIb/IIIa inhibitors in acute coronary syndromes. *JAMA* 2007;297(6):591–602.
41. Giugliano RP, White JW, Bode C, et al. Early versus delayed, provisional eptifibatide in acute coronary syndromes. *N Engl J Med* 2009;360(21):2176–90.
42. Keeley EC, Boura JA, Grines CL. Comparison of primary and facilitated percutaneous coronary interventions for ST-elevation myocardial infarction: quantitative review of randomised trials. *Lancet* 2006;367:579–88.
43. Ellis SG, Tendera M, de Belder MA, et al. Facilitated PCI in patients with ST-elevation myocardial infarction. *N Engl J Med* 2008;358(21):2205–17.
44. The CAPTURE investigators. Randomised placebo-controlled trial of abciximab before and during coronary intervention in refractory unstable angina: the CAPTURE study. *Lancet* 1997;349:1429–35.
45. Kastrati A, Mehilli J, Neumann FJ, et al. Abciximab in patients with acute coronary syndromes undergoing percutaneous coronary intervention after clopidogrel pretreatment. *JAMA* 2006;295(13):1531–8.
46. Ottervanger JP, Armstrong P, Barnathan ES, et al. Long-term results after the glycoprotein IIb/IIIa inhibitor abciximab in unstable angina: one-year survival in the GUSTO IV-ACS (global use of strategies to open occluded coronary arteries IV—acute coronary syndrome) trial. *Circulation* 2003;107:437–42.

47. Eikelboom JW, Anand SS, Malmberg K, et al. Unfractionated heparin and low-molecular-weight heparin in acute coronary syndrome without ST elevation: a meta-analysis. *Lancet* 2000;355:1936–42.
48. Cohen M, Demers C, Gurfinkel EP, et al. A comparison of low-molecular weight heparin with unfractionated heparin for unstable coronary artery disease. *N Engl J Med* 1997;337(7):447–52.
49. Antman EM, McCabe CH, Gurfinkel EP, et al. Enoxaparin prevents death and cardiac ischemic events in unstable angina/non-Q-wave myocardial infarction: results of the thrombolysis in myocardial infarction (TIMI) 11B trial. *Circulation* 1999;100:1593–601.
50. Blazing MA, de Lemos JA, White HD, et al. Safety and efficacy of enoxaparin vs unfractionated heparin in patients with non-ST-segment elevation acute coronary syndromes who receive tirofiban and aspirin: a randomized controlled trial. *JAMA* 2004;292(1):55–64.
51. Peterson JL, Mahaffey KW, Hasselblad V, et al. Efficacy and bleeding complications among patients randomized to enoxaparin or unfractionated heparin for antithrombin therapy in non-ST-segment elevation acute coronary syndromes: a systemic overview. *JAMA* 2004;292(1):89–96.
52. Montalescot G, Zeymer U, Silvain J, et al. Intravenous enoxaparin or unfractionated heparin in primary percutaneous coronary intervention for ST-elevation myocardial infarction: the international randomised open-label ATOLL trial. *Lancet* 2011;378:693–703.
53. Stone GW, Witzenbichler B, Guagliumi G, et al. Bivalirudin during primary PCI in acute myocardial infarction. *N Engl J Med* 2008;358(21):2218–30.
54. Kastrati A, Neumann FJ, Schulz S, et al. Abciximab and heparin versus bivalirudin for non-ST-elevation myocardial infarction. *N Engl J Med* 2011;365(21):1980–9.
55. Valgimigli M, Frigoli E, Leonardi S, et al. Bivalirudin or unfractionated heparin in acute coronary syndromes. *N Engl J Med* 2015;373(11):997–1009.
56. Stone GW, McLaurin BT, Cox DA, et al. Bivalirudin for patients with acute coronary syndromes. *N Engl J Med* 2006;355(21):2203–16.
57. Shahzad A, Kemp I, Mars C, et al. Unfractionated heparin versus bivalirudin in primary percutaneous coronary intervention (HEAT-PPCI): an open-label, single centre, randomised controlled trial. *Lancet* 2014;384:1849–58.
58. Cavender MA, Sabatine MS. Bivalirudin versus heparin in patients planned for percutaneous coronary intervention: a meta-analysis of randomised controlled trials. *Lancet* 2014;384:599–606.
59. Yusuf S, Mehta SR, Chrolavicius S, et al. Comparison of fondaparinux and enoxaparin in acute coronary syndromes. *N Engl J Med* 2006;354(14):1464–76.
60. Mehta SR, Cannon CP, Fox KA, et al. Routine vs selective invasive strategies in patients with acute coronary syndromes: a collaborative meta-analysis of randomized trials. *JAMA* 2005;293(23):2908–17.
61. O'Donoghue M, Boden WE, Braunwald E, et al. Early invasive vs conservative treatment strategies in women and men with unstable angina and non-ST-segment elevation myocardial infarction: a meta-analysis. *JAMA* 2008;300(1):71–80.
62. Fox KA, Clayton TC, Damman P, et al. Long-term outcome of a routine versus selective invasive strategy in patients with non-ST-segment elevation acute coronary syndrome a meta-analysis of individual patient data. *J Am Coll Cardiol* 2010;55(22):2435–45.
63. Fox KA, Dabbous OH, Goldberg RJ, et al. Prediction of risk of death and myocardial infarction in the six months after presentation with acute coronary syndrome: prospective multinational observational study (GRACE). *BMJ* 2006;333:1091–4.
64. Elbarouni B, Goodman SG, Yan RT, et al. Validation of the global registry of acute coronary event (GRACE) risk score for in-hospital mortality in patients with acute coronary syndrome in Canada. *Am Heart J* 2009;158(3):392–9.
65. Goldberg RJ, Spender FA, Fox KA, et al. Prehospital delay in patients with acute coronary syndromes (from the global registry of acute coronary events [GRACE]). *Am J Cardiol* 2009;103(5):598–603.
66. Keely EC, Boura JA, Grines CL. Primary angioplasty versus intravenous thrombolytic therapy for acute myocardial infarction: a quantitative review of 23 randomised trials. *Lancet* 2003;361:13–20.
67. Wang TY, Peterson ED, Ou FS, et al. Door-to-balloon times for patients with ST-segment elevation requiring interhospital transfer for primary percutaneous coronary intervention: a report from the national cardiovascular data registry. *Am Heart J* 2011;161(1):76–83.
68. Fibrinolytic therapy trialists' collaborative group. Indications for fibrinolytic therapy in suspected acute myocardial infarction: collaborative overview of early mortality and major morbidity results from all randomised trials of more than 1000 patients. *Lancet* 1994;343:311–22.
69. Goldman LE and Eisenberg MJ. Identification and management of patients with failed thrombolysis after acute myocardial infarction. *Ann Int Med* 2000;132:556–65.

Approach to the Patient with Syncope

James Matthew Freer

GENERAL PRINCIPLES

Definition

- **Syncope** is defined as a sudden, brief loss of consciousness and postural tone due to cerebral hypoperfusion. It is characterized by rapid and complete recovery.
- Syncope is a common disorder, occurring in 11% of the Framingham Study registry over 17 years of follow-up.[1]
- The cumulative lifetime incidence of syncope may be as high as 35%.[2] It is responsible for a sizable percentage of emergency visits and 1% of all hospital admissions.[3]
- The presence of cardiovascular disease and elderly age are strong risk factors for syncope, though syncope is more common in adolescence and young adulthood than in middle age.[1]
- **Presyncope** refers to symptoms that do not result in loss of consciousness; controversy exists regarding the relationship between presyncopal symptoms and true syncope in a patient experiencing both.

Etiology

Causes of syncope are detailed in Table 5-1.

- **Neurocardiogenic (also referred to as vasovagal, reflex, or vasodepressor)** syncope is the most common form of syncope in most patient populations.
  - It is defined as a failure of the autonomic nervous system to sustain blood pressure (BP) and/or heart rate sufficient for cerebral perfusion.
  - A number of mechanisms, such as prolonged standing, strong emotion or stress, venous pooling, hacking cough, defecation, and micturition, among others, can activate mechanoreceptors that paradoxically cause bradycardia and vasodilation, resulting in syncope.
  - Syncope related to cough, defecation, and micturition is referred to as **situational syncope**. Vasovagal syncope is generally a benign condition; in the Framingham cohort, the long-term mortality of patients with vasovagal syncope was identical to patients who never experienced syncope.[1]
- **Carotid sinus hypersensitivity** causes syncope via vagal activation and, therefore, can be considered another type of reflex syncope. This entity is much more common in elderly patients, particularly males, whereas neurocardiogenic syncope is more common in the young.
- **Cardiac** causes of syncope include the following:
  - Bradyarrhythmias
  - Conduction abnormalities (i.e., heart block)
  - Ventricular tachycardia
  - Supraventricular tachycardias
  - Outflow tract obstruction (e.g., aortic stenosis or hypertrophic cardiomyopathy)
  - Myocardial ischemia
  - Pulmonary hypertension and pulmonic stenosis

TABLE 5-1 CAUSES OF SYNCOPE

Cardiac (ischemia, arrhythmia, valvular disease, etc.)	9.5% of cases
Unknown	36.6%
Neurologic (stroke/TIA)	4.1%
Seizure	4.9%
Neurocardiogenic ("vasovagal")	21.2%
Orthostasis	9.4%
Medication related	6.8%
Other (psychiatric, carotid sinus hypersensitivity, etc.)	7.5%

Adapted from Soteriades ES, Evan JC, Larson MG, et al. Incidence and prognosis of syncope. *N Engl J Med* 2002;347:878–85.

- Patients with cardiac causes of syncope have increased mortality as compared to those with noncardiac causes. When syncopal patients with congestive heart failure (CHF) and/or coronary artery disease (CAD) are matched to patients without syncope, outcomes are identical.[4] Thus, the presence or absence of CHF and/or CAD is responsible for the increased mortality, not the symptom of syncope.
- **Orthostatic** hypotension can result from volume depletion, various medications, secondary autonomic failure from diabetes or amyloidosis, primary autonomic failure, alcohol, or often a combination of these factors.
- **Seizure** is technically not syncope, although the two are often confused and some patients with "unknown" causes of syncope do have seizures after extensive testing.
- **Pulmonary embolism** is a rare cause of syncope.
- Syncope is almost never the only manifestation of **stroke**. A posterior circulation stroke or transient ischemic attack (TIA) may manifest as vertigo, which may be confused with presyncope.
- **Psychiatric** causes of syncope include depression, anxiety, panic disorder, somatization, and drug abuse. This is sometimes referred to as **pseudosyncope**, as most patients do not experience cerebral hypoperfusion during the attack. The loss of consciousness in these patients may be due to hyperventilation or medication side effects. Psychiatric causes of syncope are much more common in young patients.

DIAGNOSIS

Clinical Presentation

History

A thorough history should be obtained from the patient and any bystanders.

- The timing and frequency of syncopal episodes can be important; numerous episodes occurring over a span of years are likely to be benign in nature, while those occurring more recently and increasing in frequency are more likely to have a serious cause.
- A prodrome of warmth, light-headedness, sweating, or nausea is often seen prior to **neurocardiogenic/vasovagal syncope**; vasovagal episodes are also common during urination, defecation, and paroxysms of cough.
- An aura, incontinence during the episode, longer duration of unconsciousness, or postevent confusion is suggestive of seizure.

- Chest pain, dyspnea, or palpitations prior to syncope suggest a **cardiac cause** or **pulmonary embolism**, as does syncope during exercise. Syncope after exercise, conversely, is often neurocardiogenic.
- A recent history of diarrhea, vomiting, excessive exposure to heat, or medication changes is suggestive of **orthostasis**.
- The patient should be asked about any focal neurologic symptoms that could be suggestive of **TIA or stroke**.
- **Carotid sinus hypersensitivity** is suspected in the patient with an event while shaving, wearing a tight shirt collar, or turning the neck suddenly.
- The past medical history should focus on the presence or absence of underlying cardiac and neurologic disease.
- A complete medication and social history should be obtained, and the family history should focus on any history of sudden cardiac death.

Physical Examination

Perform a careful physical examination on all patients, with special focus on the cardiovascular and neurologic exams.

- Vital signs should be recorded, including the documentation of orthostatic BP and pulse (drop of systolic BP by ≥20 mm Hg or increase in heart rate by ≥30, 3–5 minutes after standing).
- Such findings as an irregular pulse, brady- or tachycardia, cardiac murmur, or focal neurologic signs can suggest an etiology of syncope, or a diagnosis other than syncope, and guide further management.
- The presence or absence of carotid bruits should be documented, as carotid sinus massage is not recommended in the presence of a bruit.

Diagnostic Testing

The goals of the diagnostic workup in syncope are twofold:

- **First,** it should be determined if the event was truly syncope or presyncope, versus sudden cardiac death, seizure, vertigo, intoxication, or drop attack (loss of postural tone without loss of consciousness).
  - If the patient's event is consistent with syncope, a thorough history and physical exam (as above), along with an electrocardiogram (ECG), should be obtained to offer prognostic information as well as to guide further workup.
  - The history and physical exam will reveal a likely diagnosis in 45% of cases.[5]
  - An ECG will increase the diagnostic yield by only 5%, but it is an inexpensive and noninvasive test that may also reveal the presence of underlying cardiac disease.[5]
  - Further diagnostic tests can be obtained based on this initial workup. In large series, the underlying cause of syncope varies based on the patient population, but the etiology may remain unclear in >1/3 of patients even after exhaustive workup.[1,6]
- **Second,** the patient can be risk stratified based on historical information, the presence or absence of underlying cardiac disease, and the ECG to determine the need for hospital admission. The European Society of Cardiology and the American College of Emergency Physicians have published guidelines on the need for hospitalization in patients with syncope.[7,8]
  - In general, older patients (especially those >65 years of age) and patients with known or suspected congestive or ischemic heart disease should be admitted for further testing and telemetry monitoring (see Table 5-2).
  - In a patient <45 years with a normal EKG and no history of CHF or ventricular arrhythmia, the risk of death from any cause at 1 year is <2%, and the risk of arrhythmia at 1 year is ~5%.[9]

TABLE 5-2 INDICATIONS FOR HOSPITAL ADMISSION IN PATIENTS WITH SYNCOPE

Known or suspected CHF or CAD
Symptoms suggestive of arrhythmia or cardiac ischemia
Syncope during exercise
Advanced age (especially >65)
Hematocrit < 30
Abnormal ECG
Syncope causing severe injury
Family history of sudden cardiac death
Significant electrolyte disturbances

Adapted from Huff JS, Decker WW, Quinn JV, et al. Clinical policy: critical issues in the evaluation and management of adult patients presenting to the emergency department with syncope. *Ann Emerg Med* 2007;49:431–44; Moya A, Sutton R, Ammirati F, et al. Guidelines for the diagnosis and management of syncope. *Eur Heart J* 2009;30:2631–71.

- An etiology of syncope will be apparent in up to one-half of patients after a thorough history, physical exam, and ECG. In these patients, confirmatory testing may be indicated and treatment should be aimed at the underlying disorder. In the remainder, a decision must be made regarding the necessity and timing of further workup.
- Figure 5-1 outlines a suggested diagnostic algorithm.
- **Patients without evidence of underlying heart disease by history and ECG:**
  - **Neurocardiogenic and psychiatric** causes of syncope are common in younger patients without underlying heart disease.
  - Further testing in these patients is generally not indicated unless the circumstances of the event were serious (e.g., leading to significant trauma), the episodes are frequent,

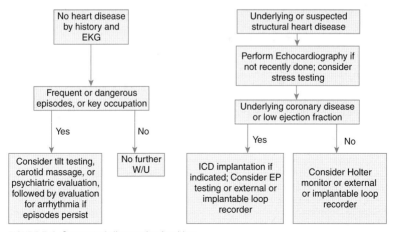

FIGURE 5-1 Suggested diagnostic algorithm.

or repeated episodes of syncope would be especially dangerous (e.g., syncope in a trucker or pilot).
- **Tilt-table testing was traditionally performed to confirm vasovagal syncope.** However, tilt-table testing has poor reproducibility and cannot be compared to a true gold standard test. For this and other reasons, tilt-table testing has conflicting recommendations in expert guidelines.[8,10]
- In the event of a negative tilt-table test (if performed) and repeated syncope, either external or internal cardiac loop recording to monitor for arrhythmia can be considered. Carotid sinus massage should be utilized in older patients with unexplained syncope.
- An echocardiogram may also be indicated in older patients to screen for underlying cardiac or valvular disease, even with a negative history and normal ECG.
- **Patients with underlying heart disease**
  - Patients with underlying heart disease and syncope are at increased risk of mortality as compared to patients with syncope and no cardiac disease. Viewed in a vacuum, an **echocardiogram** will only reveal a specific cause of syncope in 3% of patients.[11]
  - The echocardiogram is useful for risk stratification, however, as a normal echo makes arrhythmia, particularly ventricular arrhythmia, less likely. Findings on echo that may guide further workup include valvular abnormalities, a reduced ejection fraction (EF), evidence of hypertrophic cardiomyopathy, and focal wall-motion abnormalities.
  - A **stress test** should be considered in patients with structural heart disease and especially in those with symptoms during exercise or symptoms suggestive of ischemia. Causes of syncope discovered on echocardiography or stress testing should be treated accordingly.
  - Arrhythmias are a major diagnostic consideration in patients with syncope and underlying heart disease. The standard ECG will rarely delineate a specific arrhythmic cause of syncope; these should be treated accordingly. Usually, further testing is needed to reveal an underlying arrhythmia; these options are detailed below.
  - Finally, an electrophysiologic (EP) study may be considered, and an implantable defibrillator may be indicated in some patients with a low EF even in the absence of documented arrhythmia.

Laboratories
- Basic labs such as a complete blood count and basic metabolic profile are rarely useful in the workup of syncope but may occasionally reveal contributing factors such as anemia, infection, renal failure, or electrolyte abnormalities.
- A fingerstick blood glucose should be obtained by paramedics at the scene or in the emergency department to exclude hypoglycemia.

Electrocardiography
As stated above, an ECG will yield a diagnosis in only about 5% of patients but is still recommended. Helpful abnormalities on an ECG include the presence of brady- or tachyarrhythmias, atrioventricular block, bundle-branch block, a prolonged QT interval, left ventricular hypertrophy, old signs of myocardial infarction, or signs of active myocardial ischemia. Alternatively, a normal ECG makes arrhythmia less likely, though certainly not impossible.

Imaging
- **Neurologic imaging**—computed tomography (CT) of the head, magnetic resonance imaging (MRI)/magnetic resonance angiography, and cerebral angiography—is extremely low yield in unselected patients with syncope. It is indicated only in patients with focal neurologic signs or symptoms or in those with significant head trauma.
- **Carotid Dopplers** reveal stenosis in a significant percentage of older patients with syncope, but in the vast majority of these patients, the carotid stenosis was not felt to be the cause of syncope.[12] Carotid Dopplers are not indicated in the routine evaluation of syncope.

- Ventilation/perfusion scanning or CT pulmonary angiography is indicated in the rare patient suspected of having a pulmonary embolism.
- **Echocardiography** may reveal a variety of underlying myocardial and valvular diseases, as discussed above.

Diagnostic Procedures
- **Electroencephalography (EEG)** is indicated only for those with **possible seizure** or witnessed seizure-like activity. An EEG produces useful information in very few unselected patients with syncope.
- **Carotid sinus massage** can be performed at the bedside in those with suspected **carotid sinus hypersensitivity** and no evidence of carotid bruit or history of recent stroke, myocardial infarction, or ventricular tachycardia. Vigorous pressure is applied unilaterally with a circular movement to the carotid artery just below the angle of the jaw for 6–10 seconds, with ECG and noninvasive BP monitoring. Carotid massage is considered positive if symptoms are reproduced or a sinus pause of ≥3 seconds is provoked. Complications are serious but rare, with neurologic complications in <0.2%.
- **Stress testing** may reveal the presence of **coronary artery disease** and is also useful in reproducing symptoms in patients with syncope during exercise.
- **Passive, head-up tilt-table testing** is a provocative test for **neurocardiogenic/vasovagal syncope**, involving a table that quickly brings the patient from supine to erect and holds this position for 10–45 minutes. ECG and noninvasive BP monitoring are performed throughout the test, and pharmacologic agents (isoproterenol, nitrates, and adenosine) can be administered if there is no response initially. The test is positive if there is loss of consciousness or posture with a significant fall in BP or heart rate. The reported sensitivity of tilt-table testing varies widely, and the specificity is ~90%.[10] Between 50% and 62% of patients with unexplained syncope will have a positive tilt-table test. The reproducibility of repeated tilt-table testing is good for those with an initial negative result but poor for those with a positive test.[13] Interpreting the operating characteristic of this test is challenging as there is no true gold standard test.
- **Psychiatric evaluation** should be considered in young patients in otherwise good health with recurrent syncope.
- **Evaluation for arrhythmia:** Several options are available to assess for arrhythmia as the cause of syncope. Patients in whom admission is deemed necessary should first be monitored on continuous telemetry during their hospital stay. The goal of inpatient or outpatient cardiac rhythm monitoring is to correlate a syncopal episode with the cardiac rhythm (i.e., symptom–rhythm correlation), thus ruling in or out arrhythmia as the etiology.
  - **Ambulatory ECG (Holter) monitoring**: This consists of continuous monitoring of the cardiac rhythm for 24–48 hours. Prior inpatient telemetry monitoring usually obviates the need for an outpatient Holter. This type of monitoring is best suited for patients with very frequent episodes of syncope or palpitations. The yield is low, generally <20%, with few patients actually experiencing a syncopal episode during the monitoring period.[8]
  - **Continuous external cardiac monitoring (i.e., event recorder):** External loop recorders allow monitoring for a longer period of time, usually 30–60 days. Patients must apply telemetry leads every morning, and the patient or a witness then triggers the device during an event; the device then stores the rhythm strip from several minutes prior to the activation to 30–60 seconds following activation. These recorders are useful in patients who have events at least once per month. In general, loop recorders have a higher diagnostic yield than do Holter monitors; one paper showed symptom–rhythm correlation in 63% of patients, though other studies have not been as favorable.[8,14]

- **Implantable loop recorders** are devices that are implanted in a patient's subcutaneous tissue and sense the cardiac rhythm. There are no transvenous leads, and thus the risk of bloodstream infection is negligible. They are capable of recording cardiac rhythm for as long as 3 years. A recording is activated by the patient or a bystander, and the preceding and subsequent rhythms are then recorded. Newer devices automatically record significant arrhythmias as well, and telemetry information can be transmitted to the provider frequently via telephone. The device may be explanted once a diagnosis is made or the battery fails. Several studies have demonstrated that, in carefully selected patients, the device is both useful (symptom–rhythm correlation as high as 90%, though results have varied widely) and cost-effective.[8,11,15]
- **Electrophysiologic (EP) testing** involves the insertion of a transvenous catheter into the heart to assess susceptibility to various arrhythmias as well as sinus and atrioventricular nodal function. EP testing may reveal ventricular tachycardia, supraventricular tachycardia, or bradycardia as the probable cause of syncope, though it is relatively insensitive for the detection of bradyarrhythmias. EP testing is most helpful in patients with underlying cardiac. The yield is low in the absence of structural heart disease. EP studies are currently performed less frequently in the workup of syncope, as event monitors and implantable loop recorders have gained favor, and indications for ICD implantation have expanded, thus obviating the need for EP testing in many patients.

TREATMENT

Treatment is aimed at the underlying disorder, with the goal being to improve mortality (e.g., in patients with ventricular tachycardia as the underlying mechanism) or to improve quality of life and avoid injury in those with more benign causes of syncope. Treatment of arrhythmia, depending on the mechanism, may include ablation of an accessory or irritable pathway or pacemaker or ICD implantation. Though ICD implantation may be indicated to prevent sudden cardiac death, it often does not decrease the frequency of syncopal episodes. Treatment of other causes of syncope is discussed below.

- **Neurocardiogenic syncope**
  - First-line treatment for neurocardiogenic/vasovagal syncope involves **behavioral therapy** and **physical counterpressure maneuvers** (PCMs).
  - The patient and family should be educated regarding predisposing factors, and patients should be instructed to lie down at the beginning of symptoms and to avoid provocative situations.
  - Fluid and salt intake should be increased (cautiously in patients with hypertension or CHF).
  - PCMs are designed to augment venous return BP; at the beginning of an attack, patients should perform isometric exercises such as leg crossing or hand and arm clinching. Several studies have documented a decrease in syncopal episodes with these maneuvers.[16–18]
  - **Pharmacologic therapy** has generally proved disappointing at preventing vasovagal syncope.
  - Tilt-table conditioning, as patients are gradually subjected to longer intervals of upright posture, may be useful in motivated patients
  - **Pacemaker** therapy may be considered for patients with severe, recurrent vasovagal syncope refractory to other treatments, especially those with severe bradycardia or asystole on tilt-table testing or documented by event monitor or implantable loop recorder.
- **Carotid sinus hypersensitivity:** Patients with carotid sinus hypersensitivity also benefit from **behavioral modification** aimed at avoiding syncopal triggers, such as wearing shirts with tight collars, shaving while standing, etc. **Pacemaker** therapy is effective for patients with asystole of ≥3 seconds during carotid sinus massage.

- **Orthostatic hypotension**
  - Volume depletion, if present, should be corrected, and offending medications should be stopped or adjusted (e.g., diuretics, antihypertensives, some psychiatric medications, etc.).
  - Patients should be advised to increase their salt and water intake (assuming that there is no contraindication) and to spend as much time upright during the day as possible.
  - Patients should also rise from lying or sitting slowly so as to allow for equilibration of BP.
  - Lower extremity compression stockings are helpful in preventing venous pooling.
  - Midodrine or fludrocortisone can be used if behavioral therapies are ineffective.

REFERENCES

1. Soteriades ES, Evans JC, Larson MG, et al. Incidence and prognosis of syncope. *N Engl J Med* 2002;347:878–85.
2. Ganzeboom KS, Mairuhu G, Reitsma JB, et al. Lifetime cumulative incidence of syncope in the general population: a study of 549 Dutch subjects aged 35–60 years. *J Cardiovasc Electrophysiol* 2006;17:1172–76.
3. Kapoor WN. Evaluation and outcome of patients with syncope. *Medicine* 1990;69:160–76.
4. Kapoor WN, Hanusa BH. Is syncope a risk factor for poor outcomes? Comparison of patients with and without syncope. *Am J Med* 1996;100:646–55.
5. Linzer M, Yang EH, Estes NA, et al. Clinical guideline: diagnosing syncope: part 1: value of history, physical examination, and electrocardiography. *Ann Intern Med* 1997;126:989–96.
6. Getchall WS, Larsen GC, Morris CD, McAnulty JH. Epidemiology of syncope in hospitalized patients. *J Gen Intern Med* 1999;14:677–87.
7. Huff JS, Decker WW, Quinn JV, et al. Clinical policy: critical issues in the evaluation and management of adult patients presenting to the emergency department with syncope. *Ann Emerg Med* 2007;49:431–44.
8. Moya A, Sutton R, Ammirati F, et al. Guidelines for the diagnosis and management of syncope. *Eur Heart J* 2009;30:2631–71.
9. Martin TP, Hanusa BH, Kapoor WN. Risk stratification of patients with syncope. *Ann Emerg Med* 1997;29:459–66.
10. Strickberger SA, Benson DW, Biaggioni I, et al. AHA/ACCF scientific statement on the evaluation of syncope. *Circulation* 2006;113:316–27.
11. Krahn AD, Klein GJ, Yee R, Manda V. The high cost of syncope: cost implications of a new insertable loop recorder in the investigation of recurrent syncope. *Am Heart J* 1999;137:870–77.
12. Scott JW, Schwartz AL, Gates JD, et al. Choosing wisely for syncope: low-value carotid ultrasound use. *J Am Heart Assoc* 2014;3:e001063.
13. Sagrista-Sauleda J, Romero B, Permanyer-Miralda G, et al. Reproducibility of sequential head-up tilt testing in patients with recent syncope, normal EKG, and no structural heart disease. *Eur Heart J* 2002;23:1706–13.
14. Rockx MA, Hoch JS, Klein GJ, et al. Is ambulatory monitoring for 'community-acquired' syncope economically attractive? A cost-effectiveness analysis of a randomized trial of external loop recorders. *Am Heart J* 2005;150:1065.
15. Parry SW, Matthews IG. Implantable loop recorders in the investigation of unexplained syncope: a state of the art review. *Heart* 2010;96:1611–16.
16. Brignole M, Croci F, Menozzi C, et al. Isometric arm counter-pressure maneuvers to abort impending vasovagal syncope. *J Am Coll Cardiol* 2002;40:2053–59.
17. Krediet CT, van Dijk N, Linzer M, et al. Management of vasovagal syncope: controlling or aborting faints by leg crossing and muscle tensing. *Circulation* 2002;106:1684–89.
18. Van Dijk N, Quartieri F, Blanc JJ, et al. Effectiveness of physical counterpressure maneuvers in preventing vasovagal syncope: the physical counterpressure manoeuvres trial (PC-Trial). *J Am Coll Cardiol* 2006;48:1652–57.

Management of Heart Failure

6

Mark A. Gdowski

Chronic Heart Failure and Cardiomyopathy

GENERAL PRINCIPLES

Chronic heart failure (HF) is a clinical syndrome in which either functional or structural abnormalities of the heart impair its ability to fill with or eject blood, resulting in symptoms such as dyspnea, fatigue, and fluid retention.[1]

Classification

HF may be classified according to several factors, including the following:

- **Functional**: Abnormalities in myocardial contraction (**systolic dysfunction**), ventricular relaxation and filling (**diastolic dysfunction**), or both.
- Etiology
  - **Ischemic**: Coronary artery disease is the most common cause of HF in the United States. Other risk factors with high population attributable risk include tobacco use, hypertension, diabetes, and obesity.[2]
  - **Nonischemic**: Valvular heart disease, toxin induced (alcohol, cocaine), myocarditis (infectious, autoimmune), infiltrative (amyloidosis, hemochromatosis), familial, peripartum, and hypertrophic cardiomyopathy.
- **Anatomic**: **Right-sided** versus **left-sided** HF can often be distinguished.
- **Severity**: Can be classified according to the New York Heart Association (NYHA) Functional Class (Table 6-1).

Epidemiology

- Over 5.7 million people are living with HF in the United States with ~870,000 new cases of HF diagnosed each year.[2]
- HF accounts for over 1 million hospitalizations each year and the estimated 1-year and 5-year mortality are 30% and 50%, respectively.[2]

Pathophysiology

- HF begins with an initial insult leading to myocardial injury, which leads to pathologic remodeling and increases in left ventricular (LV) volume (dilatation) and/or mass (hypertrophy).
- Compensatory mechanisms like activation of the renin–angiotensin–aldosterone system (RAAS) and vasopressin, which increase sodium retention and peripheral vasoconstriction, and activation of the sympathetic nervous system, which increases levels of catecholamines, will result in increased myocardial contractility.
- Over time, however, these neurohormonal pathways lead to cellular toxicity, fibrosis, arrhythmias, and ultimately pump failure.

TABLE 6-1 NEW YORK HEART ASSOCIATION (NYHA) FUNCTIONAL CLASSIFICATION

NYHA Class	Symptoms
I (mild)	No symptoms or limitations while performing ordinary physical activity
II (mild)	Mild symptoms (shortness of breath, fatigue, and/or angina) and slight limitation during ordinary physical activity
III (moderate)	Marked limitation in activity due to symptoms, even during less than ordinary activity (e.g., walking short distances). Comfortable only at rest
IV (severe)	Severe limitations with symptoms even while at rest. Mostly bedbound patients

DIAGNOSIS

Clinical Presentation

History

The degree of clinical manifestations of HF varies depending on the rapidity of the patient's cardiac decompensation, underlying etiology, age, and comorbidities. Historically, patients may complain of fatigue, exercise intolerance/dyspnea with exertion, orthopnea, and paroxysmal nocturnal dyspnea. Presyncope, palpitations, and angina may be present in varying circumstances.

Physical Examination

The physical examination may be significant for signs of chronic pulmonary and systemic venous congestion, including pulmonary crackles, peripheral edema, elevated jugular venous pressure, pleural and pericardial effusions, hepatic congestion, and ascites. In systolic dysfunction, a third (S3) or fourth (S4) heart sound may be present.

Diagnostic Testing

Laboratories

- **B-type natriuretic peptide (BNP)** is synthesized by right ventricular (RV) and LV myocytes and released in response to stretch, volume overload, and elevated filling pressures. Serum levels of BNP are elevated in patients with asymptomatic LV dysfunction as well as symptomatic HF.
  - BNP levels have been shown to correlate with HF severity and to predict survival.[3]
  - A serum BNP level of >400 pg/mL is consistent with HF, though specificity is reduced in patients with renal dysfunction.
- **Cardiac enzymes** (i.e., troponin I or troponin T) should be considered to evaluate for ongoing myocardial ischemia.
- Additional laboratory abnormalities may include elevated levels of blood urea nitrogen (BUN) and creatinine, hyponatremia, anemia, and elevated hepatic enzymes.
- In patients with new-onset HF without CAD, diagnostic tests for HIV, hepatitis, and hemochromatosis should be obtained.

Electrocardiography

An ECG should be performed to look for evidence of ischemia (ST segment and T wave abnormalities, Q waves), previous myocardial infarction (MI), hypertrophy (increased voltage), infiltration (reduced voltage), and arrhythmias.

Imaging
- **Chest radiograph** abnormalities may include cardiomegaly and evidence of pulmonary vascular redistribution.
- **Ventricular function** should be assessed via transthoracic echocardiography, radionuclide ventriculography, or cardiac catheterization with left ventriculography.

TREATMENT

Chronic HF management has several goals: improve long-term survival, reduce symptoms, increase functional capacity, reduce hospitalizations, and prevent (and reverse) deleterious cardiac remodeling.

Medications
- The general principle of pharmacologic therapy involves the antagonism of neurohormones that are increased in patients with HF and have deleterious effects on the myocardium and the peripheral vasculature. Afterload reduction, vasodilator therapy and β-adrenergic blockade are the cornerstone of therapy for patients with chronic HF. Diuretics are reserved for relieving volume overload. Most patients will require a regimen that includes multiple medications to control symptoms and prolong survival (Table 6-2).
- **Minimization of medications with deleterious effects** in HF should be attempted. Specifically, negative inotropes (e.g., verapamil, diltiazem) should be avoided in patients with impaired ventricular contractility, as should over-the-counter β-stimulants. Nonsteroidal anti-inflammatory drugs (NSAIDs), which antagonize the effects of angiotensin-converting enzyme (ACE) inhibitors and diuretic therapy, should be avoided if possible.
- **β-Adrenergic receptor antagonists (β-blockers)**
  - β-adrenergic receptor antagonists are critical components of HF pharmacotherapy that block the effects of chronic adrenergic stimulation on the heart.
  - Large randomized trials have documented the beneficial effects of β-adrenergic antagonists on functional status and survival in patients with NYHA class II to IV symptoms.
  - Improvement in ejection fraction (EF), exercise tolerance, and functional class are common after the institution of a β-blocker.[4] Typically, 2–3 months of therapy is required to observe significant effects on LV function, but reduction of cardiac arrhythmia and incidence of sudden cardiac death may occur much earlier.[5]
  - β-adrenergic antagonists should be instituted at a low dose and titrated with careful attention to BP and heart rate. Some patients experience volume retention and worsening HF symptoms that typically respond to transient increases in diuretic therapy.
  - Individual β-adrenergic antagonists have unique properties and their beneficial effect in HF may not be a class effect. Therefore, one of three β-blockers with proven effects on patient survival in large clinical trials should be used.
    - **Carvedilol** is the best studied β-adrenergic antagonist in HF.[6-8] It has been shown to be superior to metoprolol tartrate for chronic treatment.[9]
    - Bisoprolol[10]
    - Metoprolol succinate[11]
- **ACE inhibitors** attenuate vasoconstriction, vital organ hypoperfusion, hyponatremia, hypokalemia, and fluid retention attributable to the compensatory activation of the renin–angiotensin system. Treatment with ACE inhibitors decreases afterload while increasing cardiac output.
  - Large clinical trials have clearly demonstrated that ACE inhibitors improve symptoms and survival in patients with LV systolic dysfunction.[1] They may also prevent the development of HF in patients with asymptomatic LV dysfunction and in those at high risk of developing structural heart disease or HF symptoms (CAD, diabetes mellitus, HTN).

TABLE 6-2 DRUGS COMMONLY USED FOR TREATMENT OF HEART FAILURE

Drug	Initial Does	Target
Angiotensin-Converting Enzyme Inhibitors		
Captopril	6.25–12.5 mg q6–8 h	50 mg tid
Enalapril	2.5 mg bid	10 mg bid
Fosinopril	5–10 mg daily; can use bid	20 mg daily
Lisinopril	2.5–5.0 mg daily; can use bid	10–20 mg bid
Quinapril	2.5–5.0 mg bid	10 mg bid
Ramipril	1.25–2.5 mg bid	5 mg bid
Trandolapril	0.5–1.0 mg daily	4 mg daily
Angiotensin Receptor Blockers		
Valsartan[a]	40 mg bid	160 mg bid
Losartan	25 mg daily; can use bid	25–100 mg daily
Irbesartan	75–150 mg daily	75–300 mg daily
Candesartan[a]	2–16 mg daily	2–32 mg daily
Olmesartan	20 mg daily	20–40 total mg daily
Thiazide Diuretics		
HCTZ	25–50 mg daily	25–50 mg daily
Metolazone	2.5–5.0 mg daily or bid	10–20 total mg daily
Loop diuretics		
Bumetanide	0.5–1.0 mg daily or bid	10 mg total daily (maximum)
Furosemide	20–40 mg daily or bid	400 total mg daily (maximum)
Torsemide	10–20 mg daily or bid	200 total mg daily (maximum)
Aldosterone Antagonists		
Eplerenone	25 mg daily	50 mg daily
Spironolactone	12.5–25.0 mg daily	25 mg daily
β-Blockers		
Bisoprolol	1.25 mg daily	10 mg daily
Carvedilol	3.125 mg q12 h	25–50 mg q12 h
Metoprolol succinate	12.5–25.0 mg daily	200 mg daily
Digoxin	0.125–0.25 mg daily	0.125–0.25 mg daily

[a]Valsartan and Candesartan are the only US Food and Drug Administration–approved angiotensin II receptor blockers in the treatment of heart failure.

HCTZ, hydrochlorothiazide.

- Currently, no consensus has been reached regarding the optimal dosing of ACE inhibitors in HF, although one study suggested that higher doses decrease morbidity without improving overall survival.[12]
- Absence of an initial beneficial response to treatment with an ACE inhibitor does not preclude long-term benefit.
- Most ACE inhibitors are excreted by the kidneys, necessitating careful dose titration in patients with renal insufficiency. Acute renal insufficiency may occur in patients with bilateral renal artery stenosis. Additional adverse effects include rash, angioedema, dysgeusia, increases in serum creatinine, proteinuria, hyperkalemia, leukopenia, and cough.
- A rise in serum creatinine up to 30% above baseline may be seen when initiating an ACE inhibitor and should not result in reflexive discontinuation of the medication.[13]
- **ACE inhibitors are contraindicated in pregnancy.** Enalapril and captopril may safely be used by breastfeeding mothers.
- Oral potassium supplements, potassium salt substitutes, and potassium-sparing diuretics should be used with caution during treatment with an ACE inhibitor.
- **Angiotensin II receptor blockers (ARBs)** inhibit the renin–angiotensin system via specific blockade of the angiotensin II receptor. In contrast to ACE inhibitors, they do not increase bradykinin levels, which may be responsible for adverse effects such as cough.
  - ARBs reduce mortality and morbidity associated with HF in patients who are not receiving an ACE inhibitor and therefore should be used when ACE inhibitors are not tolerated.[14]
  - Caution should be exercised when ARBs are used in patients with renal insufficiency and bilateral renal artery stenosis because hyperkalemia and acute renal failure can develop. Renal function and potassium levels should be periodically monitored.
  - ARBs are contraindicated in pregnancy.
- **Aldosterone receptor antagonists** attenuate aldosterone-mediated sodium retention, vascular reactivity, oxidant stress, inflammation, and fibrosis.
  - **Spironolactone** is an aldosterone receptor antagonist that should be considered in NYHA class III to IV patients with low EF and has been shown to improve survival and decrease hospitalizations in these patients.[15]
  - **Eplerenone**, a selective aldosterone receptor antagonist without the estrogenic side effects of spironolactone, is FDA approved for the treatment of HTN and HF. It has proven beneficial in patients with HF following MI[16] and in less symptomatic HF patients (NYHA Class II) with reduced EF.[17]
  - The potential for development of life-threatening hyperkalemia exists with the use of these agents. Serum potassium must be monitored closely after initiation; concomitant use of ACE inhibitors and NSAIDs in the presence of renal insufficiency (creatinine >2.5 mg/dL) increases the risk of hyperkalemia.
  - Gynecomastia may develop in 10–20% of men treated with spironolactone; eplerenone should be used in this case.
- **Vasodilator therapy** is another mainstay of treatment in patients with HF. Arterial vasoconstriction (afterload) and venous vasoconstriction (preload) occur in patients with HF as a result of activation of the RAAS system and adrenergic nervous system.
  - **Hydralazine** acts directly on arterial smooth muscle to produce vasodilation and reduce afterload.
  - **Nitrates** are predominantly venodilators and help relieve symptoms of venous and pulmonary congestion. They reduce myocardial ischemia by decreasing ventricular filling pressures and directly dilating coronary arteries. Nitrate therapy may precipitate hypotension in patients with reduced preload.
  - A combination of hydralazine and isosorbide dinitrate (starting dose: 37.5/20 mg three times daily) when added to standard therapy with β-blockers and ACE inhibitors has been shown to reduce mortality in African American patients.[18]

- In the absence of ACE inhibitors, ARBs, aldosterone receptor antagonists, and β-blockers, the combination of nitrates and hydralazine improves survival in patients with systolic HF and should be considered when patients are unable to tolerate RAAS blockade.[19]
- Reflex tachycardia and increased myocardial oxygen consumption may occur, requiring cautious use in patients with ischemic heart disease.
- **Digitalis glycosides** increase myocardial contractility and may attenuate the neurohormonal activation associated with HF.
  - Digoxin decreases the number of HF hospitalizations without altering overall mortality.[20]
  - Digoxin has a narrow **therapeutic index**, and serum levels should be followed closely, particularly in patients with unstable renal function.
  - The usual daily dose is 0.125–0.25 mg and should be decreased in patients with renal insufficiency. Clinical benefits may not be related to the serum levels; although serum digoxin levels of 0.8–2.0 ng/mL are considered "therapeutic," toxicity can occur in this range.
  - Discontinuation of digoxin in patients who are stable on a regimen of digoxin, diuretics, and an ACE inhibitor may result in clinical deterioration.
- **Calcium channel blockers** have no favorable effects on mortality in HF.
  - Dihydropyridine calcium channel blockers such as amlodipine may be used in hypertensive HF patients already on maximal medical therapy, but do not improve mortality.[21]
  - Nondihydropyridine calcium channel blockers should be avoided because their negative inotropic effects may potentiate worsening HF.
- **Diuretic therapy** often leads to clinical improvement in patients with symptomatic HF. Frequent assessment of the patient's weight along with careful observation of fluid intake and output is essential during initiation and maintenance of therapy. Frequent complications of therapy include hypokalemia, hyponatremia, hypomagnesemia, volume contraction alkalosis, intravascular volume depletion, and hypotension. Serum electrolytes, BUN, and creatinine levels should be followed after institution of diuretic therapy. Hypokalemia may be life threatening in patients who are receiving digoxin or in those who have severe LV dysfunction that predisposes them to ventricular arrhythmias. Potassium supplementation or a potassium-sparing diuretic should be considered in addition to careful monitoring of serum potassium levels.
  - **Thiazide** diuretics (**hydrochlorothiazide, chlorthalidone**) can be used as initial agents in patients with normal renal function in whom only a mild diuresis is desired. **Metolazone**, unlike other thiazides, exerts its action at the proximal as well as the distal tubule and may be useful in combination with a loop diuretic in patients with a low glomerular filtration rate and diuretic resistance.
  - **Loop diuretics (furosemide, torsemide, bumetanide, ethacrynic acid)** should be used in patients who require significant diuresis and in those with markedly decreased renal function. Furosemide reduces preload acutely by causing direct venodilation when administered IV, making it useful for managing severe HF or acute pulmonary edema. Use of loop diuretics may be complicated by hyperuricemia, hypocalcemia, ototoxicity, rash, and vasculitis. Furosemide, torsemide, and bumetanide are sulfa derivatives and may rarely cause drug reactions in sulfa-sensitive patients; ethacrynic acid can be used in these patients.
  - **Sacubitril/valsartan** is a combination of the neprilysin inhibitor sacubitril and the ARB valsartan and was recently approved for use in patients with systolic HF and NYHA class II–IV symptoms. In a large trial, this agent was shown to be superior to enalapril in reducing death and rehospitalization among NYHA class II–IV patients with systolic HF.[22]

TABLE 6-3 INOTROPIC AGENTS[a]

Drug	Dose	Mechanism	Effects/Side Effects
Dopamine	1–3 µg/kg/min	Dopaminergic receptors	Splanchnic vasodilation
	2–8 µg/kg/min	β_1-Receptor agonist	+Inotropic
	7–10 µg/kg/min	α-Receptor agonist	↑ SVR
Dobutamine	2.5–15.0 µg/kg/min	$\beta_1 > \beta_2$ > α-Receptor agonist	+ Inotropic, ↓ SVR, tachycardia
Epinephrine	0.05–1 µg/kg/min; titrate to desired mean arterial pressure. May adjust dose every 10–15 min by 0.05–0.2 µg/kg/min to achieve desired blood pressure goal	$\beta_1 > \alpha$ Low doses = β High doses = α	+ Inotropic, ↑ SVR
Milrinone[b]	50-µg/kg/bolus IV over 10 min, 0.375–0.75 µg/kg/min	↑ cAMP	↓ SVR, +inotropic

[a]Increased risk of atrial and ventricular tachyarrhythmias.
[b]Needs does adjustment for creatinine clearance.
cAMP, cyclic adenosine monophosphate; SVR, systemic vascular resistance; ↑, increased; ↓, decreased.

- **Inotropic agents**
  - Sympathomimetic agents are potent parenteral drugs primarily used to treat severe HF (Table 6-3). Beneficial and adverse effects are mediated by stimulation of myocardial β-adrenergic receptors. The most important adverse effects are related to the arrhythmogenic nature of these agents and the potential for exacerbation of myocardial ischemia. Treatment should be guided by careful hemodynamic and ECG monitoring. Patients with refractory chronic HF may benefit symptomatically from continuous ambulatory administration of IV inotropes as palliative therapy or as a bridge to mechanical ventricular support or cardiac transplantation. However, this strategy may increase the risk of life-threatening arrhythmias or indwelling catheter–related infections.[1]
  - **Norepinephrine, rather than dopamine**, should be used for stabilization of the hypotensive HF patient. Although a large randomized trial found no difference in mortality between dopamine and norepinephrine, there were more adverse events (primarily arrhythmogenic) in the dopamine group and subgroup analysis of those with cardiogenic shock showed an increased rate of death at 28 days in the dopamine group.[23]
  - **Dobutamine** is a synthetic analog of dopamine with predominantly β-adrenoreceptor activity. It increases cardiac output, lowers cardiac filling pressures, and generally has a neutral effect on systemic blood pressure. Dobutamine has no significant role in the treatment of HF resulting from diastolic dysfunction or a high-output state.

- **Phosphodiesterase inhibitors** increase myocardial contractility and produce vasodilation by increasing intracellular cyclic adenosine monophosphate. **Milrinone** is currently available for clinical use and is indicated for treatment of refractory HF. Hypotension may develop in patients who receive vasodilator therapy or have intravascular volume contraction or both.
- **Nitroglycerin** is a potent vasodilator with effects predominantly on the venous and, to a lesser extent, arterial vascular beds. It relieves pulmonary and systemic venous congestion and is an effective coronary vasodilator. It is the preferred vasodilator for treatment of HF in the setting of acute MI or unstable angina.
- **Sodium nitroprusside** is a direct arterial vasodilator with less potent venodilatory properties. Its predominant effect is to reduce afterload and is effective in patients with HF who are hypertensive and who have severe aortic or mitral valvular regurgitation.

Other Nonpharmacologic Therapies

- **Coronary revascularization** reduces ischemia and may improve systolic function in patients with CAD.
- **Implantable cardioverter–defibrillator (ICD)** placement is recommended in patients with persistent LV dysfunction (EF < 35%) for the prevention of sudden cardiac death.[24]
  - Patients should receive at least 3–6 months of optimal medical therapy and discontinuation of proarrhythmic drugs prior to reassessment of EF and implantation of an ICD.
  - Following an acute MI or revascularization, EF should be assessed after 40 days of optimal medical therapy prior to ICD implantation.
- **Cardiac resynchronization therapy (CRT)** or **biventricular pacing** can improve quality of life and reduce risk of death in patients with an EF of <35%, NYHA class II–IV HF, and conduction abnormalities (left bundle-branch block and atrioventricular delay).[25,26]
- An **intra-aortic balloon pump (IABP)** can be considered for temporary hemodynamic support in patients who have failed pharmacologic therapy and have transient myocardial dysfunction or awaiting a definitive procedure such as a left ventricular assist device (LVAD) or cardiac transplantation.

Surgical Management

- **Ventricular assist devices (VADs)** are surgically implanted devices that draw blood from the left ventricle (LV), energize flow through a motor unit, and deliver the energized blood to the aorta, resulting in augmented cardiac output and lower intracardiac filling pressures.
  - Temporary support is indicated for patients with severe HF after cardiac surgery or individuals with intractable cardiogenic shock after acute MI.
  - Durable support is indicated as a bridge to transplantation for patients awaiting heart transplant or as destination therapy for select patients who are ineligible for transplant with refractory end-stage HF and a HF-related life expectancy with therapy of <2 years.[1]
- **Cardiac transplantation** is an option for selected patients with severe end-stage HF that has become refractory to aggressive medical therapy and for whom no other conventional treatment options are available.
  - Candidates considered for transplantation should be <65 years of age (although selected older patients may also benefit), have advanced HF, have a strong psychological support system, have exhausted all other therapeutic options, and be free of irreversible extracardiac organ dysfunction that would limit functional recovery or predispose them to posttransplantation complications.[27]
  - Survival rates after heart transplantation are ~90%, 70%, and 50% at 1, 5, and 10 years, respectively.

- In general, functional capacity and quality of life improve significantly after transplantation.
- Posttransplant complications include acute and chronic rejection, typical and atypical infections, and adverse effects of immunosuppressive agents. Surgical complications and acute rejection are the major causes of death in the first posttransplant year. Cardiac allograft vasculopathy (CAD/chronic rejection) and malignancy are the leading causes of death after the first posttransplant year.

Lifestyle/Risk Modification
- **Exercise** training is recommended in stable HF patients. Ideally, it should be started slowly in a monitored outpatient setting and reach a target of 20–45 minutes a day for 3–5 days per week for a total of 8–12 weeks. Short-term effects of exercise training in patients with chronic stable HF are additive to pharmacologic treatment and are associated with a decrease in neurohormonal activation.[28]
- Patients enrolled in exercise training programs notice increased exercise capacity, decreased symptoms, increased quality of life, and decreased hospitalization rate. The effects of long-term exercise training on survival are not defined.
- **Dietary counseling for sodium and fluid restriction** should be provided. Daily intake of 2 g of sodium per day is recommended. Excessive restriction (<1.5 g/d of sodium) may be harmful.
- Smoking cessation and abstinence from alcohol are strongly encouraged.

Acute Heart Failure and Cardiogenic Pulmonary Edema

GENERAL PRINCIPLES

Acute HF is the sudden development of signs and symptoms of insufficient cardiac output. This may occur in patients with chronic HF as well as patients with a previously functional and morphologically normal LV. Acute HF accounts for a substantial number of inpatient hospitalizations and incurs significant morbidity and mortality. The diagnosis must be made rapidly, reversible causes identified, and treatment instituted expeditiously.

Etiology
- Potential inciting factors include acute myocardial ischemia, arrhythmia (e.g., atrial fibrillation), infection, hypertension, acute or progressive valvular dysfunction, renal failure, and exposure to myocardial toxins.
- In patients with chronic compensated HF, acute HF may result from medication nonadherence or dietary indiscretion (i.e., increased sodium and fluid intake).
- Other factors that may contribute to acute HF presentations include postoperative status, peripartum status, and iatrogenic hypervolemia.
- Acute right-sided HF may result from pulmonary embolism (PE).

Pathophysiology
- Cardiogenic pulmonary edema (CPE) occurs when the pulmonary capillary pressure exceeds the forces that maintain fluid within the vascular space (serum oncotic pressure and interstitial hydrostatic pressure).
- Increased pulmonary capillary pressure may be caused by LV failure, obstruction to transmitral flow (e.g., mitral stenosis, atrial myxoma), or, rarely, pulmonary venoocclusive disease.
- Accumulation of fluid in the pulmonary interstitium is followed by alveolar flooding and impairment of gas exchange.

DIAGNOSIS

Clinical Presentation
- Clinical manifestations of CPE may occur rapidly and include dyspnea, orthopnea, anxiety, and restlessness. The patient may expectorate pink frothy fluid.
- It is important to delineate the onset and severity of symptoms. Patients should be carefully questioned regarding the precipitating factors above.
- Physical signs of decreased peripheral perfusion, pulmonary congestion, use of accessory respiratory muscles, and wheezing are often present. Physical exam may demonstrate pulmonary crackles, an S3 gallop, and peripheral edema. Elevated jugular venous distention is the most specific and reliable physical exam indicator of right-sided volume overload and generally representative of left-sided filling pressures.

Diagnostic Testing

Laboratories
- B-type natriuretic peptide (BNP) (please see section on lab evaluation under "Chronic Heart Failure and Cardiomyopathy").
- **Cardiac enzymes** (i.e., troponin I or troponin T) should be obtained to evaluate for ongoing myocardial ischemia.[29]
- Additional laboratory abnormalities may include elevated levels of BUN and creatinine, hyponatremia, anemia, and elevated hepatic enzymes.

Electrocardiography
Abnormalities in the ECG are common and include supraventricular and ventricular arrhythmias, conduction delays, and nonspecific ST–T segment changes.

Imaging
Chest radiograph abnormalities include cardiomegaly, interstitial and perihilar vascular engorgement, Kerley B lines, and pleural effusions. The radiographic abnormalities may follow the development of symptoms by several hours, and their resolution may be out of phase with clinical improvement. A normal chest radiograph does not rule out LV dysfunction or HF.

TREATMENT

- Continuous pulse oximetry and telemetry should be initiated. Vital signs need to be assessed frequently. IV access should be obtained.
- Supplemental oxygen should be administered initially to increase arterial oxygen content to >60 mm Hg. Mechanical ventilation is indicated if oxygenation is inadequate by noninvasive means or if hypercapnia coexists.[30]
- Placing the patient in a sitting position improves pulmonary function.
- Bed rest, pain control, and relief of anxiety can decrease cardiac workload.
- Precipitating factors should be identified (e.g., severe hypertension, myocardial ischemia, new-onset arrhythmias, volume overload) and corrected. Resolution of pulmonary edema can often be accomplished with correction of the underlying process.

Medications
- **Loop diuretics**
  - **Furosemide** is a venodilator that decreases pulmonary congestion within minutes of IV administration well before its diuretic action begins.
  - An initial dose of 20–80 mg IV should be given over several minutes and can be increased, based on response, to a maximum of 200 mg in subsequent doses. Patients who regularly take furosemide and/or have chronic kidney disease often need higher doses to achieve the same diuretic effect.

- **Nitrates**
  - **Nitroglycerin** is a potent venodilator that can potentiate the effect of furosemide. It relieves pulmonary and systemic venous congestion and is an effective coronary vasodilator.
  - Nitroglycerin is the preferred vasodilator for treatment of HF in the setting of acute MI or unstable angina. Intravenous administration is preferable to oral and transdermal forms as it can be rapidly titrated, although sublingual nitroglycerin (in pill or spray form) can be administered quickly, even before obtaining IV access.
  - IV nitroglycerin can be started at 5–10 mcg/min and increased every few minutes to desired effect or a maximum of 300 mcg/min.
- **Morphine sulfate**
  - **Morphine sulfate** reduces anxiety and dilates pulmonary and systemic veins.
  - Morphine, 2–4 mg IV, can be given over several minutes and can be repeated every 10–25 minutes until an effect is seen.
- **Nitroprusside** is an effective adjunct medication that is useful in CPE resulting from acute valvular regurgitation or hypertension. Pulmonary and systemic arterial catheterization should be considered to guide titration of nitroprusside therapy.
- **Inotropic agents** (Table 6-3), such as dobutamine or milrinone, may be helpful after initial treatment of CPE in patients with concomitant hypotension or shock.

SPECIAL CONSIDERATIONS

- **Right heart catheterization** (e.g., Swan-Ganz catheter) may be helpful in cases where a prompt response to therapy does not occur. The pulmonary artery catheter allows differentiation between cardiogenic and noncardiogenic causes of pulmonary edema via measurement of central hemodynamics and cardiac output. It may then be used to guide subsequent therapy. The routine use of right heart catheterization in acute HF patients is not beneficial.[31]
- **Acute hemodialysis** and **ultrafiltration** may be effective, especially in the patient with significant renal dysfunction and diuretic resistance but is not a first-line therapy.[32]

REFERENCES

1. Yancy CW, Jessup M, Bozkurt B, et al. 2013 ACCF/AHA guideline for the management of heart failure: a report of the American College of Cardiology Foundation/American Heart Association Task Force on practice guidelines. *Circulation* 2013;128:e240–327.
2. Mozaffarian D, Benjamin E, Go A, et al. Heart disease and stroke statistics—2015 update. *Circulation* 2015;131:e29–322.
3. Maisel A, Krishnaswamy P, Nowak R, et al. Rapid measurement of B-type natriuretic peptide in the emergency diagnosis of heart failure. *N Engl J Med* 2002;347:161.
4. Krum H, Sackner-Bernstein J, Goldsmith R, et al. Double-blind, placebo-controlled study of long-term efficacy of carvedilol in patients with severe chronic heart failure. *Circulation* 1995;92(6):1499.
5. Krum H, Roecker E, Mohasci P, et al. Effects of initiating carvedilol in patients with severe chronic heart failure. *JAMA* 2003;289:712–8.
6. Bristow MR, Gilbert EM, Abraham WT, et al. Carvedilol produces dose-related improvements in left ventricular function and survival in subjects with chronic heart failure. MOCHA Investigators. *Circulation* 1996;94:2807–16.
7. Dargie HJ. Effect of carvedilol on outcome after myocardial infarction in patients with left-ventricular dysfunction: the CAPRICORN randomized trial. *Lancet* 2001;357:1385–90.
8. Packer M, Fowler MD, Roecker EB, et al. Effect of carvedilol on the morbidity of patients with severe chronic heart failure: results of the carvedilol prospective randomized cumulative survival (COPERNICUS) study. *Circulation* 2002;106:2194–9.
9. Poole-Wilson PA, Swedberg K, Cleland JG, et al. Comparison of carvedilol and metoprolol on clinical outcomes in patients with chronic heart failure in the carvedilol or metoprolol european trail (COMET): randomized controlled trial. *Lancet* 2003;362:7–13.

10. CIBIS Investigators and Committees. The Cardiac Insufficiency Bisoprolol Study II (CIBIS II): a randomised trial. *Lancet* 1999;353:9–13.
11. Hjalmarson A, Goldstein S, Fagerberg B, et al. Effects of controlled-release metoprolol on total mortality, hospitalizations, and well-being in patients with heart failure: the metoprolol CR/XL randomized intervention trial in congestive heart failure (MERIT-HF). *JAMA* 2000;283:1295–302.
12. Packer M, Poole-Wilson PA, Armstrong PW, et al. Comparative effects of low and high doses of the angiotensin-converting enzyme inhibitor, lisinopril, on morbidity and mortality in chronic heart failure. ATLAS study group. *Circulation* 1999;100:2312–8.
13. Palmer BF. Renal dysfunction complicating the treatment of hypertension. *N Engl J Med* 2002;347:1256–61.
14. Cohn JN, Tognoni G. A randomized trial of the angiotensin-receptor blocker valsartan in chronic heart failure. *N Engl J Med* 2001;345:667–75.
15. Pitt B, Zannad F, Remme WJ, et al. The effect of spironolactone on morbidity and mortality in patients with severe heart failure. Randomized Aldactone Evaluation Study Investigators. *N Engl J Med* 1999;341:709–17.
16. Pitt B, Remme W, Zannad F, et al. Eplerenone, a selective aldosterone blocker, in patients with left ventricular dysfunction after myocardial infarction. *N Engl J Med* 2003;348:1309–21.
17. Zannad F, McMurray J, Krum H, et al. Eplerenone in patients with systolic heart failure and mild symptoms. *N Engl J Med* 2011;364:11–21.
18. Taylor AL, Ziesche S, Yancy C, et al. Combination of isosorbide dinitrate and hydralazine in blacks with heart failure. *N Engl J Med* 2004;351:2049–57.
19. Cohn JN, Archibald DG, Ziesche S, et al. Effect of vasodilator therapy on mortality in chronic congestive heart failure. Results of a Veterans Administration Cooperative Study. *N Engl J Med* 1986;314:1547–52.
20. Digitalis Investigation Group. The effect of digoxin on mortality and morbidity in patients with heart failure. *N Engl J Med* 1997;336:525–33.
21. Packer M, O'Connor C, Ghali J, et al. Effect of amlodipine on morbidity and mortality in severe chronic heart failure. *N Engl J Med* 1996;335:1107–14.
22. McMurray J, Packer M, Desai A, et al. Angiotensin-neprilysin inhibition versus enalapril in heart failure. *N Engl J Med* 2014;371:993–1004.
23. De Backer D, Biston P, Devriendt J, et al. Comparison of dopamine and norepinephrine in the treatment of shock. *N Engl J Med* 2010;362:779–89.
24. Bardy GH, Lee KL, Mark DB, et al. Amiodarone or an implantable cardioverter–defibrillator for congestive heart failure. *N Engl J Med* 2005;352:225–37.
25. Cleland JG, Daubert JC, Erdmann E, et al. The effect of cardiac resynchronization on morbidity and mortality in heart failure. *N Engl J Med* 2005;352:1539–49.
26. Bristow MR, Saxon LA, Boehmer J, et al. Cardiac-resynchronization therapy with or without an implantable defibrillator in advanced chronic heart failure. *N Engl J Med* 2004;350:2140–50.
27. Mehra M, Kobashigawa J, Starling R, et al. Listing criteria for heart transplantation: International society for heart and lung transplantation guidelines for the care of cardiac transplant candidates—2006. *J Heart Lung Transplant* 2006;25:1024–42.
28. O'Connor C, Whellan D, Lee K, et al. Efficacy and safety of exercise training in patients with chronic heart failure. *JAMA* 2009;301:1439–50.
29. Horwich TB, Patel J, MacLellan WR, et al. Cardiac troponin I is associated with impaired hemodynamics, progressive left ventricular dysfunction, and increased mortality rates in advanced heart failure. *Circulation* 2003;108:833–8.
30. Masip J, Roque M, Sanchez B, et al. Noninvasive ventilation in acute cardiogenic pulmonary edema. *JAMA* 2005;294:3124–30.
31. Binanay C, Califf RM, O'Connor CM, et al. Evaluation study of congestive heart failure and pulmonary artery catheterization effectiveness: the ESCAPE trial. *JAMA* 2005;294:1625–33.
32. Costanzo MR, Guglin M, Saltzberg M, et al. Ultrafiltration versus intravenous diuretics for patients hospitalized for acute decompensated heart failure. *J Am Coll Cardiol* 2007;49:675.

Atrial Fibrillation

Kelly M. Carlson

GENERAL PRINCIPLES

Atrial fibrillation (AF) is a **supraventricular** arrhythmia in which the atria contract rapidly, irregularly, and independently of the ventricles. It is the most common sustained arrhythmia and strongly associated with increasing age affecting 0.5% of the population aged 50–59 years and almost 10% of the population >80 years of age. AF confers a fivefold increase in the **risk of stroke** and doubles the mortality rate.

Classification

- **Paroxysmal AF**: ≥2 episodes, lasting ≤7 days, often self-terminating within 24 hours
- **Persistent AF**: lasts >7 days and fails to self-terminate. Persistent AF requires medical and/or electrical intervention to achieve sinus rhythm. Persistent AF may be the first presentation, the culmination of several episodes of paroxysmal AF, or **long-standing persistent AF** (>1 year).
- **Permanent AF**: continuous AF where cardioversion has failed or has not been attempted lasting >1 year. It also refers to those when the decision is made to not pursue restoration of sinus rhythm by any means, including ablation.
- **Lone AF**: paroxysmal, persistent, or permanent AF in younger patients (<60 years old) with a structurally normal heart

Etiology

The exact mechanism of atrial fibrillation remains an area of intense study. Many conditions are associated with an increased risk of AF and it is strongly associated with increasing age.[1]

- **Structural heart disease**: valvular heart disease (i.e., mitral valve stenosis or prolapse, mitral annular calcification), hypertrophic or dilated cardiomyopathy, and coronary artery disease (CAD)
- **Other arrhythmias**: sick sinus (tachy–brady) syndrome and Wolff-Parkinson-White syndrome
- **Acute conditions**: acute myocardial infarction (MI), pulmonary embolism (PE), pericarditis, alcohol intoxication (holiday heart), cardiac surgery, and infections
- **Systemic illnesses**: hypertension, diabetes mellitus, hyperthyroidism, or hypothyroidism
- **Drugs**: anticholinergic and sympathomimetic drugs, theophylline
- **Echocardiographic correlates**: left ventricular (LV) hypertrophy, left atrial enlargement, reduced LV ejection fraction, and mitral valve abnormalities
- **"Lone atrial fibrillation"**: 10–15% of patients have no identifiable risk factors for thromboembolism or cardiac structural abnormality.

Risk Factors

- Age > 65
- Previous stroke or transient ischemic attack (TIA)
- Hypertension
- Diabetes mellitus

- Congestive heart failure (CHF)
- CAD
- Thyrotoxicosis
- In addition, echocardiographic risk factors include **left atrial enlargement** and a **reduced left LV ejection fraction**.

DIAGNOSIS

Clinical Presentation

History
- Patients present with a **wide variety of symptoms**, determined to a large extent by underlying cardiac function, comorbidities, and patient perception, though many are asymptomatic.
- **Common complaints** include palpitations, dizziness, fatigue, chest pain, dyspnea, or presyncope. Most symptoms result from tachycardia. It is unusual for patients to have dizziness or dyspnea from rate-controlled AF alone, and these patients should be evaluated for other causes of their symptoms.
- Patients may present with **unstable angina** in the setting of significant CAD; CHF with orthopnea, lower extremity edema, and dyspnea; focal **neurologic deficits** (in the setting of an embolic stroke); severe **abdominal or extremity pain** (in the setting of peripheral embolization with mesenteric or limb ischemia); or frank **syncope (sick sinus)**.

Physical Examination
- Usually, there is a rapid, **irregularly irregular** pulse, S1 of varying intensity, and absence of S4 or A waves.
- Examination should also focus on identifying signs of CHF including lower extremity edema, dyspnea, crackles and/or wheezing on pulmonary exam, and elevated jugular venous pressure (JVP) though the A wave may be absent thus this is less sensitive.
- **Other possible findings** include goiter, hyperthyroid signs, wheezing (underlying pulmonary disease), focal neurologic deficits, or evidence of peripheral embolization (a cold extremity or absent pulse).

Diagnostic Testing

Laboratories
- Thyroid function test should be obtained.
- Serial cardiac enzymes if acute MI suspected, or if the patient has known CAD, or multiple CAD risk factors.
- Arterial blood gas (ABG) sampling if PE is suspected.
- A complete blood count can help assess for anemia or infection.
- A complete metabolic panel will help assess electrolyte abnormalities.
- Blood cultures and further infectious workup should be performed if an underlying infection is suspected.

Electrocardiography
ECG reveals the absence of P waves with an irregular ventricular rhythm and an irregularly irregular **ventricular rhythm, or atrial fibrillation with rapid ventricular response is usually at a rate of 110–170 beats per minute (bpm)**. The QRS complexes are usually narrow though the ventricular response (QRS morphology) varies according to different properties of AV node and conduction system, vagal/sympathetic tone, and presence of accessory pathway.

Imaging
- **CXR** can detect any underlying pulmonary pathology and measure the cardiac silhouette.
- **Transthoracic echocardiography (TTE)** is a useful tool to evaluate for valvular or other cardiac structural abnormality and to measure left atrial size, left ventricular size.

- **Transesophageal echocardiography (TEE)** can be employed to identify thrombi in the left atrium prior to cardioversion.
- If PE is expected, lower extremity venous Doppler studies and ventilation/perfusion scan or CT scan may be necessary.
- Brain imaging should be obtained if neurologic deficits are present.

Diagnostic Procedures
Cardiac stress testing may be indicated if the patient has known CAD or multiple CAD risk factors.

TREATMENT

The therapeutic approach to AF is best divided into three broad areas:

- Control of the ventricular rate
- Restoration and maintenance of sinus rhythm
- Reduction of the risk of thromboembolic complications

Ultimately, the specific approach to management of AF will vary for individual patients and will depend to a large extent on concomitant illnesses/conditions, patient preferences, and severity of symptoms/complications. **If symptoms are severe or if the patient is hemodynamically unstable, the treatment of choice is urgent synchronized DC cardioversion without anticoagulation (120–200 J biphasic or 200 J monophasic).**[1]

Rate Control

- Usually, the **ventricular rate is 110–170 bpm** in the absence of drug therapy or conduction system disease. If the rapid rate persists, patients are at an increased risk of hemodynamic instability, tachycardia associated cardiomyopathy, and increase in symptoms given decreased ventricular filling and increased myocardial demand.
- There is no benefit with strict rate control (<80 bpm at rest or <110 bpm during 6-minute walk) compared to lenient rate control (resting heart rate <110 bpm) in patients with persistent AF.[2]
- Correcting reversible causes including hypoxia, infection, and thyroid illnesses have been shown to improve success of rate control.
- **Pharmacologic rate control**: In the absence of significant symptoms, IV medications are unnecessary and best avoided in favor of oral preparations, which carry less risk of hypotension and symptomatic bradycardia.
  - **Beta adrenergic blockers (β-blockers)** blunt atrioventricular (AV) nodal conduction and slow ventricular response. **They are the agents of choice when AF is associated with thyrotoxicosis, acute myocardial infarction (MI), or postoperatively.** If acutely needed, metoprolol may be given starting at 5 mg IV over 2–3 minutes and repeated twice more until desired heart rate is achieved. This should be followed by an oral dose of metoprolol, 25–50 mg PO bid. β-blockers should be avoided in patients with acute decompensated heart failure and hypotension and used with caution in those with reactive airway disease.
  - **Calcium channel blockers** are available in both IV and PO preparations. The **nondihydropyridines** (e.g., diltiazem, verapamil) **are effective rate-control** agents. Diltiazem 5–10 mg IV over 2 minutes may be given and repeated in 15 minutes if desired rate is not achieved; it can also be followed with 5–15 mg/h IV drip for <24 hours. Calcium channel blockers should also be avoided in hypotension and acute decompensated heart failure. Oral preparations may be used for long-term rate control.

- **Digoxin** slows the ventricular response by increasing vagal tone and blunting AV nodal conduction.
  - The onset of action is significantly delayed compared with other agents, and rate control is often lost with increased sympathetic tone (e.g., exercise). It is therefore most effective in controlling resting heart rate and less effective for ambulatory patients. Unlike its inotropic effects, rate control is not seen until serum levels are >1.4 ng/mL.
  - It is **best suited for patients with coexisting symptomatic LV dysfunction** (given its positive inotropic effect), as an adjunct to β-blocker or calcium channel blocker therapy or as an alternative for intolerant patients.
  - Avoid digoxin in cases of acute or chronic renal dysfunction.
- **Amiodarone** is a class III antiarrhythmic that has AV nodal–blocking properties along with sympatholytic and calcium channel antagonist properties. It is a secondary agent, used primarily for refractory rate control or in patients in acute decompensated heart failure or hypotensive. It may convert a patient to sinus rhythm, thus increasing the risk of thromboembolism in patients with prolonged AF who are not anticoagulated. **Amiodarone increases digoxin levels and inhibits warfarin metabolism, so appropriate adjustments to those medications should be made.**

Restoration and Maintenance of Sinus Rhythm

- No studies have demonstrated a survival benefit or a reduction in thromboembolic events with chronic rhythm control over the alternate strategy of ventricular rate control and long-term anticoagulation, particularly in patients prone to persistent or chronic AF.
- In large trials with mostly older patients with asymptomatic persistent AF, there was no mortality benefit to a rhythm-control strategy as compared with a rate-control strategy (AFFIRM, RACE trials). In fact, there were trends toward improved survival and stroke risk with the rate-control strategy.[3,4]
- Most patients with symptomatic AF prefer a rhythm-control strategy to achieve sinus rhythm.
- The differences in quality of life between the two strategies were not demonstrable in the AFFIRM trial.[3]
- **Cardioversion can be performed with synchronized direct current cardioversion (DCC) and/or antiarrhythmic medications**. Because of the increased risk of thromboembolic events in the first few weeks after cardioversion, elective cardioversions should generally be performed with anticoagulation and continued for a minimum of 4 weeks afterward.
  - If the patient is hemodynamically unstable, urgent synchronized DCC starting at 200 J is warranted without anticoagulation.
  - Cardioversion can also be performed without anticoagulation in the setting of short-duration AF (<48 hours) or after a TEE demonstrates absence of a left atrial thrombus.
  - In the stable form, if the AF has lasted >48 hours, is of unknown duration, or is with coexisting mitral stenosis or a history of a thromboembolism, cardioversion should be delayed until anticoagulation can be maintained at appropriate levels (international normalized ratio [INR] of 2.0–3.0) for 3–4 weeks or until evaluation for thrombi of the left atrial appendage by TEE is performed.
- **Pharmacologic agents**
  - Pharmacologic agents for restoration and maintenance of sinus rhythm are shown in Table 7-1.[1]
  - Although the conversion rate with drugs is significantly lower than with electrical cardioversion, these agents are commonly used as either alternatives to DCC, adjuncts to DCC, or as salvage therapy in case of failed DCC.
  - Some research demonstrates evidence that pretreatment with antiarrhythmic medications can improve the success of DC cardioversion.[1]

TABLE 7-1 PHARMACOLOGIC AGENTS USED TO TREAT ATRIAL FIBRILLATION

Medication	Indication	Dosing
Amiodarone	Conversion and maintenance in patients with normal or reduced LV function	Oral load: 300 mg PO bid–tid for 1–3 wk, then maintain at 200–300 mg PO qd. Check baseline thyroid, liver, and pulmonary function tests.
		IV load: 150 mg IV over 10 min, then 1 mg/min for 6 h, then 0.5 mg/min for 18 h, followed by oral maintenance
Flecainide	Conversion and maintenance with patients with reduced LV function	Maintenance: start 50 mg PO bid.
	For paroxysmal atrial fibrillation with normal left ventricular function and no coronary artery disease	
Propafenone	For structurally normal hearts and no coronary artery disease	Conversion: 600 mg PO once
		Maintenance: start 150–300 mg PO bid.
Sotalol	For maintenance only	Starting dose: 80 mg PO bid
		Follow QT interval for excessive prolongation (daily for ≥3 d) and should be initiated as an inpatient with monitoring.
		Must have renal dosing.

Data from January CT, Wann L, Alpert JS, et al. 2014 AHA/ACC/HRS guideline for the management of patients with atrial fibrillation: executive summary: a report of the American College of Cardiology/American Heart Association Task Force on Practice Guidelines and the Heart Rhythm Society. *J Am Coll Cardiol* 2014;64(21):2246–80.

- Do not pharmacologically cardiovert a patient whom you would not be comfortable cardioverting electrically based on embolic risk.
- **If an antiarrythmic is being considered, a cardiologist should be consulted to assist in choosing the appropriate medication and monitoring for side effects and potential organ toxicity.**
- **Nonpharmacologic methods** of restoring/maintaining sinus rhythm exist.
  - The **Cox-Maze** procedure is a cardiac operation in which a sternotomy is performed and a series of carefully placed incisions are made in the atria to channel the erratic electrical activity to the AV node. Anticoagulation is continued initially after the procedure, and the decision to discontinue is individualized for each patient.[5]
  - Percutaneous approaches, including **pulmonary vein isolation and ablation**, are used in specialized settings.
  - The focus of **atrial flutter** may be destroyed by **radiofrequency ablation**, often resulting in restoration of normal sinus rhythm. Many of these patients will be left with AF, however.

TABLE 7-2 STROKE RISK IN PATIENTS WITH NONVALVULAR ATRIAL FIBRILLATION

CHADS$_2$ Risk Criteria	Score
Congestive heart failure (any previous history)	1
Hypertension (controlled or uncontrolled)	1
Age $\geq$ 75 y	1
Diabetes (controlled or uncontrolled)	1
Stroke/TIA (any previous history)	2

CHADS$_2$ Score	Recommended Therapy
0	Aspirin 81/325 mg daily or no therapy[a]
1	Aspirin 81/325 mg daily or oral anticoagulation[b]
$\geq$2	Oral anticoagulation[b]

[a]For patients <65 years old and without heart disease (lone AF).
[b]Warfarin, INR goal 2.0–3.0, target 2.5; if mechanical valve, target INR 2.5–3.5.

Adapted from Gage BF, Van Walravn C, Pearce L, et al. Selecting patients with atrial fibrillation for anticoagulation: stroke risk stratification in patients taking aspirin. *Circulation* 2004;110:2287–92; Gage BF, Waterman AD, Shannon W, et al. Validation of clinical classification schemes for predicting stroke: results from National Registry of Atrial Fibrillation. *JAMA* 2001;285:2864–70.

Thromboembolic Risk Reduction: Stroke Prevention

There is a significant risk of stroke in patients with AF due to the formation of thrombi. Risk factors for thromboembolic events related to AF and yearly risk of stroke without anticoagulation can be estimated using the CHADS$_2$ scoring system that is detailed in Table 7-2.[6,7] A more expanded scoring system, the CHA$_2$DS$_2$-VASc scoring system, detailed in Table 7-3, includes female gender, vascular disease, and age 65–74 years as risk factors and increases the value of age >75 years.[8] Including the additional risk factors can help clinicians further risk stratify those patients with a CHADS$_2$ score of 1 as research has demonstrated that for those patients with a CHADS$_2$ score of 0–1 but a CHADS-VASc score of 1–2, there is a significant increased risk for events (mortality) in those not anticoagulated.[9] The overall goal of preventing thromboembolic events must be weighed against the risk of bleeding complications with anticoagulation. The recent development of the HAS-BLED score (detailed in Table 7-4) helps clinicians risk stratify both initiating and continuing antociagulation.[10] For patients with a **lower risk** for stroke (CHADS$_2$ score 0), the risks of anticoagulation outweigh the benefit; therefore. aspirin is reasonable. Patients with "lone AF" can be managed with aspirin alone. Those with an intermediate score of 1, aspirin or anticoagulation may be used. Those at the highest risk for bleeding based on the scoring system, it is recommended to regularly review and use overall caution with anticoagulation.[11–13] Thus, a history of GI bleeding, hemorrhagic stroke, fall risk, renal insufficiency, etc. should all be considered when choosing one anticoagulant over another. Specific anticoagulants are detailed below:

- **Warfarin** inhibits the synthesis of vitamin K–dependent clotting factors.
  - The anticoagulant effect of warfarin is highly variable with genetic polymorphisms, oral intake of vitamin K, interaction with medications, liver dysfunction, and current antibiotic use.

TABLE 7-3. STROKE RISK IN PATIENTS WITH NONVALVULAR ATRIAL FIBRILLATION

CHA$_2$DS$_2$-VASc Risk Criteria	Score
Congestive heart failure (any previous history)	1
Hypertension (controlled or uncontrolled)	1
Age > 75 y	2
Diabetes mellitus (controlled or uncontrolled)	1
Stroke, TIA, thromboembolism	2
Vascular disease (peripheral, coronary artery disease, aortic plaque, prior MI)	1
Age 65–74	1
Sex (female)	1

CHA$_2$DS$_2$-VASc Score	Recommended Therapy
0	No therapy
1	ASA 81–325 mg or oral anticoagulation[a]
≥2	Oral antigcoagulation[a]

[a]Warfarin, INR goal 2.0–3.0, target 2.5; if mechanical valve, target INR 2.5–3.5.

Adapted from Lip GY, Halperin JL. Improving stroke risk stratification in atrial fibrillation. *Am J Med* 2010;123(6):484–8.

TABLE 7-4. HAS-BLED SCORING SYSTEM TO DETERMINE 1-YEAR RISK FOR MAJOR BLEEDING[a] IN PATIENTS WITH ATRIAL FIBRILLATION

Risk Factors	Score
Hypertension (uncontrolled, >160 systolic)	1
Abnormal renal function (dialysis, transplant, Cr >2.6 mg/dL or >200 μmol/L)	1
Abnormal liver function (cirrhosis or bilirubin >2× normal or AST/ALT/AP >3× normal)	1
Stroke history	1
History of major **B**leeding or predisposition to bleeding	1
History of **L**abile INR (time if therapeutic range <60%)	1
Elderly, age >65 y	1
Current "excess" use of alcohol (≥8 **D**rinks a week)	1
Currently taking antiplatelet **D**rug(s) or NSAID(s)	1

Risk Factors	Score
HAS-BLED Score	**Bleeding Risk (% Bleeds Per 100 Patient-Years)**
0–1	Low risk (1.1%)
2	Intermediate risk (1.9%)
≥3	High risk (4.9%)[b]

[a]Any bleeding requiring hospitalization, causing a decrease in hemoglobin level > 2 g/L, and/or requiring blood transfusion that was not hemorrhagic stroke.

[b]Risk score of ≥3 indicates increased risk for bleeding in 1 year with recommendations for regular review and overall caution with anticoagulation use.

Adapted from Lip GY, Deirfre L. Use of the CHA_2DS_2-VASc and HAS-BLED scores to aid decision making for thromboprophylaxis in nonvalvular atrial fibrillation. *Circulation* 2012;126:860–5; Granger CB, Alexander JH, McMurray JJ, et al. Apixaban versus warfarin in patients with atrial fibrillation. *N Engl J Med* 2011;365(11):981–92; Patel MR, Mahaffey KW, Garg J, et al. Rivaroxaban versus warfarin in nonvalvular atrial fibrillation. *N Engl J Med* 2011;365(10): 883–91; Guigliano RP, Ruff CT, Braunwald E, et al. Edoxaban versus warfarin in patients with atrial fibrillation. *N Engl J Med* 2013;369:2093–104.

- Warfarin's anticoagulation effect is monitored with the INR, a standardized report of prothrombin time (PT). The goal INR for most indications is 2.0–3.0, though some clinical situations require different goals.[1]
- Given the individual variable response to warfarin, the INR should be checked every week with dose adjustments until a steady state is reached. Once this is achieved, INR blood tests can be checked less frequently.
- It is important to ask the patient about missed doses, overall compliance, consistent diet, recent antibiotic use, and new or change in medications if the INR level suddenly changes or is difficult to achieve therapeutic level.
- **Warfarin may be reversed with oral or IV vitamin K with effect in 24 hours and 8–12 hours, respectively. Additional reversal agents include fresh frozen plasma (FFP), prothrombin complex concentrate (PCC), or recombinant factor VIIa** with immediate effect in the case of over anticoagulation and life-threatening bleeding.[14]
- **Novel oral anticoagulants** (NOACs)
  - Because the risk/benefit ratio for anticoagulation is unique to each individual, variation exists in recommended anticoagulation strategies. These new alternatives to warfarin are being offered as anticoagulation that tailors to the individual's preferences, medical history, and risks factors.
  - A major benefit of the NOACs is that they do not require monitoring with blood tests like warfarin adding convenience for the patient and physician.
  - NOACs must be adjusted for renal insufficiency; if a patient develops kidney injury, overanticoagulation may occur and result in life-threatening bleeding.
  - It is important to note that NOACs have limited options for reversal agents at present.
  - **Dabigatran** is a direct thrombin inhibitor. It reduces the risk of stroke and systemic embolism in those with nonvalvular AF as demonstrated in the RE-LY trial, which demonstrated superiority to warfarin with the 150 mg bid dose with similar bleeding rates and noninferiority to warfarin with the 110 mg bid dose with lower bleeding rates.[15]
    - Dabigatran is dosed as 150 mg PO bid for patients with CrCl >30 mL/min and 75 mg PO bid for those with a CrCl 15–30 mL/min.[16] It is 85% renally cleared

with a mean half-life of 14–17 hours and should be stopped in patients who develop acute kidney injury.[16]
- It is not approved for use with mechanical heart valves.
- A common side effect of dabigatran is dyspepsia or gastric ulcers.
- Dabigatran is currently the only NOAC with an FDA-approved reversal agent, though there are reversal agents for other NOACs currently under investigation. **A humanized monoclonal fragment antigen binding (Fab) to dabigatran, idarucizumab, recently became the first FDA-approved NOAC-specific reversal agent.**[17] A recombinant human factor Xa agent is under investigation and may be approved in the future once the risk of immediate thrombosis with reversal is further studied.[18]

○ **Apixaban** is a factor Xa inhibitor and is approved for stroke prophylaxis and prevention of systemic embolism in patients with nonvalvular atrial fibrillation.
  - Apixaban demonstrated superiority to warfarin for stroke prophylaxis with lower bleeding rates and improvement in overall mortality in the ARISTOTLE trial.[19]
  - It is typically dosed as 5 mg PO bid or 2.5 mg PO bid for patients with ≥2 of the following: ≥80 years of age, ≤60 kg body weight, and Cr ≥1.5 mg/dL.[16] It is about 27% renally cleared and is not recommended for patient with severe hepatic impairment; the mean half-life is ~12 hours.[16]
  - The most common side effect is bleeding complications. There is an increased risk for stroke when stopped, and thus, another anticoagulant should be considered for at least 1 week.
  - Again, no factor Xa reversal agents are FDA approved at this time.

○ **Rivaroxaban** is a factor Xa inhibitor that is approved for stroke prophylaxis and the prevention of systemic embolism in patients with nonvalvular atrial fibrillation. It has also been approved for DVT/PE treatment.
  - The ROCKET AF trial demonstrated noninferiority to warfarin for nonvalvular atrial fibrillation with similar overall bleeding events though fewer intracranial and fatal bleeding events.[20]
  - Rivaroxaban is dosed once daily as either 15 mg for patients with CrCl 15–50 mL/min and 20 mg for patients with CrCl >50 mL/min.[16] It is about 33% renally cleared and not recommended for those with moderate or severe hepatic impairment or coagulopathy from liver disease. The mean half-life is 5–13 hours.[16]
  - Similar to apixaban, the most common side effect is bleeding complications and an increased risk of stroke when the medication is stopped, thus another anticoagulant should be considered for at least 1 week once it is stopped.[16]
  - There are no factor Xa reversal agents that are FDA approved at this time.

○ **Edoxaban** is a direct Xa factor inhibitor that is FDA approved for nonvalvular atrial fibrillation and DVT/PE.
  - The ENGAGE AF-TIMI 48 trial demonstrated superiority to warfarin at the 60 mg dosing and noninferiority with the 30 mg dosing. The study demonstrated significantly fewer major bleeding events and fewer overall cardiovascular-related deaths at both dosages.[21]
  - **It is not recommended in patients with a CrCl >95 mL/min** as these patients had an increased rate of ischemic stroke with edoxaban 60 mg once daily compared to patients treated with warfarin.[16]
  - A 50% dose reduction in patients with features that are known to increase edoxaban drug levels including renal dysfunction (CrCl 30–50 mL/min), low body weight (≤60 kg), or concomitant use of medication with P-glycoprotein interaction prevents excess drug interaction and optimizes risk of ischemic and bleeding events.[22]
  - As noted above, there are no FDA-approved factor Xa reversal agents at this time.

REFERENCES

1. January CT, Wann L, Alpert JS, et al. 2014 AHA/ACC/HRS guideline for the management of patients with atrial fibrillation: executive summary: a report of the American College of Cardiology/American Heart Association Task Force on Practice Guidelines and the Heart Rhythm Society. *J Am Coll Cardiol* 2014;64(21):2246–80.
2. Van Gelder IC, Gorenveld HF, Crijns HJ, et al. Lenient versus strict rate control in patients with atrial fibrillation. *N Engl J Med* 2010;362:1363–73.
3. Wyse DG, Waldo AL, DiMarco JP, et al. A comparison of rate control and rhythm control in patients with atrial fibrillation. *N Engl J Med* 2002;347:1825–33.
4. Van Gelder IC, Hagens VE, Bosker HA, et al. A comparison of rate control and rhythm control in patients with recurrent persistent atrial fibrillation. *N Engl J Med* 2002;347:1834–40.
5. Ad N, Henry L, Shuman DJ, Holmes S. A more specific anticoagulation regimen is required for patients after the Cox-Maze procedure. *Ann Thorac Surg* 2014;98:1331–8.
6. Gage BF, Van Walravn C, Pearce L, et al. Selecting patients with atrial fibrillation for anticoagulation: stroke risk stratification in patients taking aspirin. *Circulation* 2004;110:2287–92.
7. Gage BF, Waterman AD, Shannon W, et al. Validation of clinical classification schemes for predicting stroke: results from National Registry of Atrial Fibrillation. *JAMA* 2001;285:2864–70.
8. Lip GY, Halperin JL. Improving stroke risk stratification in atrial fibrillation. *Am J Med* 2010;123(6):484–8.
9. Lip GY, Skjoth F, Rasmussen H, Larsen TB. Oral anticoagulation, aspirin, or no treatment in patients with nonvalvular atrial fibrillation with 0 or 1 stroke risk factor based on the CHA_2DS_2-VASc score. *J Am Coll Cardiol* 2015;65(14):1385–94.
10. Lip GY, Deirfre L. Use of the CHA_2DS_2-VASc and HAS-BLED scores to aid decision making for thromboprophylaxis in nonvalvular atrial fibrillation. *Circulation* 2012;126:860–5.
11. Camm AJ, Kirhhof P, Lip GY, et al. Guidelines for management of atrial fibrillation. *Eur Heart J* 2010;31(19):2369–429.
12. Pisters R, Lane DA, Nieuwlaat R, et al. A novel user-friendly score (HAS-BLED) to assess 1-yr risk of major bleeding in patients with atrial fibrillation: the Euro Heart Survey. *Chest* 2010;138:1093–100.
13. Lip GY, Andreotti F, Fauchier L, et al. Bleeding risk assessment and management in atrial fibrillation patients: a position document from the European Heart Rhythm Association, endorsed by the European Society of Cardiology Working Group on Thrombosis. *Europace* 2011;13:723–46.
14. Garcia DA, Crowther MA. Reversal of warfarin. *Circulation* 2012;125:2944–7.
15. Connolly SJ, Ezekowitz MD, Yusuf S, et al. Dabigatran versus warfarin in patients with atrial fibrillation. *N Engl J Med* 2009;361:1139–51.
16. Heidbuchel H, Verhamme P, Alings M, et al. EHRA practical guide on the use of new oral anticoagulants in patients with non-valvular atrial fibrillation: executive summary. *Eur Heart J* 2013;34:2094–106.
17. Pollack CV, Reilly PA, Eikelboom J, et al. Idarucizumab for dabigatran reversal. *N Engl J Med* 2015;373:511–20.
18. Gosselin RC, Adcock D, Hawes EM, et al. Evaluating the use of commercial drug-specific calibrators for determining PT and APTT reagent sensitivity to dabigatran and rivaroxaban. *Thromb Haemost* 2015;113:931–42.
19. Granger CB, Alexander JH, McMurray JJ, et al. Apixaban versus warfarin in patients with atrial fibrillation. *N Engl J Med* 2011;365(11):981–92.
20. Patel MR, Mahaffey KW, Garg J, et al. Rivaroxaban versus warfarin in nonvalvular atrial fibrillation. *N Engl J Med* 2011;365(10):883–91.
21. Giugliano RP, Ruff CT, Braunwald E, et al. Edoxaban versus warfarin in patients with atrial fibrillation. *N Engl J Med* 2013;369:2093–104.
22. Ruff CT, Giugliano RP, Braunwald E, et al. Association between edoxaban dose, concentration, anti-Factor Xa activity and outcomes: an analysis of data from the randomised, double-blind ENGAGE AF-TIMI 48 trial. *Lancet* 2015;385:2288–95.

Anticoagulation and Surgery

Happy D. Thakkar and Mark S. Thoelke

GENERAL PRINCIPLES

- Leading indications for anticoagulation are venous thromboembolic (VTE) disease (deep venous thrombosis [DVT] or pulmonary embolism [PE]), atrial fibrillation (AF), and mechanical heart valves.
- Temporary interruption of anticoagulation for procedures occurs over 250,000 times a year in the United States, introducing a small but significant risk of thrombosis.[1]
- Continuing oral anticoagulation (OAC) or bridging with heparinoids leads to increased risk of periprocedural bleeding.
- The novel oral anticoagulants ([NOACs]; e.g., dabigatran, rivaroxaban, apixaban, and edoxaban) raise further concerns for managing periprocedural bleeding, as most lack routine methods for urgently reversing their effect.
- The role of the consultant is to weigh the risk of thrombotic complications associated with interrupting OAC against the risk of bleeding complications.

DETERMINING RISK

Risk of Major Bleeding

The first step should be to determine the bleeding risk for the procedure.

- **Procedures at low risk for major bleeding**
  - These procedures include dental, dermatologic, ophthalmologic, arthroscopic, bronchoscopic, and endoscopic (without biopsy).
  - Cholecystectomy and other laparoscopic procedures are also considered low risk (although some surgeons may disagree).
  - **These procedures may be undertaken without discontinuing OAC, although resistance to proceeding as such is relatively common.**
  - Dental patients with bleeding should use mouthwash containing tranexamic or epsilon-aminocaproic acid.
  - Pacemaker and implantable cardioverter–defibrillator procedures can also be undertaken without interrupting warfarin therapy, as heparin bridging may pose up to a fivefold greater risk of device-pocket hematomas.[2]
- **Most other surgical procedures carry a high risk for major bleeding**, estimated at about 2%, and warrant period of anticoagulation interruption.[3]
  - The literature is hindered by the lack of a consensus definition for major bleeding, though generally includes intracranial bleeding, bleeding that results in admission, or bleeding requiring two or more units of packed red blood cells to correct.
  - Major bleeds occur most frequently in the gastrointestinal and urinary tracts and are accompanied by up to 10% risk of mortality.[4]
- **Bleeding risk also depends on patient comorbidities and age.** Scoring systems have been developed to help incorporate such factors into the bleeding risk assessment for AF patients on warfarin. The HAS-BLED score (please see Chapter 7) has been the most predictive of these systems, although it has yet to be externally validated.[5]

- Overaggressive postoperative anticoagulation may paradoxically lead to increased risk of thrombosis, as bleeding or oozing may delay resumption of OAC.
- **It should be noted that regional or epidural anesthesia carries a risk of hematoma formation and resultant cord compression. Low molecular weight heparins (LMWHs) are not FDA approved for patients receiving epidural anesthesia.**

Risk of Thrombosis

Second, the risk of thrombosis from the interruption of OAC should be assessed. This risk is determined largely by the underlying indication for anticoagulation.[6]

- **VTE patients** are at high risk for thromboembolic complications if they are <3 months from the index event or if they carry the diagnosis of an active cancer. Patients >12 months removed from a VTE event are at low risk.
- **AF patients** are considered high risk for stroke based on a $CHADS_2$ (please see Chapter 7) score of ≥5 or history of systemic embolism within the past 12 weeks. Those with $CHADS_2$ scores ≤2 are at low risk.
- **Mechanical heart valve patients** are at high risk for thromboembolic events with any mitral valve prosthesis, older (e.g., caged-ball or tilting-disk) aortic valve prosthesis, multiple valve prostheses, or a history of cardioembolic events. Low-risk patients are those with bileaflet aortic valve prostheses and no other risk factors (e.g., AF or history of cardioembolic event).
- As indicated by the common practice of admitting patients for subtherapeutic internationalized normalized ratios (INRs), the risk of thrombosis during interruption of anticoagulation therapy is probably overestimated by clinicians.
  ○ A patient with a St. Jude bileaflet mitral valve, for instance, has a yearly risk of thrombosis off anticoagulation of 23%.[7] Thus, for 4 days of interrupted anticoagulation, the risk of thrombosis would be 0.25% (4/365 × 0.23).
  ○ Anticoagulation reduces the risk of thrombosis by 75%,[8] so the absolute risk reduction (ARR) of bridging with parenteral anticoagulation during these 4 days would be 0.19% (0.25% × 0.75).
  ○ The number needed to treat (NNT) to prevent one thrombotic event by bridging is thus 526 (NNT = 1/ARR).
  ○ The observed data for perioperative stroke rate, at 0.4%, is higher than these calculations.[6] This may be because the surgical milieu leads to a prothrombotic state itself or because the abrupt discontinuation of OAC theoretically leads to a rebound hypercoagulable state. While surgery clearly increases risk of venous thrombosis, this observed increase may be presumptive evidence for increased arterial thrombosis as well.
- However infrequent, perioperative thrombotic complications may be catastrophic, with a 9–14% all-cause mortality rate at 30 days post procedure.[9]

DISEASE-SPECIFIC PERIOPERATIVE ANTICOAGULATION MANAGEMENT

Venous Thromboembolism

Risk factors for VTE are many and varied (Table 8-1).

- **Risk of VTE recurrence** depends on risk factors, circumstances precipitating initial DVT, and time treated with OAC. In the 1st month after a DVT, each day without anticoagulation increases the absolute recurrence risk by 1%. Recurrence after discontinuing anticoagulation after 4 weeks is 8–10%, and after 3 months is 4–5%.[11]
- **For patients with a newly diagnosed DVT, delay surgery if at all possible** for at least 1 month. Surgery within 3 months of a DVT event should be treated as high risk with

TABLE 8-1 VENOUS THROMBOEMBOLISM RISK FACTORS

Major surgery (abdomen, pelvis, or lower extremities)	Prolonged immobility/paralysis (multiple trauma, spinal cord injury)
Acute medical illness (e.g., MI, CVA)	Heart or respiratory failure
Trauma (major or lower extremity)	Inflammatory bowel disease
Malignancy or cancer therapy	Nephrotic syndrome
Prior DVT or PE	Myeloproliferative disorders
Age >40 y	Paroxysmal nocturnal hemoglobinuria
Pregnancy/postpartum	Obesity
Estrogen use	Varicose veins
Central venous catheterization	Inherited or acquired thrombophilia

CVA, cerebrovascular accident; DVT, deep venous thrombosis; MI, myocardial infarction; PE, pulmonary embolism.

Adapted from Geerts WH, Pineo GF, Heit JA, et al. Prevention of venous thromboembolism: the Seventh ACCP Conference on Antithrombotic and Thrombolytic Therapy. *Chest* 2004;126:338S–400S. Ref.[10]

bridging therapy (see below). If interruption of anticoagulation is absolutely necessary before 1 month of anticoagulation, an inferior vena cava filter (possibly retrievable) should be considered.

Atrial Fibrillation

- Nonvalvular AF has a 4.5% risk per year of systemic embolization. Perioperatively, this risk is about 1.2%.[12] In the 30 days after an arterial embolic event, the risk is 0.5% per day. Risk can be better stratified using tools such as the $CHADS_2$ or CHA_2DS_2VASc (please see Chapter 7) scores, though these have not been validated for perioperative settings.[13]
- OAC with warfarin provides a 66% yearly relative risk reduction of systemic embolization with nonvalvular AF.[14]
- AF without risk factors is considered low risk, with no need for bridging therapy. Indeed, the 2014 American College of Cardiology/American Heart Association/Heart Rhythm Society (ACC/AHA/HRS) guidelines for atrial fibrillation no longer recommend even long-term aspirin prophylaxis for many of these patients.[15]
- Patients with multiple risk factors qualify as intermediate or high risk by the 2012 American College of Chest Physicians (ACCP) guidelines.[1]
  - These guidelines recommend bridging anticoagulation during OAC interruption for high-risk patients and to consider bridging for intermediate-risk patients.
  - More recently, findings from the BRIDGE study indicate that forgoing bridging anticoagulation perioperatively for AF patients is noninferior to bridging with LMWH and decreases the risk of major bleeding threefold.[16] However, this trial included only 58 patients with a $CHADS_2$ score of ≥ 5 and excluded certain high-risk procedures.
  - More studies will be necessary to inform future guidelines for recommendations on better risk stratifying these patients.
- **Recent embolic stroke should lead to consideration of delaying procedures until risk returns to baseline. If the procedure is necessary, however, these patients should be treated as high risk.**

Prosthetic Heart Valves
- The annual rate of major thrombotic events for mechanical valves without anticoagulation is 8% and is highest in the first 3 months after valve surgery.[17]
- Anticoagulation decreases this risk by 75%.[18]
- Risk factors for thromboembolic events include AF, severe left ventricular dysfunction (ejection fraction <30%), prior embolic events, mitral versus aortic valve, and hypercoagulable states.
- Bileaflet aortic valve replacements (AVR) without any of these risk factors are considered low risk by both the ACCP and the ACC/AHA guidelines and require no bridging therapy.[1,18]
- **Bridging anticoagulation is recommended for high-risk prosthetic valve patients by multiple society guidelines**, though there is disagreement on which patients fall into this high-risk group. **In general, bileaflet AVR with any of the risk factors above, older generation valve prostheses, and all mechanical mitral valves are considered higher risk and should receive bridging therapy.**
- Temporary interruption of OAC for surgery may be bridged with either unfractionated heparin (UFH) or LMWH.
- OAC should be resumed as soon as possible postoperatively, based on adequate achievement of hemostasis and bleeding risk. In emergency situations requiring reversal of warfarin therapy, fresh frozen plasma (FFP) is preferred over vitamin K as it is less likely to trigger hypercoagulability.

TREATMENT

Please see summary of thromboembolic risk and possible treatments based on risk highlighted in Table 8-2.

- **Bridging with UFH versus LMWH**
  - LMWH has been shown to be at least as comparable to UFH in treatment of thrombosis and embolism.[19]
  - The benefits of LMWH include the lack of need for monitoring, decreased bleeding risk, and potential outpatient use.
  - The major drawback of LMWH is its relative lack of reversibility with protamine.
  - Obese patients may need anti-Xa monitoring.
  - The use of LMWH in pregnant patients with mechanical valves came into question due to a 2002 Food and Drug Administration (FDA) warning against its use.[20] This warning stemmed from deaths in pregnant women with mechanical valves. Subsequently, there have been more data supporting the use of LMWH than UFH in patients with mechanical valves, and its use in this situation is now supported by the 2012 ACCP[1] as well as the 2014 ACC/AHA[18] guidelines.
- **Timing of bridging and anticoagulation interruption**
  - **Patients on warfarin:** For patients requiring interruption of warfarin therapy, the ACCP guidelines recommend stopping warfarin 5 days prior to the procedure, allowing INR to drift to near normal, and initiating bridging anticoagulation with a heparin product 3 days prior to the procedure.[1] Warfarin can be resumed the evening after the procedure given no bleeding concerns. **The patient's input regarding risk of complications may be helpful.**
  - **Patients on NOACs:** The NOACs include the direct thrombin inhibitor dabigatran as well as the direct factor Xa inhibitors rivaroxaban, apixaban, and edoxaban.
    - These agents have gained approval for and widespread clinical use in prevention of stroke in AF as well as prophylaxis and treatment of VTE.[21]
    - They have short half-lives, rapid onset and offset of action (1–3 hours), and renal clearance.

TABLE 8-2 THROMBOEMBOLIC RISK AND TREATMENT

Low Risk	Intermediate Risk	High Risk
Bileaflet AVR without risk factors	Bileaflet AVR with risk factors	Any mitral valve replacement (MVR) or older model AVR
AF without stroke and CHADS$_2$ score <2	AF with CHADS$_2$ score 3 or 4	AF CHADS$_2$ score >5
VTE >12 mo after therapy	VTE within past 3–12 mo	Recent (<3 mo) CVA/TIA or VTE <3 mo
Treatment	**Treatment**	**Treatment Patients on Warfarin**
No preprocedure bridging needed	Pre- and postprocedural low-dose UFH or LMWH	Hold warfarin 5 d before procedure; start full-dose UFH or LMWH 3 d before procedure as INR drifts down.
Postprocedural low-dose UFH or LMWH is indicated by procedure.		Stop UFH 5 h before procedure; alternatively, stop LMWH 12–24 h before procedure.
		Postprocedural bridging with full-dose UFH or LMWH until INR is therapeutic

Treatment Patients on NOACs

Hold NOAC 1–4 d before procedure depending on renal function and bleeding risk.

Consider bridging anticoagulation with UFH or LMWH in patients at high risk for thrombotic events and requiring extended NOAC therapy interruption (e.g., patients unable to take oral medications post-op).

Resume NOAC therapy after adequate hemostasis has been achieved following the procedure.

As most NOACs lack urgent reversal strategies, use caution with resumption and consider heparin products to bridge if concerned about postprocedural bleeding.

AVR, aortic valve replacement; CVA/TIA, cerebrovascular accident/transient ischemic attack; INR, international normalized ratio; LMWH, low molecular weight heparin; MVR, mitral valve replacement; NOAC, novel oral anticoagulants; UFH, unfractionated heparin; VTE, venous thromboembolism.

- Importantly, NOACs cannot be monitored for anticoagulation efficacy with routine tests (e.g., INR), and most lack methods for urgently reversing their effect.
- Idarucizumab, a monoclonal antibody fragment against dabigatran, recently became the first FDA-approved NOAC-specific reversal agent.[22]
- Interruption of anticoagulation for patients on NOACs is largely based on pharmacokinetic studies and best practice models rather than well-designed clinical trials.
- Depending on the patient's renal function and the procedural bleeding risk, NOAC therapy should be held 1–2 days prior to procedures.[23]
- For patients with significant renal impairment (creatinine clearance <50 mL/min) or those undergoing procedures with high bleeding potential (e.g., cardiovascular surgery or spinal anesthesia), consider holding NOAC therapy 2–4 days prior.
- Bridging anticoagulation is generally not required for patients on NOACs because, unlike warfarin, these agents do not require the levels of their target factors to reaccumulate over several days. However, bridging anticoagulation should be considered for patients at high risk for thrombotic events who require an extended interruption of NOAC therapy.[24]

REFERENCES

1. Douketis J, Spyropoulos AC, Spencer FA, et al. Perioperative management of antithrombotic therapy: Antithrombotic Therapy and Prevention of Thrombosis, 9th ed: American College of Chest Physicians Evidence-Based Clinical Practice Guidelines. *Chest* 2012;141:e326S–50S.
2. Birnie DH, Healey JS, Wells GA, et al. Pacemaker or defibrillator surgery without interruption of anticoagulation. *N Engl J Med* 2013;368:2084–93.
3. Tafur AJ, McBane R, Wysokinski WE, et al. Predictors of major bleeding in peri-procedural anticoagulation management. *J Thromb Haemost* 2012;10:261–7.
4. Guerrouij M, Uppal CS, Alklabi A, Douketis JD. The clinical impact of bleeding during anticoagulation therapy: assessment of morbidity, mortality and post-bleed anticoagulant management. *J Thromb Thrombolysis* 2011;31:419–23.
5. Omran H, Bauersachs R, Rübenacker S, et al. The HAS-BLED score predicts bleedings during bridging of chronic oral anticoagulation. Results from the national multicentre BNK Online bRiDging REgistRy (BORDER). *Thromb Haemost* 2012;108:65.
6. Baron TH, Kamath PS, McBane RD. Management of antithrombotic therapy in patients undergoing invasive procedures. *N Engl J Med* 2013;368:2113–24.
7. Salem D, Stein P, Al-Ahmed A, et al. Antithrombotic therapy in valvular heart disease—native and prosthetic. *Chest* 2004;126:457S–82S.
8. Dunn A, Turpie A. Perioperative management of patients receiving oral anticoagulants. *Arch Intern Med* 2003;163:901–8.
9. Majeed A, Hwang HG, Connolly SJ, et al. Management and outcomes of major bleeding during treatment with dabigatran or warfarin. *Circulation* 2013;128:2325–32.
10. Geerts WH, Pineo GF, Heit JA, et al. Prevention of venous thromboembolism: the Seventh ACCP Conference on Antithrombotic and Thrombolytic Therapy. *Chest* 2004;126:338S–400S.
11. Kearon C. Long-term management of patients after venous thromboembolism. *Circulation* 2004;110:10–8.
12. Healey JS, Eikelboom J, Douketis J, et al. Periprocedural bleeding and thromboembolic events with dabigatran compared with warfarin: results from the Randomized Evaluation of Long-Term Anticoagulation Therapy (RE-LY) randomized trial. *Circulation* 2012;126:343.
13. Lip GY, Nieuwlaat R, Pisters R, et al. Refining clinical risk stratification for predicting stroke and thromboembolism in atrial fibrillation using a novel risk factor-based approach: the euro heart survey on atrial fibrillation. *Chest* 2010;137:263–72.
14. Furie KL, Kasner SE, Adams RJ, et al. Guidelines for the prevention of stroke in patients with stroke or transient ischemic attack. *Stroke* 2011;42:227–76.
15. January CT, Wann LS, Alpert JS, et al. 2014 AHA/ACC/HRS guideline for the management of patients with atrial fibrillation. *J Am Coll Cardiol* 2014;64:2246–80.
16. Douketis JD, Spyropoulos AC, Kaatz S, et al. Perioperative bridging anticoagulation in patients with atrial fibrillation. *N Engl J Med* 2015;373:823–33.

17. Cannegieter SC, Rosendaal FR, Briet E. Thromboembolic and bleeding complications in patients with mechanical heart valve prostheses. *Circulation* 1994;89:635–41.
18. Nishimura RA, Otto CM, Bonow RO, et al. 2014 AHA/ACC guideline for the management of patients with valvular heart disease. *J Am Coll Cardiol* 2014;63:e57–185.
19. Spyropoulos AC, Turpie AG, Dunn AS, et al. Perioperative bridging therapy with unfractionated heparin or low-molecular-weight heparin in patients with mechanical prosthetic heart valves on long-term oral anticoagulants (from the REGIMEN Registry). *Am J Cardiol* 2008;102:883–9.
20. American College of Obstetricians and Gynecologists. ACOG Committee Opinion: safety of Lovenox in pregnancy. *Obstet Gynecol* 2002;100:845–6.
21. Caldeira D, Rodrigues FB, Barra M, et al. Non-vitamin K antagonist oral anticoagulants and major bleeding-related fatality in patients with atrial fibrillation and venous thromboembolism: a systematic review and meta-analysis. *Heart* 2015;101:1204–11.
22. Pollack CV, Reilly PA, Eikelboom J, et al. Idarucizumab for dabigatran reversal. *N Engl J Med* 2015;373:511–20.
23. Schulman S, Crowther M. How I treat with anticoagulants in 2012: new and old anticoagulants, and when and how to switch. *Blood* 2012;119:3016–23.
24. Beyer-Westendorf J, Gelbricht V, Förster K, et al. Peri-interventional management of novel oral anticoagulants in daily care: results from the prospective Dresden NOAC registry. *Eur Heart J* 2014;35:1888–96.

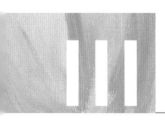

Pulmonary

Dyspnea

Rachel H. Bardowell and Adam V. Meyer

GENERAL PRINCIPLES

- Dyspnea is the sensation of difficulty breathing. Patients use various descriptors (e.g., "tight," "heavy," "hard to breathe," "hunger for air," "cannot get enough air," etc.) that may correspond to specific causes.
- Up to 50% of patients admitted to tertiary care hospitals are affected by this often debilitating symptom.[1]
- When patients with dyspnea first present to the hospital, priority should be placed on determining the underlying process leading to the symptom as well as optimizing oxygenation. Many patients will have a previously known cardiac, respiratory, or neuromuscular condition, which can lead to dyspnea. It may be challenging to determine if there is worsening of a previously known condition or the onset of a new condition.
- Dyspnea is subjective and distinct from the laboratory finding of hypoxia.
- The medical consultant is frequently called to evaluate an inpatient who experiences the sudden onset of dyspnea. In this situation, a reasonable, rapid differential includes the following (even before seeing the patient): pulmonary embolism (PE), pneumothorax, pneumonia, airflow obstruction (mainly chronic obstructive pulmonary disease [COPD] and/or asthma), pulmonary edema, angioedema or anaphylaxis, myocardial ischemia/infarction, arrhythmias, and anxiety.
- Of course, once the patient is evaluated, this initial differential should quickly be refined. Anxiety is common in patients with dyspnea. Dyspnea may also be a manifestation of an underlying anxiety disorder. Psychogenic dyspnea is common in patients presenting to the hospital, and there is significant cost associated with their evaluation.[2] These patients may have associated depression or pain. Patients may describe progressive anxiety culminating in dyspnea (rather than progressive dyspnea resulting in anxiety). They may also describe perioral or extremity numbness.
- Metabolic acidosis is compensated by tachypnea with large tidal volumes and a respiratory alkalosis. This rarely leads to dyspnea unless the acidosis is severe or there is underlying pulmonary pathology.
- Abdominal distention from ascites, pregnancy, or morbid obesity may also lead to dyspnea, but this is less likely to present acutely.
- Table 9-1 reviews the differential diagnosis in more general terms for the acute setting. The list of potential specific causes is enormous. Further details on many of the elements in the differential are discussed in other chapters.

DIAGNOSIS

Clinical Presentation

History

The history should include the following:

- Onset, quality, severity, duration, and ameliorating/exacerbating factors

TABLE 9-1 DIFFERENTIAL DIAGNOSIS OF DYSPNEA

Pulmonary: bronchospasm (e.g., COPD, asthma, anaphylaxis), aspiration, pneumonia, ARDS, pneumothorax, pulmonary embolism, pleural effusion, pulmonary hemorrhage, pulmonary hypertension

Cardiac: heart failure, pulmonary edema, right-to-left shunts, cardiac tamponade, acute myocardial ischemia, valvular dysfunction, arrhythmia

Hematologic: significant anemia, toxins resulting in impaired O_2–Hgb association or dissociation (e.g., CO)

CNS or neurologic: increased intracranial pressure (Cushing response), neuromuscular disease (i.e., respiratory muscle weakness)

Miscellaneous: severe metabolic acidosis, deconditioning, abdominal distention (e.g., morbid obesity, pregnancy, ascites), psychogenic (diagnosis of exclusion)

ARDS, acute respiratory distress syndrome; CNS, central nervous system; COPD, chronic obstructive pulmonary disease.

- Associated symptoms such as fevers, chills, sweats, orthopnea, paroxysmal nocturnal dyspnea, wheezing, edema, chest pain, cough, sputum production, hemoptysis, palpitations, nausea, anxiety, dizziness, orthostasis, and weakness
- History of pulmonary, cardiac, neuromuscular/neurologic, renal, hepatic, and coagulopathic disorders
- Risk factors for deep venous thrombosis/PE[3]
- Ingestion of drugs, medications, toxic substances, and administration of IV fluids
- Smoking and environmental exposures

Physical Examination

The exam should focus on the cardiovascular and respiratory systems.[4-6]

- Respiratory rate, effort, and pattern of breathing should be carefully observed.
- Auscultate for adventitious lung sounds such as rales/crackles, rhonchi, and wheezes as well as for assessing the quality of airflow.
- Auscultate for murmurs, rubs, and gallops as well as note the rhythm and rate.
- Evaluate for signs of pulmonary consolidation, hyperresonance, and pleural effusion (e.g., egophony, changes in tactile fremitus, dullness to percussion).
- Evaluate jugulovenous pulsations and edema.
- Palpate the chest wall for tenderness, heaves, abnormal apical impulse, or crepitus.
- Evaluate for signs of deep venous thrombosis (e.g., asymmetric edema).
- Consider measurement of the pulsus paradoxus.

Diagnostic Testing

Testing should be directed based on results of history, physical exam, and vital signs, including pulse oximetry. The sometimes tenuous correlation between SaO_2 by pulse oximetry and measured PaO_2 must be recognized, particularly in the clinically important range of percentages in the 80s to low 90s.

Laboratories
- Anemia is rapidly ruled out with a complete blood count (CBC).
- Consider checking arterial blood gases (ABG) in all patients being evaluated for dyspnea. The ABG can provide a great deal of information. A patient can have a normal SaO_2, but an ABG may reveal a wide A–a gradient—an indication of lung pathology.

- A simple but useful approach to interpreting the blood gas is to consider a low PaO_2 to be the result of pulmonary parenchymal or airspace disease, right-to-left shunts, ventilation/perfusion mismatching, or a dramatic increase in oxygen consumption with respect to delivery.
- An elevated $PaCO_2$ is almost invariably the result of decreased alveolar ventilation or decreased exchange of gas between atmosphere and the alveolus. Most commonly, this is due to disease of the airways (COPD or asthma), but it may also be caused by chest wall disease or weakness of the respiratory muscles.
- Central causes of elevated PCO_2 include central nervous system lesions, obesity, hypoventilation, and hypothyroidism.
- With psychogenic causes, the ABG often reveals respiratory alkalosis with normal O_2 transfer.
- The A–a gradient is calculated as follows: A–a gradient = $PAO_2 - PaO_2$ where the $PA = [(760 - 47) \times FiO_2] - (PaCO_2/0.8)$.

- Consider where appropriate, but not in all patients: B-type natriuretic peptide (BNP),[7] troponin I (or troponin T), and D-dimer.
  - Maintain a high degree of suspicion for PE, or you will miss the diagnosis. A normal D-dimer can be useful to exclude a PE in patients with low pretest probability[8] but is less useful in older patients and patients who have been hospitalized for more than 3 days.[9]
  - Similarly, a BNP can exclude the diagnosis of heart failure but will not replace clinical and imaging correlation if elevated.[10,11]

Electrocardiography
An electrocardiogram should be obtained.[11]

Imaging
- A chest radiograph should be obtained.[11] Most causes of acute onset dyspnea are apparent after evaluating with a CXR and ECG.
- Bedside lung ultrasound, when available, can improve diagnostic accuracy in the evaluation of acute onset dyspnea.[12] This requires some degree of specialized training, however.
- Where appropriate, consider additional imaging studies including:
  - If PE is highly suspected, additional imaging including venous Doppler, ventilation–perfusion scanning, or computed tomography scan of the chest may be necessary.[3]
  - Pulmonary function testing with diffusing capacity for CO of the lung.
  - If heart failure is the suspected etiology, then echocardiography may be beneficial.

Diagnostic Procedures
Additional testing may be necessary to confirm a suspected diagnosis. Further diagnostic procedures to evaluate dyspnea can include the following: pulmonary function testing with diffusing capacity for CO (DLCO) of the lung and exercise cardiopulmonary testing and ABGs may reveal abnormalities that are not apparent at rest, particularly in patients with chronic dyspnea.[1]

TREATMENT

Treatment should focus on identifying and treating the underlying cause. Further details regarding management of specific conditions are discussed in other chapters. Psychogenic dyspnea can be controlled acutely with benzodiazepines such as lorazepam, though caution should be exercised especially in patients with concomitant pulmonary disease, due to the risk of respiratory depression and hypercapnia. Haloperidol may also be considered for its anxiolytic effect (which will not cause respiratory depression) in patients in the hospital who are delirious or psychotic.[2]

REFERENCES

1. Parshall MB, Schwartzstein RM, Adams L, et al.; American Thoracic Society Committee on Dyspnea. An official American Thoracic Society statement: update on the mechanisms, assessment, and management of dyspnea. *Am J Respir Crit Care Med* 2012;185:435–52.
2. Smoller JW, Pollack MH, Otto MW, et al. Panic anxiety, dyspnea, and respiratory disease. Theoretical and clinical consideration. *Am J Respir Crit Care Med* 1996;154:6–17.
3. Fedullo PF, Tapson VF. Clinical practice. The evaluation of suspected pulmonary embolism. *N Engl J Med* 2003;349:1247–56.
4. Metlay JP, Kapoor WN, Fine MJ. Does this patient have community-acquired pneumonia? Diagnosing pneumonia by history and physical examination. *JAMA* 1997;278:1440–5.
5. Badgett RG, Lucey CR, Mulrow CD. Can the clinical examination diagnose left-sided heart failure in adults? *JAMA* 1997;277:1712–9.
6. Panju AA, Hemmelgarn BR, Guyatt GH, Simel DL. The rational clinical examination. Is this patient having a myocardial infarction? *JAMA* 1998;280:1256–63.
7. Mueller C, Scholer A, Laule-Kilian K, et al. Use of B-type natriuretic peptide in the evaluation and management of acute dyspnea. *N Engl J Med* 2004;350:647–54.
8. Stein PD, Hull RD, Patel KC, et al. D-dimer for the exclusion of acute venous thrombosis and pulmonary embolism: a systematic review. *Ann Intern Med* 2004;140:589–602.
9. Brotman DJ, Segal JB, Jani JT, et al. Limitations of D-dimer testing in unselected inpatients with suspected venous thromboembolism. *Am J Med* 2003;114:276–82.
10. Roberts E, Ludman AJ, Dworzynski K, et al.; NICE Guideline Development Group for Acute Heart Failure. The diagnostic accuracy of the natriuretic peptides in heart failure: systematic review and diagnostic meta-analysis in the acute care setting. *BMJ* 2015;350:h910.
11. Wang CS, FitzGerald JM, Schulzer M, et al. Does this dyspneic patient in the emergency department have congestive heart failure? *JAMA* 2005;294:1944–56.
12. Filopei J, Siedenburg H, Rattner P, et al. Impact of pocket ultrasound use by internal medicine housestaff in the diagnosis of dyspnea. *J Hosp Med* 2014;9:594–7.

Chronic Obstructive Lung Disease

10

Maanasi Samant and Thomas M. Ciesielski

GENERAL PRINCIPLES

- Chronic obstructive pulmonary disease (COPD) is commonly encountered in the general inpatient setting. A systematic approach is particularly useful in evaluating those suffering from this condition. COPD is a preventable and treatable disease.[1]
- COPD is the fourth leading cause of death in the United States, behind heart disease, cancer, and cerebrovascular accidents. The burden and prevalence of COPD is expected to increase.[2]
- The economic burden of COPD is also concerning; in the United States, the estimated direct costs of the disease are $29.5 billion. COPD exacerbations account for the majority of this figure.[1]

Definition

The pulmonary component of COPD is characterized by **airflow limitation that is not fully reversible**. Significant extrapulmonary effects may be present.

Classification

- Historically, COPD has been classified as **chronic bronchitis** and/or **emphysema**.[1]
- Chronic bronchitis and emphysema are descriptive terms and may not reflect the severity of airflow limitation.[1]
- Chronic bronchitis is defined as cough productive of at least two tablespoons of sputum on most days of 3 consecutive months in 2 consecutive years.[1]
- Emphysema is defined pathologically as nonuniform enlargement of the distal airspaces with destruction of the acini, loss of lung elasticity, and absence of any fibrotic changes.[3]
- The forced expiratory volume in 1 second (FEV_1) is more reflective of the degree of airflow limitation and is used in conjunction with the patient's symptoms and physical findings to gauge the severity of disease (Table 10-1).[3]

Etiology

The airflow limitation is usually progressive and associated with an abnormal inflammatory response to noxious particles or gases. The disease is polygenic with deficiency of α_1-antitrypsin being a well-documented genetic risk factor.[4]

Pathophysiology

- Inflammation leading to repeated injury and repair leads to many structural changes throughout the lung parenchyma and airways. Airway remodeling and loss of alveolar attachments result in decreased elastic recoil.[3] These changes lead to the following:
  - Airflow limitation
  - Hypersecretion of mucus
  - Air trapping
  - Abnormal gas exchange
  - Cor pulmonale (right heart failure)[1]

TABLE 10-1 CLASSIFICATION OF COPD BASED ON POSTBRONCHODILATOR FEV_1

Severity	FEV_1/FVC	FEV_1 (% Predicted)	Symptoms
Stage I: Mild	<70	≥80	Chronic cough and sputum production may be present, but not always.
Stage II: Moderate	<70	79–50	Dyspnea on exertion, cough, and sputum production sometimes present
Stage III: Severe	<70	30–49	Increasing dyspnea, reduced exercise capacity, fatigue, and repeated exacerbations
Stage IV: Very severe	<70	<30 or <50 plus chronic respiratory failure	Respiratory failure defined as PaO_2 <60 mm Hg with or without $PaCO_2$ >50 mm Hg; respiratory failure may lead to cor pulmonale; quality of life very impaired; and exacerbations may be life threatening.

COPD, chronic obstructive pulmonary disease; FEV_1, forced expiratory volume in 1 second.
Adapted from Rabe KF, Hurd S, Anzueto A, et al. Global strategy for the diagnosis, management, and prevention of chronic obstructive pulmonary disease: GOLD executive summary. *Am J Respir Crit Care Med* 2007;176:532-55.

- **Acute exacerbations** of COPD may be related to multiple factors including the following:
  ○ Viral infections (more common)
  ○ Bacterial infections (less common)
  ○ Poor air quality (fine particulates, NO_2, SO_2, ozone)
  ○ Nonadherence to medical therapy[3]

Risk Factors

- **Cigarette smoking** is the most common risk factor for the development of COPD.[4]
- Only a minority of smokers (about 15%) develop clinically significant COPD.[1]
- Other risk factors include hereditary deficiency of α_1-antitrypsin, inhalation exposure to occupational dusts and chemicals, as well as exposure to indoor pollution from the burning of biomass fuels in confined spaces.[3]

DIAGNOSIS

Clinical Presentation

History

COPD should be considered in those with known exposure to risk factors. There is considerable variability in the clinical course of individual patients with COPD. In most patients, the course is usually progressive, especially if exposure to noxious insults has not ceased. Hallmark clinical symptoms consist of the following:

- Chronic cough: Cough is usually the initial symptom, occurring in the fifth decade of life.
- Dyspnea that is gradually progressive over time. Dyspnea on exertion (DOE) generally presents in the sixth to seventh decades of life.

- Sputum production[3]
- When COPD becomes severe, weight loss may occur, though malignancy needs to be excluded.
- Obstructive lung disease in the absence of a significant smoking history should bring other pathologies into consideration.
- An **acute exacerbation of COPD** may be indicated by increased dyspnea, increased cough, and increased sputum production and/or sputum purulence.[2] The severest exacerbations are characterized by the presence of all three and mild exacerbations by only one.

Physical Examination
- Acute exacerbation
  - Vitals signs are essential. Admit to an intensive care unit (ICU) those with unstable vital signs and those who require assisted ventilation.
  - Altered mental status may be a result of hypercarbia or hypoxemia.
  - Fever may be suggestive of an infection.
  - Inspection of the respiratory status (pursed-lip breathing, prolonged expiration, accessory muscle use, nasal flaring, paradoxical abdominal movements, cyanosis) is helpful in identifying those in distress.
  - Pulmonary auscultation may reveal prolonged expiration, expiratory wheezes, rales, or bronchial breath sounds. In severe exacerbations, breath sounds may be barely audible.
- Chronic findings of COPD should be evaluated.
  - Signs of cor pulmonale may be present (right ventricular heave, jugular venous distention, and lower extremity edema).
  - Cachexia may be present, but malignancy and other causes of weight loss should be ruled out.[1]
  - Clubbing is generally not a feature of COPD; its presence should prompt an evaluation for etiologies such as lung cancer.

Differential Diagnosis

Other diagnoses should be considered in evaluating those suspected of suffering from COPD, as signs and symptoms may overlap significantly with other diseases, such as:

- Asthma
- Congestive heart failure (CHF)
- Bronchiectasis
- Obliterative bronchiolitis
- Diffuse panbronchiolitis
- Tuberculosis

Diagnostic Testing

The diagnosis of COPD should be supported by spirometry in those with the signs and symptoms suggestive of the disease. Spirometry is the "gold standard" for measuring airflow limitation.[1]

Laboratories
- Arterial blood gases (ABGs) must be checked in order to assess the PaO_2 and $PaCO_2$. Pulse oximetry provides no information about $PaCO_2$. Reliance solely on pulse oximetry during an acute exacerbation can result in life-threatening hypercarbia.[1]
- A complete blood count (CBC) may reveal polycythemia if chronic hypoxemia is present.[1]
- Blood chemistries may indicate an increased concentration of bicarbonate if chronic hypercapnea is present.
- An ECG may show signs of cor pulmonale, myocardial ischemia, or an arrhythmia.[3]

Imaging
- CXR may show signs of hyperinflation/air trapping: flattened diaphragms; bullae; increased retrosternal clear space; long, narrow heart shadow; and hyperlucency. These findings have a limited sensitivity for a diagnosis of COPD.[1]
- Pulmonary edema, pneumonia, and pneumothorax can cause increased dyspnea and should be evaluated and treated appropriately if present.[1]

Diagnostic Procedures
- Spirometry is the primary method for diagnosing COPD, but its use is of limited value during acute exacerbations in patients with known COPD.[2]
- A postbronchodilator FEV_1/forced vital capacity (FVC) of <0.70 confirms the presence of airflow limitation. The FEV_1 defines the severity of expiratory airflow obstruction and is an important predictor of prognosis and mortality (Table 10-1).[3]
- Total lung capacity (TLC), residual volume (RV), and functional residual capacity (FRC) are typically elevated and are indicative of hyperinflation.[1]

TREATMENT

The global initiative for chronic obstructive lung disease (GOLD) was formed in 1998 to bring more attention to the prevention and management of COPD. The first consensus report in 2001 created a staging system of severity that has been used to assist in management of COPD.

Treatment of Stable COPD
- After diagnosis of COPD, treatment should aim to relieve symptoms and prevent exacerbations. The GOLD report suggests a treatment approach that is based on the GOLD stage classification of severity of COPD (Table 10-1) along with exacerbations, hospitalizations, and other symptom scores, including the Modified British Medical Research Council (mMRC) Questionnaire, which primarily rates breathlessness and the COPD assessment test (CAT) and looks at health status impairment with COPD.[1] The following treatment approach takes into account these factors[1]:
    - Low-risk patients with low symptom scores (GOLD stage I or II with few if any exacerbations or other limitations): PRN short-acting anticholinergic or short-acting β_2-adrenergic agonists (SABA)
    - Low-risk patients with more symptoms (GOLD stage I or II with more exacerbations but not hospitalizations, some symptoms/limitations): long-acting anticholinergic and/or long-acting β_2-adrenergic agonists (LABA)
    - High-risk patients with low symptom scores (GOLD stage III or IV, exacerbations with hospitalizations, symptoms/limitations): inhaled corticosteroid (ICS) + long-acting anticholinergic or LABA
    - High-risk patients with more symptoms (GOLD stage III or IV, exacerbations with hospitalizations, significant symptoms/limitations): ICS + long-acting anticholinergic and/or LABA
- **Supplemental oxygen** therapy has been shown to decrease mortality and improve physical and mental functioning in hypoxemic patients with COPD. Long-term oxygen therapy should be prescribed for those who qualify and are willing to comply with its use. Oxygen therapy is indicated for the following:
    - Oxygen needs should be reassessed at least yearly and adjustments made as warranted.
    - Any patient with a $PaO_2 \leq 55$ mm Hg or $SaO_2 \leq 88\%$.[4]
    - Patients with evidence of pulmonary hypertension, polycythemia (hematocrit > 55%), or heart failure and $PaO_2 \leq 59$ mm Hg or $SaO_2 \leq 89\%$.

- **Smoking cessation** should be encouraged, with referral to a counselor if available. Discuss and prescribe smoking cessation aids (nicotine replacement therapy, bupropion, or varenicline) if needed.[1]
- **Phosphodiesterase 4 inhibitor (roflumilast)** can be offered to patients with severe COPD who are at risk for severe exacerbations despite treatment with ICS, LABA, and tiotropium.[5]
- **Azithromycin** can be considered in patients at increased risk of exacerbation (on continuous supplemental oxygen or with one exacerbation in the past year). However, baseline cardiovascular risk must be considered before starting treatment.[6]
- **Pulmonary rehabilitation** improves quality of life and exercise tolerance and should be offered.[4]
- **Influenza and pneumococcal vaccines** should be kept current.[4]
- Adherence with therapies along with correct usage (particularly inhaled therapies) should be reviewed.[1]

Treatment of Acute Exacerbations of COPD

If patients are presenting with increased cough, sputum production, and worsening dyspnea and there is concern for acute exacerbation, the following therapies are available:

- **Supplemental oxygen** is frequently needed and should be provided in order to achieve a $PaO_2 > 60$ mm Hg or $SaO_2 > 90\%$. Hypercarbia may result from overzealous oxygen administration; an ABG should be obtained if this is suspected, with subsequent adjustments in FiO_2 as indicated.[2]
- **Bronchodilators** administered via nebulizer or metered-dose inhalers are the mainstay of therapy. Inhaled $β_2$-adrenergic agonists and anticholinergics are the bronchodilators of choice. Both are similarly effective for acute exacerbations. Combined therapy may also be used.[2]
- **Systemic steroids** are indicated to shorten recovery time, improve lung function, and reduce the risk of relapse.[1]
  - The REDUCE trial demonstrated that a 5-day course of 40 mg of prednisone was noninferior with respect to re-exacerbations to a 14-day course of prednisone.[7] Thus, the GOLD committee recommends a 5-day course of 40 mg of prednisone.[1]
  - Inhaled corticosteroids do not have a role in treating exacerbations.
- **Antibiotics** are indicated in those patients who suffer from pneumonia, severe exacerbations (requiring assisted ventilation), or moderate exacerbations with increased sputum purulence as one of the presenting symptoms.
  - The course of mild exacerbations is unlikely to be altered by antibiotic therapy.[8]
  - Antibiotics should be chosen based on local resistance patterns.[1]
  - Pneumonia should be treated following the appropriate guidelines.[1]
  - The most common bacterial pathogens are *Streptococcus pneumoniae*, *Haemophilus influenzae*, and *Moraxella catarrhalis*.[9] Patients with more severe exacerbation have a higher incidence of infection with gram-negative bacilli including *Pseudomonas aeruginosa*.[1]
  - For moderate to severe exacerbations, recommended antibiotics include a macrolide, amoxicillin/clavulanate, a second- or third-generation cephalosporin, or quinolones with enhanced activity against penicillin-resistant *S. pneumoniae*.[1]
  - Patients requiring mechanical ventilation should receive antibiotic therapy that also covers *P. aeruginosa*.[1]
  - Duration of antibiotics therapy is typically 5–10 days depending on the specific clinical scenario and the agent used.[1]
- **Noninvasive ventilation** (NIV) has been shown to decrease length of hospital stay, endotracheal intubation rates, and mortality.[10]

- Indications for NIV include respirations > 25 breaths per minute, pH < 7.35, and/or $PaCO_2$ > 45 mm Hg and moderate to severe dyspnea with signs of distress.[1]
- Contraindications to NIV include craniofacial trauma, cardiovascular instability, respiratory arrest, uncooperative patient, high aspiration risk, and extreme obesity.[2]
- **Mechanical ventilation** is indicated when there is a contraindication to NIV or failure to respond to NIV. Risks of mechanical ventilation include ventilator-associated pneumonia, barotrauma, and failure to wean.[1]
- **Smoking cessation** should be encouraged.[2]
- **Methylxanthines** (e.g., aminophylline and theophylline) are not indicated in acute exacerbations owing to the significant risk for side effects.[2]

OUTCOME/PROGNOSIS

- The BODE index may be useful in assessing the risk of death. The BODE index consists of the following[11]:
  - **B**ody-mass index (BMI)
  - airway **O**bstruction (FEV_1)
  - **D**yspnea (as measured by the Medical Research Council dyspnea score)
  - **E**xercise capacity (6-minute-walk distance)
- BODE index scores can range from 0 to 10. For each quartile increase in the BODE score, there was a statistically significant increase in the associated mortality rate. At the highest quartile (BODE score 7–10), there was a mortality rate of 80% at 52 months. For the lowest quartile (BODE score 0–2), the rate was ~ 20% at 52 months. While the study does have limitations, the BODE index appears to be a better predictor than the FEV_1 alone of the risk of death due to any cause and also respiratory causes.[11]

REFERENCES

1. Global Initiative for Chronic Obstructive Lung Disease (GOLD). *Global Strategy for the Diagnosis, Management and Prevention of COPD, Updated 2015.* Available at: http://www.goldcopd.org/uploads/users/files/GOLD_Report_2015_Apr2.pdf (last accessed 1/30/16).
2. Stoller JK. Clinical practice. Acute exacerbations of chronic obstructive pulmonary disease. *N Engl J Med* 2002;346:988–94.
3. Rabe KF, Hurd S, Anzueto A, et al. Global strategy for the diagnosis, management, and prevention of chronic obstructive pulmonary disease: GOLD executive summary. *Am J Respir Crit Care Med* 2007;176:532–55.
4. Sutherland ER, Cherniack RM. Management of chronic obstructive pulmonary disease. *N Engl J Med* 2004;350:2689–97.
5. Martinez FJ, Calverley PM, Goehring UM, et al. Effect of roflumilast on exacerbations in patients with severe chronic obstructive pulmonary disease uncontrolled by combination therapy (REACT): a multicentre randomised controlled trial. *Lancet* 2015;385:857–66.
6. Albert RK, Connett J, Bailey WC, et al. Azithromycin for prevention of exacerbations of COPD. *N Engl J Med* 2011;365:689–98.
7. Leuppi JD, Schuetz P, Bingisser R, et al. Short-term vs conventional glucocorticoid therapy in acute exacerbations of chronic obstructive pulmonary disease: the REDUCE randomized clinical trial. *JAMA* 2013;309:2223–31.
8. Anthonisen NR, Manfreda J, Warren CP, et al. Antibiotic therapy in exacerbations of chronic obstructive pulmonary disease. *Ann Intern Med* 1987;106:196–204.
9. Sethi S, Evans N, Grant BJ, Murphy TF. New strains of bacteria and exacerbations of chronic obstructive pulmonary disease. *N Engl J Med* 2002;347:465–71.
10. Caples SM, Gay PC. Noninvasive positive pressure ventilation in the intensive care unit: a concise review. *Crit Care Med* 2005;33:2651–8.
11. Celli BR, Cote CG, Marin JM, et al. The body-mass index, airflow obstruction, dyspnea, and exercise capacity index in chronic obstructive pulmonary disease. *N Engl J Med* 2004;350:1005–12.

Asthma

Jaimie E. Bolda and Walter B. Gribben

GENERAL PRINCIPLES

Worldwide, ~300 million people suffer from asthma; the highest prevalence is in developed countries. About 11% of the US population has asthma. Prevalence, hospitalization rates, morbidity, and mortality attributable to asthma have all increased significantly over the last few decades. Factors conjectured to be causative for the increased prevalence include exposure to tobacco smoke and air pollution, dietary influences, obesity, and lack of exposure to infections and microbial products early in life. Hospital admission rates are higher in nonwhites. In the United States, there are approximately 5000 deaths due to asthma per year. Many of these deaths are likely preventable. Death rates are higher among African Americans, Hispanics, those with lower levels of education, inhabitants of large cities, and the poor. The economic burden of asthma is enormous.[1]

Definition

- The National Asthma Education and Prevention Program (NAEPP) Expert Panel Report 3 (EPR3) defines asthma as "a common chronic disorder of the airways that is complex and characterized by variable and recurring symptoms, airflow obstruction, bronchial hyperresponsiveness, and an underlying inflammation."[2]
- The more descriptive definition from the prior NAEPP EPR2 (1997) still remains entirely valid. "Asthma is a chronic inflammatory disorder of the airways in which many cells and cellular elements play a role. In particular, mast cells, eosinophils, T lymphocytes, macrophages, neutrophils, and epithelial cells. In susceptible individuals, this inflammation causes recurrent episodes of wheezing, breathlessness, chest tightness, and coughing, particularly at night or in the early morning. These episodes are usually associated with widespread but variable airflow obstruction that is often reversible either spontaneously or with treatment. The inflammation also causes an associated increase in the existing bronchial hyperresponsiveness to a variety of stimuli. Reversibility of airflow limitation may be incomplete in some patients with asthma."[3]

Classification

The **classification of the severity of asthma** in adults who are not currently taking long-term control medications is presented in Table 11-1. Specific forms of asthma include four types:

- **Cough-variant asthma**, where coughing is the predominant or sole symptom; the diagnosis is confirmed by resolution of the cough with antiasthmatic treatment.[4,5]
- **Exercise-induced bronchoconstriction (EIB) or asthma** describes patients with bronchoconstriction primarily or solely in association with exercise (generally after exercise). Such patients should derive benefit from pretreatment with a β2-agonist. About 10% of the general population has EIB. However, it is important to note that EIB occurs in up to 90% of all asthmatics and is, therefore, a strong trigger for symptoms.[6]
- **Occupational asthma** consists of bronchoconstriction, bronchial hyperresponsiveness, and airway inflammation caused by exposure to workplace asthmagens. Triggers may be immunogenic or nonimmunogenic. In the latter situation, the condition may be

TABLE 11-1 CLASSIFICATION OF ASTHMA SEVERITY IN ADULTS

	Mild Intermittent	Mild Persistent	Moderate Persistent	Severe Persistent
Symptoms	≤2 days per week	>2 days per week but not daily	Daily	Throughout the day
Nighttime awakenings	<2 per month	3–4 per month	More than once a week but not nightly	Often seven times a week
Short-acting β_2-agonist use for symptom control	≤2 days per week	>2 days per week but not more than once a day	Daily	Several times a day
Interference with normal activity	None	Minor limitation	Some limitation	Extremely limited
Lung function	Normal FEV_1 between exacerbations $FEV_1 > 80\%$ predicted FEV_1/FVC normal	$FEV_1 > 80\%$ predicted FEV_1/FVC normal	$FEV_1 > 60\%$ but $<80\%$ predicted FEV_1/FVC reduced 5%	$FEV_1 < 60\%$ predicted FEV_1/FVC reduced >5%
Recommended step at which to initiate treatment	Step 1	Step 2	Step 3	Step 4 or 5

Adapted from National Asthma Education and Prevention Program Expert Panel. *Report 3 (EPR3): Guidelines for the Diagnosis and Management of Asthma. Full Report 2007.* National Institutes of Health. Publication No. 08-4051. Bethesda: National Heart, Lung, and Blood Institute, 2007.

referred to as **reactive airways dysfunction syndrome (RADS)** or **irritant-induced asthma**. There are hundreds of known stimulants and occupations at risk. Preexisting asthma worsened by the patient's occupation without clear substantiation for a diagnosis of independent occupational asthma is sometimes called **work-aggravated asthma**.[7]

- **Nocturnal asthma** is the nighttime worsening of asthma symptoms and is relatively common among asthmatics. Its occurrence is associated with inadequate control and increased morbidity. It is unclear if nocturnal asthma is a clinically distinct diagnosis or merely a marker for uncontrolled or more severe asthma.[8]

Pathophysiology

Airflow limitation is caused by multiple factors in the airways, including the following:

- Bronchoconstriction (bronchial smooth muscle contraction)
- Airway edema

- Excessive secretion of mucus and plugging
- Airway hyperresponsiveness (excessive bronchoconstrictor response to stimuli)
- Airway remodeling (subepithelial fibrosis, thickening of the subbasement membrane, smooth muscle hypertrophy/hyperplasia, blood vessel proliferation/dilation, and mucous gland hyperplasia)
- **Airway inflammation** appears to be a crucial underlying aspect of asthma pathophysiology.
  - Multiple **inflammatory cells** participate: eosinophils, mast cells, lymphocytes (particularly Th2 cells), neutrophils, dendritic cells (important antigen-presenting cells), macrophages, smooth muscle cells, and epithelial cells.
  - A wide array of **inflammatory mediators** contribute to the inflammatory response: chemokines (e.g., eotaxin), cytokines (e.g., the interleukins IL-1β, IL-4, IL-5, and IL-13; tumor necrosis factor α [TNF-α]; and granulocyte–macrophage colony-stimulating factor [GM-CSF]), leukotrienes, and nitric oxide.
  - **Immunoglobulin E** (IgE) is also important in the pathophysiology of asthma. High-affinity IgE receptors are found on mast cells, basophils, dendritic cells, and lymphocytes. When mast cells are activated, they release many mediators that cause bronchoconstriction and promote inflammation.
- The factors that render certain individuals susceptible and those that initiate and perpetuate the inflammatory process are not precisely known. It does appear, however, that the interactions of environmental exposures at crucial times during immune development and host characteristics are particularly important. There are clearly aspects of asthma that are inheritable, and multiple genes have been associated with asthma. Obviously, though, asthma is not a single gene-related disease. Airborne allergens (e.g., dust mites and cockroaches) and viral infections are also thought to play key roles in the pathogenesis of asthma, especially when exposure occurs at vulnerable times in immunologic development. Precise mechanisms are not known, and some data are conflicting.[2,9]

Risk Factors

Risks for the development of asthma include the following factors:

- In childhood, male sex; in adulthood, female sex
- Family history (i.e., genetic susceptibility)
- Airway hyperreactivity
- Atopy and allergies
- Obesity
- Environmental exposures (i.e., allergens, pollution, cigarette smoking and exposure to secondhand smoke, infections, occupational exposures)[2]

DIAGNOSIS

Clinical Presentation

History

- The quintessential symptoms of asthma are wheezing, chest tightness, breathlessness, and coughing.
- In determining the severity of asthma, pertinent history includes the frequency of symptoms and use of a rescue metered-dose inhaler (MDI), presence of nocturnal symptoms, peak expiratory flow rates (PEFs), and degree to which everyday activities are limited (see Table 11-1).
- The patient should also be questioned regarding how well rescue MDIs work and how well controlled his or her asthma has been, if at all. Other factors include a history of frequent emergency department (ED) visits, prior admissions to an intensive care unit (ICU) and/or prior mechanical ventilation, recent oral corticosteroid therapy, and history of psychosocial problems, including medical noncompliance.

- It is important to identify aggravating factors or "triggers" for asthma. A careful allergy history should be obtained, including the presence of atopy, pets, active or passive smoke inhalation, and home/work/school environments. Be aware of the common allergens in your geographic area during each season.[2,10]

Physical Examination

The physical examination should focus on the patient's vital signs, general appearance, and pulmonary system. Between exacerbations, the exam may be completely normal.

- Check vital signs, which may reveal tachypnea and tachycardia (often from high doses of β2-agonist). A decreasing respiratory rate may indicate respiratory muscle fatigue rather than improvement in airway obstruction.
- Watch for decreasing mental status, which may represent hypercarbia or hypoxia.
- Examine the head, ears, eyes, nose, and throat to assess for signs of chronic allergic disease, including conjunctivitis, nasal polyps, rhinorrhea, and sinus tenderness.
- Observe for signs of respiratory fatigue or failure. These include inability to speak (words, phrases, sentences), inability to lie down, accessory muscle use, paradoxical abdominal movements, and pulsus paradoxus.
- Auscultate for inspiratory/expiratory wheezing, prolonged expiratory phase, and diminished general air movement. In patients with audible inspiratory/expiratory wheezes over the upper airways or neck, rule out other causes of airway obstruction, including vocal cord dysfunction, foreign bodies, and upper airway tumors.
- Beware of the patient with no wheezing and poor air movement, as these findings may signify severe asthma and respiratory failure.
- Assess for signs of chronic corticosteroid use such as thin skin, easy bruising, cushingoid facies, central obesity, and proximal muscle weakness.

Differential Diagnosis

The differential diagnosis of asthma could potentially include all differential items for dyspnea, cough, wheezing, and chest tightness. A more limited differential diagnosis is presented in Table 11-2.

Diagnostic Testing

Diagnostic Procedures

- In stable patients, the diagnosis and severity of asthma are confirmed by **pulmonary function tests** (PFTs). In general, there is evidence of obstructive lung disease with a reduced forced expiratory volume in 1 second (FEV_1) and FEV_1/forced vital capacity (FVC) ratio. In addition, a postbronchodilator improvement in FEV_1 by at least 12% and 200 mL should be seen, indicative of reversible airway disease. Lung volumes will often show increased residual volume and a normal diffusion capacity of CO. The latter differentiates asthma from chronic obstructive pulmonary disease (COPD). Some asthmatics will have normal PFTs between attacks. During acute exacerbations, PEF should be routinely checked before and 15–20 minutes after administration of bronchodilators to assess the efficacy of therapy.[2,11]
- **Bronchial challenge testing** can be used to identify patients with abnormal airway hyperresponsiveness. Pharmacologic testing using methacholine has varying sensitivity and specificity based on the state of symptoms at the time of testing. In general, a positive test is indicated by a reduction in the FEV_1 of 20% or by a reduced specific airway conductance of 35–45% from baseline. This test simply indicates airway hyperresponsiveness, but does not give information about the etiology (i.e., COPD, cystic fibrosis, etc.). Many asthmatics have exercise-induced airway changes, even in the absence of exercise-induced symptoms. PFTs obtained before and after treadmill testing may therefore reveal the variability in FEV_1.[2,12]

TABLE 11-2 DIFFERENTIAL DIAGNOSIS OF ASTHMA IN ADULTS

Laryngopharyngeal Causes

Upper airway cough syndrome (UACS, previously known as postnasal drip syndrome)

Postinfectious cough

Gastroesophageal reflux disease (GERD)

Laryngopharyngeal reflux (LPRD)

Tonsillar hypertrophy

Peritonsillar abscess or mass

Retropharyngeal abscess or mass

Vocal cord dysfunction syndrome

Laryngocele

Vocal cord paralysis

Cricoarytenoid arthritis (e.g., rheumatoid arthritis)

Epiglottitis

Laryngostenosis

Large Airway[a] Causes

Foreign bodies

Tumors (malignant and benign and intrinsic and extrinsic)

Tracheal stenosis

Tracheomalacia

Tracheobronchitis (e.g., herpetic)

Goiter

Acute bronchitis

Postinfectious cough

Small Airway[a]/Parenchymal Causes

Postinfectious cough

Acute bronchitis

Chronic bronchitis without COPD

Chronic obstructive pulmonary disease (COPD)

Congestive heart failure (CHF)

Pulmonary embolism (PE)

Bronchiectasis

Bronchiolitis

Nonasthmatic eosinophilic bronchitis (NAEB)

Pulmonary infiltration with eosinophilia (PIE)

Respiratory bronchiolitis–interstitial pneumonia (RB-ILD)

Interstitial lung disease (ILD)

Chronic fungal and mycoplasmal infections

Other Causes

Drug-induced cough (e.g., secondary to angiotensin-converting enzyme inhibitors)

Carcinoid syndrome

"Ear cough" (Arnold reflex)

Deconditioning

Psychogenic

[a]The distinction between large and small and upper and lower airways is not always precise.

- **Allergy testing**: Skin allergy testing can be considered for patients with persistent asthma and those who are exposed to indoor allergens.

Laboratories
- **For acute asthma exacerbations**, measurement of **arterial blood gases** (ABGs) is not routinely indicated in every acute exacerbation.
  - However, ABGs should be strongly considered in patients who fail to respond to initial therapy with persistently diminished PEF and/or $FEV_1 \leq 25\%$ of predicted and those in severe respiratory distress or suspected of hypoventilation.
  - During the course of an exacerbation, tachypnea usually results in a below-normal $PaCO_2$. The presence of normal or increased $PaCO_2$ may indicate impending respiratory failure.[13]
- **For chronic asthma, in vitro allergy testing** can be considered for patients with persistent asthma and those who are exposed to indoor allergens.

Imaging
Chest radiography is not routinely needed but should be obtained if there is a suspicion of conditions such as congestive heart failure, pneumonia, pneumothorax, or pneumomediastinum.[2]

TREATMENT

The NAEPP EPR3 provides detailed treatment guidelines for asthma exacerbations and the chronic management of asthma.

Treatment of Acute Exacerbations of Asthma
- All patients should be taught to recognize the early warning signs of worsening asthma and have an **asthma action plan** for home management of asthma exacerbations. Patients should monitor their symptoms and PEFs. Exacerbations should be treated as early as possible. All patients should attempt to remove environmental factors that may be precipitating or contributing to the exacerbation.
- Patients with severe symptoms, those with PEF < 50% of predicted or personal best, and those at high risk for death should simultaneously initiate treatment with a short-acting β_2-agonist (SABA) and seek immediate medical attention. Risk factors for death from asthma include the following:
  - Prior severe exacerbations
  - Two or more asthma admissions in the previous year
  - Three or more ED visits for asthma in the previous year
  - Admission or ED visit for asthma in the previous month
  - Use of more than two MDIs of SABA a month
  - Low socioeconomic status
  - Inner-city dwelling
  - Illicit drug use
  - Major psychosocial issues, or major comorbidities (cardiovascular, pulmonary, and psychiatric)[2]
- **Mild and some moderate exacerbations** may be manageable at home per the patient's asthma action plan. A **moderate exacerbation** is indicated by FEV_1 and/or PEF 40–69% with moderate symptoms. Initial treatment should be SABA (e.g., albuterol MDI 4–8 puffs or 2.5–5 mg by nebulizer), up to two treatments 20 minutes apart.
  - If the symptomatic response is **good** and the PEF is ≥80%, the patient may continue SABA q3–4 hours for 24–48 hours. A short course of oral systemic corticosteroids can be considered. The patient should contact the physician for further instructions.

- If the response is **incomplete** (PEF still 50–79%, the patient still dyspneic and/or wheezing), SABA (e.g., albuterol MDI 4–8 puffs q20 minutes up to 4 hours or 2.5–5 mg by nebulizer q20 minutes for a total of three doses, then q1–4 hours) should be continued and oral systemic corticosteroids started (e.g., prednisone 40–60 mg daily for 5–10 days). The physician should be urgently contacted for instructions.
- If the response is **poor** (PEF < 50%, marked dyspnea and/or wheezing), SABA should be repeated, oral systemic corticosteroids started, and immediate medical attention sought.[2]
• **More significant moderate and all severe exacerbations** should be managed in the ED. A **severe exacerbation** is indicated by FEV_1 and/or PEF < 40%, severe symptoms at rest, accessory muscle use, high-risk patients (see above), and no improvement after initial treatment. Such patients should receive O_2, nebulized SABA, ipratropium every hour, and oral corticosteroids (if not already done). Adjunctive therapies such as magnesium sulfate (2 g IV) and heliox may be considered. If there is any evidence of impending or actual respiratory failure, the patient should be immediately intubated, mechanically ventilated, and admitted to the ICU. It is better to err on the side of caution in this context, as patients can deteriorate very rapidly. A rapid initial assessment should include a brief history and physical and an objective measurement of lung function (e.g., PEF and/or FEV_1) if possible. Pulse oximetry is indicated for patients in severe distress or those with a PEF and/or FEV_1 < 40%. Serial oximetry is superior to a one-time SaO_2 measurements.[2]
- SABA is recommended for all patients and supplemental O_2 for most patients (to maintain $SaO_2 \geq 90\%$, 95% in patients with coexisting cardiac disease or pregnancy). Repetitive doses of SABA may be given by MDI or nebulizer q20 minutes.[2] MDIs are preferred to nebulizers due to the relatively inefficient delivery system of the nebulizer device. MDIs with spacers require much lower doses of SABA to achieve a comparable improvement in lung function.[14,15]
- Inhaled ipratropium bromide may also be added (MDI 8 puffs q20 minutes up to 3 hours or 0.5 mg by nebulizer q20 minutes for three doses, then as needed). The evidence regarding ipratropium in asthma exacerbations is mixed. Use of anticholinergic therapy is typically reserved for the most severe exacerbations, and therapy is generally stopped upon hospital admission with a few exceptions (e.g., refractory asthma requiring ICU admission, patients on monoamine oxidase inhibitor therapy, and asthma that has been triggered by β-blocker therapy).[2]
- Systemic corticosteroids should be given (e.g., prednisone 40–80 mg daily or equivalent doses of IV methylprednisolone); however, the optimal dose is unknown. The effects of comparable doses of oral and intravenous glucocorticoids are nearly identical. Intravenous steroids should be given to patients with impending respiratory arrest or intolerance for oral agents; otherwise, oral steroids are just as effective. Severe exacerbations requiring hospitalization generally require 5–14 days of therapy. Tapering is not necessary if the duration of treatment is less than a week and probably not necessary for courses <10 days. ICS may be started at any time and are indicated for all hospitalized patients after discharge.[2]
- Intravenous magnesium sulfate can be used in severe exacerbations; however, routine use of this agent in mild to moderate exacerbations does not confer a significant benefit.[2,16–18] Its benefit in severe exacerbations is thought to be related to its inhibition of calcium influx leading to bronchodilation.[19] It is contraindicated in renal insufficiency.
- Other interventions such as methylxanthines, antibiotics, aggressive hydration, chest physiotherapy, mucolytics, and sedation are generally not recommended. Heliox may be considered in extremely severe exacerbations progressing toward intubation.[2,20]
- If mechanical ventilation is necessary, permissive hypercapnia is recommended.[2]
• A reassessment should be performed after initial treatment (after one dose of SABA with a severe exacerbation and after three doses in all patients), including an assessment of symptoms, a repeat physical exam, PEF and/or FEV_1, and SaO_2. The patient's response

to initial treatment, rather than his or her condition immediately on presentation, is more predictive of the subsequent need for hospitalization.
- A **good response** is indicated by FEV_1 and/or $PEF \geq 70\%$, no distress, a normal exam, and the response sustained for 60 minutes. Such patients may be discharged to home. A short course of oral corticosteroids should be continued (e.g., prednisone 40–80 mg daily for 5–10 days). Consideration should be given to initiating an inhaled corticosteroid (ICS).
- An **incomplete response** is indicated by FEV_1 and/or PEF 40–69% and continued mild to moderate symptoms. Determination of the disposition of these patients should be individualized. Those sent home can be treated as above; the others are admitted to the non-ICU hospital ward. There they should be treated with O_2, continued SABA, and systemic corticosteroids (oral or IV). Vital signs, SaO_2, and FEV_1/FVC should be monitored.
- A **poor response** is indicated by FEV_1 and/or $PEF < 40\%$, $PCO_2 \geq 42$ mm Hg, continued severe symptoms, and drowsiness/confusion. These patients should be admitted to the ICU and intubation/mechanical ventilation considered. They continue to receive SABA and systemic corticosteroids (oral or IV).[2]

Treatment of Chronic Asthma

NAEPP EPR3 and the Global Initiative for Asthma (GINA) recommend a stepwise approach to the management of chronic asthma, depending on asthma severity (Table 11-1). There are substantive differences between them, but on the whole, the approaches are similar. Importantly, both emphasize the importance of ICS as the mainstay of treatment for patients with persistent symptoms and the advice that all patients should have SABA available for quick relief. The recommendations presented here are somewhat more reflective of the EPR3. The recommended therapies by step are shown below.

- **Step 1**: SABA PRN. Appropriate only for intermittent asthma.
- **Step 2**: Low-dose ICS (Table 11-3). Less preferred alternatives include mast cell stabilizers (e.g., cromolyn or nedocromil), leukotriene modifiers (LMs) (e.g., montelukast or zileuton), and theophylline.
- **Step 3**: Low-dose ICS + long-acting β_2-agonist (LABA) or medium-dose ICS. Less preferred alternatives include low-dose ICS + either LM or theophylline.
- **Step 4**: Medium-dose ICS + LABA. Less preferred alternatives include medium-dose ICS + either LM or theophylline.
- **Step 5**: High-dose ICS + LABA. The anti-IgE agent omalizumab may be considered for those with allergies.
- **Step 6**: High-dose ICS + LABA + oral corticosteroid (lowest possible dose). The anti-IgE agent omalizumab may be considered for those with allergies.[2,10]
- Therapy should "step up" to achieve control. Once control has been achieved for at least 3 months, an attempt can be made to "step down."
- It is always valuable to remember the importance of adherence to therapy, inhaler technique, and control/elimination of environmental triggers.
- Consultation with an asthma specialist should be considered for patients requiring step 4 or higher treatment to achieve/maintain adequate control.
- The use of LABAs (e.g., salmeterol and formoterol) should be considered carefully owing to an increased risk of adverse outcomes.[21]
- The addition of desensitization immunotherapy should be considered for those with allergic asthma as an adjunct to step 2–4 therapy. Desensitization and omalizumab should be administered only by clinicians with specific knowledge who are equipped to treat anaphylaxis.[22–24]
- All patients should have an asthma action plan (see above) to deal with exacerbations and have SABA readily available for this purpose.

TABLE 11-3 INHALED CORTICOSTEROID DOSING

Drug	Low Dose (mcg/d)	Medium Dose (mcg/d)	High Dose (mcg/d)
Triamcinolone MDI (75 mcg/puff)	300–750	>750–1500	>1500
Beclomethasone HFA (40, 80 mcg/puff)	80–240	>240–480	>480
Budesonide DPI (90, 180 mcg/inhalation)	180–600	>600–1200	>1200
Flunisolide MDI (250 mcg/puff)	500–1000	>1000–2000	>2000
Flunisolide HFA (80 mcg/puff)	320	>320–640	>640
Fluticasone HFA (44, 110, 220 mcg/puff)	88–264	>264–440	>440
Fluticasone DPI (50 mcg/inhalation)	100–300	>300–500	>500
Mometasone DPI (220 mcg/dose)	220	440	>440
Budesonide/formoterol HFA (80/4.5, 160/4.5 mcg/puff)	160/9–320/18	320/18–640/18	640/18
Fluticasone/salmeterol HFA (45/21, 115/21, 230/21 mcg/puff)	90/42–180/84	180/84–460/84	460/84–920/84
Fluticasone/salmeterol DPI (100/50, 250/50, 500/50 mcg/inhalation)	200/100	500/100	1000/100

MDI, metered-dose inhaler; HFA, hydrofluoroalkane; DPI, dry powder inhaler.

Adapted from National Asthma Education and Prevention Program Expert Panel. *Report 3 (EPR3): Guidelines for the Diagnosis and Management of Asthma. Full Report 2007. National Institutes of Health. Publication No. 08-4051*. Bethesda: National Heart, Lung, and Blood Institute, 2007.

REFERENCES

1. Braman SS. The global burden of asthma. *Chest* 2006;130:S4–S12.
2. National Asthma Education and Prevention Program Expert Panel. *Report 3 (EPR3): Guidelines for the Diagnosis and Management of Asthma. Full Report 2007. NIH Publication No. 08-4051*. Bethesda: National Institutes of Health, National Heart, Lung, and Blood Institute, 2007.
3. National Asthma Education and Prevention Program Expert Panel. *Report 2 (EPR2): Guidelines for the Diagnosis and Management of Asthma. Full Report 1997. NIH Publication No. 97-4051*. Bethesda: U.S. Department of Health and Human Services; National Institutes of Health; National Heart, Lung, and Blood Institute; National Asthma Education and Prevention Program, 1997.
4. Antoniu SA, Mihaescu T, Donner CF. Pharmacotherapy of cough-variant asthma. *Expert Opin Pharmacother* 2007;8(17):3021–8.

5. Dicpinigaitis PV. Chronic cough due to asthma: ACCP evidence-based clinical practice guidelines. *Chest* 2006;129:75–9.
6. Parsons JP, Mastronarde JG. Exercise-induced bronchoconstriction in athletes. *Chest* 2005;128: 3966–74.
7. Beach J, Russell K, Blitz S, et al. A systematic review of the diagnosis of occupational asthma. *Chest* 2007;131:569–78.
8. Calhoun WJ. Nocturnal asthma. *Chest* 2003;123:399S–405S.
9. Eder W, Ege MJ, von Mutius E. The asthma epidemic. *N Engl J Med* 2006;355:2226–35.
10. Global Initiative for Asthma (GINA). *Global Strategy for Asthma Management and Prevention.* 2007.
11. Wagers S, Jaffe EF, Irvin CG. Development, structure, and physiology in normal and asthmatic lung. In: Adkinson, NF Jr, Busse WW, Yunginger JW, et al., eds. *Middleton's Allergy Principles and Practice*. 6th ed. St Louis, MO: Elsevier, 2003.
12. Birnbaum S, Barreiro TJ. Methacholine challenge testing: identifying its diagnostic role, testing, coding, and reimbursement. *Chest* 2007;131:1932–5.
13. Martin TG, Elenbaas RM, Pingleton SH. Use of peak expiratory flow rates to eliminate unnecessary arterial blood gases in acute asthma. *Ann Emerg Med* 1982;11:70.
14. Cates CJ, Welsh EJ, Rowe BH. Holding chambers (spacers) versus nebulisers for beta-agonist treatment of acute asthma. *Cochrane Database Syst Rev* 2013;(9):CD000052.
15. Newman KB, Milne S, Hamilton C, Hall K. A comparison of albuterol administered by metered-dose inhaler and spacer with albuterol by nebulizer in adults presenting to an urban emergency department with acute asthma. *Chest* 2002;121:1036.
16. Cheuk DK, Chau TC, Lee SL. A meta-analysis on intravenous magnesium sulphate for treating acute asthma. *Arch Disease Child* 2005;90:74–7.
17. Kew KM, Kirtchuk L, Michell CI. Intravenous magnesium sulfate for treating adults with acute asthma in the emergency department. *Cochrane Database Syst Rev* 2014;(5):CD010909.
18. Silverman RA, Osborn H, Runge J, et al. IV magnesium sulfate in the treatment of acute severe asthma: a multicenter randomized controlled trial. *Chest* 2002;122:489–97.
19. Skobeloff EM, Spivey WH, McNamara RM, Greenspon L. Intravenous magnesium sulfate for the treatment of acute asthma in the emergency department. *JAMA* 1989;262:1210.
20. Ho AM, Lee A, Karmakar MK, et al. Heliox vs air-oxygen mixtures for the treatment of patients with acute asthma: a systematic overview. *Chest* 2003;123:882.
21. Salpeter SR, Buckley NS, Ormiston TM, et al. Meta-analysis: effect of long-acting beta-agonists on severe asthma exacerbations and asthma-related deaths. *Ann Intern Med* 2006;144:904–12.
22. Abramson MJ, Puy RM, Weiner JM. Allergen immunotherapy for asthma. *Cochrane Database Syst Rev* 2003;(4):CD001186.
23. Marcus P. Incorporating anti-IgE (omalizumab) therapy into pulmonary medicine practice: practice management implications. *Chest* 2006;129:466–74.
24. Strunk RC, Bloomberg GR. Omalizumab for asthma. *N Engl J Med* 2006;354: 2689–95.

Solitary Pulmonary Nodule   12

Rachel K. McDonald and Thomas M. Ciesielski

GENERAL PRINCIPLES

- The solitary pulmonary nodule (SPN) is defined as a ≤3-cm isolated, spherical, well-circumscribed radiographic opacity completely surrounded by aerated lung without associated atelectasis, hilar enlargement, or pleural effusion.[1,2]
- A lesion >3 cm is referred to as pulmonary mass and should be considered malignant until proven otherwise.[1,3]
- Some authorities also distinguish subcentimeter nodules (<8 mm), which are much less likely to be malignant and are more difficult to characterize on imaging, as well as more difficult to approach with nonsurgical biopsy.[1,4]
- The large majority of SPNs are discovered incidentally on plain CXRs or CT scan of the chest obtained for other reasons.[5]
- The prevalence of SPNs is dependent on the characteristics of the population studied (e.g., age, smoking status, etc.) and the technique used (i.e., CXR or CT). It has been reported to range from 0.2% up to 20%,[2,3] and even up to 40–60% in lung cancer screening trials.[1]
- Importantly, long-term survival is dramatically better after resection of a malignant SPN compared with that for advanced lung cancer (80% at 5 years vs. <5% at 5 years, respectively).[3]
- The goal of the physician is to diagnose surgically curable malignant nodules before the disease is no longer surgically curable while at the same time avoiding surgery in patients with benign disease.[5]
- The causes of SPN are broad and are listed in Table 12-1.
- The rate of malignancy in patients with SPNs varies greatly depending on study population and methods of detection. Certain imaging characteristics increase the risk of malignancy; these are discussed below.

DIAGNOSIS

Clinical Presentation

The vast majority of patients with an SPN will be asymptomatic with regard to the nodule itself due to the fact that most SPNs are discovered incidentally on chest imaging obtained for another reason.[5]

History

- Age, smoking status, history of extrathoracic cancer ≥5 years before detection of the nodule, and hemoptysis are perhaps the most important historical features that increase the likelihood of malignancy.[5,6]
- Patients should also be asked about constitutional symptoms that may be due to malignancy or infection, such as fever, chills, sweats, weight loss, anorexia, weakness, fatigue, and malaise.

TABLE 12-1 PARTIAL DIFFERENTIAL DIAGNOSIS OF SOLITARY PULMONARY NODULE

Neoplastic

Malignant
Primary Lung Cancer
  Adenocarcinoma
  Squamous cell
  Small cell
  Large cell
  Carcinoid
  Lymphoma
Metastatic (e.g., breast, colorectal, prostate, etc.)

Benign
Hamartoma

Vascular
Arteriovenous malformation
Hemangioma
Focal hemorrhage
Pulmonary infarct

Inflammatory
Sarcoidosis
Granulomatosis with polyangiitis
Rheumatoid arthritis

Infectious

Granulomatous
Tuberculosis
Nontuberculous mycobacteria
Histoplasmosis
Coccidiomycosis
Cryptococcosis
Aspergillosis
Blastomycosis

Nongranulomatous
Parasitic (e.g., ascariasis, echinococcosis, etc.)
Round pneumonia
Lung abscess/septic embolus

Other
Healed or nonspecific granulomas
Nonspecific inflammation or fibrosis
Round atelectasis
Bronchogenic cyst
Intrapulmonary lymph node
Pulmonary sequestration
Amyloid

Physical Examination

The physical examination is usually normal with regard to the SPN. Nonetheless, a careful pulmonary examination is indicated.

Diagnostic Testing

Imaging

CXR and Chest CT findings suggestive of malignancy are as follows:

- **The likelihood of malignancy increases rapidly with size.** SPNs <1 cm are not usually malignant, but those >3 cm often are.[2,6]
- Irregular, lobulated, or spiculated margins increase the likelihood of malignancy. Smooth margins are more likely to be benign, and scalloped margins have an intermediate likelihood.[2,6,7]
- Stippled and/or eccentric calcifications are associated with malignancy.[6,7]
- Laminated, central, and diffuse calcifications suggest a granuloma (e.g., histoplasmosis or tuberculosis), while the popcorn pattern suggests hamartoma.[2]
  - Patients with obviously benign calcifications do not need to be evaluated further as benign patterns of calcification in malignant nodules are exceedingly rare.[2,6]

- The exception to this is that benign calcification patterns can sometimes be seen in pulmonary nodules in patients with a history of bone malignancies (e.g., osteosarcoma or chondrosarcoma).[2]
- The volume doubling time for malignant SPNs is usually between 20 and 300 days, often <100 days.[1] One doubling time equates to an approximately 30% increase in diameter.
- Based on these assumptions, most authorities agree that SPNs that are stable in size for 2 years are very unlikely to be malignant.[1,2] However, slowly growing bronchoalveolar cancers are known to exist, and they may subsequently become more aggressive. This seems to be particularly true of lesions with a ground-glass appearance; lengthier follow-up may be indicated in these cases (see below).[1,4]
- Because of the importance of growth rate, it is critical to compare current with previous CXRs or CTs.
- Upper lobe lesions, particularly on the right, are more likely to be malignant, whereas benign nodules have no predilection for a particular location in the lungs.[2]
- High-resolution chest CT is clearly more sensitive and specific for the detection and characterization of SPNs. The American College of Chest Physicians (ACCP) recommends that all patients with an indeterminate SPN on CXR have high-resolution CT of the chest performed.[4] Any prior chest CTs should be reviewed.
- In addition to the radiographic features discussed above, CT characteristics suggestive of malignancy include the following[2,4,6,8]:
  - A nodule that appears as either (1) pure ground glass or (2) mixed ground glass and solid is more often malignant than purely solid nodule.
  - Vascular convergence
  - Dilated bronchus leading into the nodule
  - Pseudocavitation
  - Thick (>15 mm), irregular-walled cavitation
  - Dynamic contrast enhancement >15 Hounsfield units (HU) on chest CT
  - Fat attenuation (–40 to –120 HU) is strongly suggestive of hamartoma or lipoma. Some metastatic malignancies (e.g., liposarcoma or renal cell carcinoma) may occasionally contain fat.
- Fluorodeoxyglucose positron emission tomography (^{18}F-FDG PET) may also be used to further characterize SPNs.
  - Reviews have estimated the sensitivity to be 87–96.8% and specificity 77.8–83%.[3,4,9]
  - Sensitivity is less for subcentimeter SPNs (<8–10 mm), and therefore it is not recommended to obtain PET imaging for evaluation of subcentimeter nodules.[4]
  - It is important to recognize that false negatives can occur; if clinical suspicion still exists, a biopsy should be strongly considered.
  - The ACCP recommends ^{18}F-FDG PET for patients with low to moderate pretest probability and an SPN >8–10 mm in size with indeterminate CT characteristics. Indeterminate nodules are defined as lacking benign calcification, lacking fat pathognomonic of hamartomas, and lacking a feeding artery or vein typical of an arteriovenous malformation.[4]
  - In some centers, PET and CT can be combined in a single scan. This may provide additional diagnostic information as PET imaging is more accurate for detecting regional lymph node metastases, which may be present in up to 21% of T1 stage lung cancers.[10]
- The ACCP recommends that clinicians estimate the pretest probability of malignancy before ordering further imaging studies or biopsy. This may be done qualitatively using all of the factors discussed above, as appropriate. Furthermore, the pretest probability of malignancy may be predicted quantitatively using one of several prediction models that have been developed. The Bayesian prediction model has been shown in some studies to be more accurate than expert opinion in determining whether a nodule is benign or

malignant. This model uses the radiographic characteristics of nodule size, edge, growth rate, location, and presence or absence of benign calcifications.[11] An alternative prediction model was developed by Swensen et al. In this model, the independent predictors are age, smoking (current or past), history of cancer diagnosed ≥5 years ago, nodule diameter, spiculation, and location in upper lobe.[12] Further studies using this model have found that the addition of nodule volume has enhanced the model's predictive ability.[13]

TREATMENT

Once the clinical and imaging characteristics are known, the choice of subsequent management can be a close call between risk and benefit. Alternatives include observation with serial radiographs, additional diagnostic workup (further imaging, nonsurgical biopsy, or a combination of the two), and surgery. Each of these has advantages and disadvantages that depend greatly on the likelihood of malignancy. **Most importantly, growth on subsequent imaging is presumptive of malignancy and requires further diagnostic evaluation rather than continued observation.**

- **Follow-up of subcentimeter pulmonary nodules:** In general, subcentimeter nodules have a low likelihood of malignancy and are therefore followed with serial imaging at time intervals determined by their initial size at discovery. The recommendations for continued evaluation of subcentimeter nodules are further determined according to their CT appearance (pure ground glass, pure solid, or mixed). The follow-up schedule recommended by the ACCP is outlined in Table 12-2.[4] Of note, the Fleischner Society, a thoracic imaging society, has guidelines that differ slightly from the ACCP.[14]
- **Follow-up Evaluation of SPNs >8 mm:** After estimating the pretest probability that an SPN is malignant, the decision must be made whether to further evaluate the nodule with additional imaging, nonsurgical biopsy, or surgical resection. Again, the Fleischner Society guidelines will differ slightly.[14]
  - **Observational follow-up consists of serial high-resolution CT scans at 3, 6, 12, and 24 months**. If the lesion is stable after 2 years, the risk of malignancy is very low. However, any evidence of growth is presumptive evidence of malignancy. Observation is appropriate for nodules in the following scenarios[2]:
    - Nodules with a very low likelihood of malignancy (<5%)
    - Nodules with low likelihood (<30–40%) of malignancy and a negative ^{18}F-FDG PET scan or dynamic contrast enhancement of <15 HU on chest CT
    - Nondiagnostic needle biopsy and a negative ^{18}F-FDG PET scan
    - Patients who decline aggressive evaluation
  - Biopsy is recommended for SPNs >8–10 mm in patients who would be appropriate candidates for surgical cure when[2]:
    - There is low to moderate probability of malignancy (6–28%).
    - The clinical likelihood of malignancy and results of imaging studies are not in agreement (e.g., high clinical suspicion but a negative ^{18}F-FDG PET scan).
    - A specific treatment is available for a benign diagnosis (e.g., fungal infection)
    - The patient wants biopsy confirmation prior to committing to surgery.
  - **Usually the preferred biopsy technique is CT-guided transthoracic needle aspiration (TTNA)**, especially for more peripheral lesions. The most common complication of TTNA is development of a pneumothorax. However, the reported rate of pneumothorax development is variable, ranging from 15 to 40%.[2,3] Fortunately, chest tubes are only required in 4–18% of pneumothoraces caused by TTNA.[1–3] One limitation of TTNA is that the patient must be able to lie still for >30 minutes, perform a breath hold, and withhold from coughing during the duration of the procedure.[2]

TABLE 12-2 RECOMMENDATIONS FOR FOLLOW-UP CT IMAGING OF SUBCENTIMETER PULMONARY NODULES

Nonsolid Nodules (pure ground glass)	Timing of Follow-Up	
≤5 mm	No follow-up	
>5 mm	Annual CT for 3 years	
Partly Solid Nodules (>50% ground glass)	**Timing of Follow-Up**	
≤8 mm	Repeat CT at 3, 12, and 24 mo followed by annual CT for additional 1–3 years	
>8 mm	Repeat CT at 3 mo, then PET or nonsurgical biopsy or surgical resection for nodules that persist	
Solid Nodules	**Timing of Follow-Up**	
	No Lung Cancer Risk Factors[a]	**Risk Factors for Lung Cancer Present**
≤4 mm	Optional follow-up	12 mo, none further if stable
4–6 mm	12 mo, none further if stable	6–12 mo, if stable 18–24 mo
>6–8 mm	6–12 mo, if stable 18–24 mo	3–6 mo, 9–12 mo, and 24 mo if stable

[a]Major risk factors: smoking (current or past), history of radiation therapy, environmental toxin exposure

Adapted from Gould MK, Donington J, Lynch WR, et al. Evaluation of patients with pulmonary nodules: when is it lung cancer? Diagnosis and Management of Lung Cancer, 3rd edition: ACCP evidence-based clinical practice guidelines. *Chest* 2013;143(Suppl):e93S–e120S.

- Bronchoscopic biopsy may be a viable alternative in specific situations (e.g., central lesions, lesions adjacent to a bronchus, an air bronchogram in the lesion) and when there is available expertise.[3] Electromagnetic navigation bronchoscopic biopsy is an emerging technique for peripheral lesions.

Surgical Management

Surgical management is recommended for indeterminate SPNs of >8–10 mm in appropriate surgical candidates when the clinical likelihood of malignancy is moderate to high, the ^{18}F-FDG PET is positive, a nonsurgical biopsy is suspicious for malignancy, or the patient prefers to undergo a definitive procedure.[1,4,15]

- Thoracotomy is the most definitive approach, particularly for more centrally located SPNs that are not accessible by other techniques. Operative mortality for the removal of malignant nodules is ~3–7%, although it is <1% for resection of benign nodules.[3]
- Video-assisted thoracoscopic surgery (VATS) is a minimally invasive technique with a lower mortality rate, about 1%. It is usually the preferred method for SPNs in the peripheral third of the lung. In about 12% of cases, the procedure must be converted to a traditional thoracotomy.

REFERENCES

1. Ost DE, Gould MK. Decision making in patients with pulmonary nodules. *Am J Respir Crit Care Med* 2012;185:363–72.
2. Winer-Muram HT. The solitary pulmonary nodule. *Radiology* 2006;239:34–49.
3. Ost D, Fein AM, Feinsilver SH. Clinical practice. The solitary pulmonary nodule. *N Engl J Med* 2003;348:2535–42.
4. Gould MK, Donington J, Lynch WR, et al. Evaluation of patients with pulmonary nodules: when is it lung cancer? Diagnosis and Management of Lung Cancer, 3rd edition: ACCP evidence-based clinical practice guidelines. *Chest* 2013;143(Suppl):e93S–120.
5. Swensen SJ, Silverstein MD, Edell ES, et al. Solitary pulmonary nodules: clinical prediction model versus physicians. *Mayo Clin Proc* 1999;74:319–29.
6. Gurney JW. Determining the likelihood of malignancy in solitary pulmonary nodules with Bayesian analysis. Part I. Theory. *Radiology* 1993;186:405–13.
7. Jeong YJ, Yi CA, Lee KS. Solitary pulmonary nodules: detection, characterization, and guidance for further diagnostic workup and treatment. *Am J Roentgenol* 2007;188:57–68.
8. Swensen SJ, Viggiano RW, Midthun DE, et al. Lung nodule enhancement at CT: multicenter study. *Radiology* 2000;214:73–80.
9. Wahidi MM, Govert JA, Goudar RK, et al. Evidence for the treatment of patients with pulmonary nodules: when is it lung cancer? ACCP evidence-based clinical practice guidelines, 2nd ed. *Chest* 2007;132:94S–107.
10. Gould MK, Maclean JG, Kuschner WG, et al. Accuracy of positron emission tomography for diagnosis of pulmonary nodules and mass lesions: a meta-analysis. *JAMA* 2001;285:914–24.
11. Gurney JW, Lyddon DM, McKay JA. Determining the likelihood of malignancy in solitary pulmonary nodules with Bayesian analysis. Part II. Application. *Radiology* 1993;186:415–22.
12. Swensen SJ, Silverstein MD, Ilstrup DM, et al. The probability of malignancy in solitary pulmonary nodules. Application to small radiologically indeterminate nodules. *Arch Intern Med* 1997;157:849–55.
13. Mehta HJ, Ravenel JG, Shaftman SR, et al. The utility of nodule volume in the context of malignancy prediction for small pulmonary nodules. *Chest* 2014;145:464–72.
14. MacMahon H, Austin JHM, Gamsu G, et al. Guidelines for management of small pulmonary nodules detected on CT scans: a statement from the Fleischner Society. *Radiology* 2005;237:395–400.
15. Patel VK, Naik SK, Naidich DP, et al. A Practical Algorithmic Approach to the Diagnosis and Management of Solitary Pulmonary Nodules. *Chest* 2013;143:840–6.

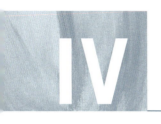

IV Gastroenterology

Approach to Nausea and Vomiting

Cheryl R. McDonough

GENERAL PRINCIPLES

- Nausea and vomiting are common complaints resulting in billions of dollars of health care expenditure yearly, as well as even higher costs in lost work productivity.[1]
- Nausea is the unpleasant subjective feeling of impending vomiting.
- Vomiting is a series of organized motor and autonomic responses resulting in the forceful expulsion of gastric contents from the stomach and out of the mouth.
- Vomiting is distinct from regurgitation, which is the passive retrograde flow of esophageal contents into the mouth and from rumination, which is the effortless regurgitation of recently ingested food into the mouth followed by rechewing and then reswallowing or spitting out.
- Vomiting can be stimulated by neuronal or humoral mechanisms, but regardless of the stimulus, the act of vomiting is coordinated by the vomiting center (or emetic center) in the medulla.
- The vomiting center can be electrically stimulated by the vagus nerve; these afferent impulses from the gastrointestinal (GI) tract are relayed to the vomiting center via the nucleus tractus solitarius.
- The vomiting center also receives afferent impulses from multiple other areas, such as the pharynx, vestibular system, heart, peritoneum, thalamus, hypothalamus, and cerebral cortex.
- The chemoreceptor trigger zone (CTZ) in the area postrema in the floor of the fourth ventricle also activates the vomiting center. The CTZ is partially outside the blood–brain barrier and is stimulated by other emetic stimuli, such as drugs, uremia, hypoxia, diabetic ketoacidosis, enterotoxin derived from gram-positive bacteria, radiation sickness, and motion sickness.
- The principle neurotransmitter receptors that mediate vomiting include muscarinic M1, dopamine D2, histamine H_1, 5-hydroxytryptamine$_3$ (5-HT_3) serotonin, and neurokinin-1 (NK-1) substance P.[2]

DIAGNOSIS

Clinical Presentation

- The American Gastroenterological Association advocates a 3-step approach to the evaluation and management of the patient with nausea and vomiting:
  - Correction of complications such as volume depletion and electrolyte abnormalities
  - Identification and elimination of the underlying etiology when possible
  - Suppression or elimination of the symptoms themselves if the primary cause cannot be identified easily and promptly eliminated[1]
- Key points in the patient's history include onset, duration, and timing of symptoms; precipitating and relieving factors; medications; travel; sick contacts; associated symptoms such as change in bowel habit; presence or absence of flatus; abdominal pain or bloating; fever; and dizziness. During the physical exam, particular attention should

be paid to volume status, abdominal exam, and extra-abdominal findings that would narrow the differential.
- Finally, if an organic etiology or motility problem is not revealed, functional nausea and vomiting should be considered, although a definitive diagnosis can be difficult to make.

History
- Acute onset of symptoms (1–2 days) suggests infection, toxin, medication-related side effect, or more serious possibilities such as obstruction, pancreatitis, appendicitis, or cholecystitis.
- Medication side effects can also be more insidious in onset. Gastroparesis, metabolic disorders, pregnancy, or gastroesophageal reflux disease can also lead to insidious onset of nausea without vomiting.
- Early-morning vomiting can be associated with pregnancy, uremia, alcohol, and increased intracranial pressure. Intracranial disorders causing increased intracranial pressure can cause projectile vomiting or vomiting without associated nausea and may, of course, be associated with other neurologic symptoms such as headache, vertigo, or focal neurologic deficits.
- Gastroparesis and gastric outlet obstruction frequently cause delayed vomiting, often more than an hour after eating. The vomitus may be partly digested. Early satiety and postprandial abdominal bloating and pain may be seen with gastroparesis.
- Bilious vomitus indicates a more distal obstruction in the small bowel rather than the gastric outlet.
- Feculent vomiting, which can be seen in intestinal obstruction, reflects bacterial degradation of intestinal contents. Abdominal pain may be severe, colicky, and temporarily improved after vomiting with small bowel obstruction. A recent change in bowel habit and lack of flatus may also be noted.
- Vomiting associated with anorexia nervosa or bulimia typically occurs during or soon after meals.
- Regurgitation of undigested food (not technically vomiting) can indicate an esophageal disorder such as Zenker diverticulum, achalasia, or esophageal stricture.
- Weight loss may result from a malignancy but could also be a result of food avoidance from another problem, such as gastric outlet obstruction secondary to peptic ulcer disease.
- Recurrent bouts of severe vomiting may indicate cyclic vomiting syndrome, particularly in the pediatric population, and if associated with chronic marijuana use and compulsive bathing likely represent the cannabis hyperemesis syndrome.[1,3]

Physical Examination
- Physical exam may show supine or orthostatic hypotension, tachycardia, dry mucous membranes, or decreased skin turgor as a result of hypovolemia.
- Signs of an associated endocrine disorder, such as thyrotoxicosis or Addison disease, should be sought.
- Collagen vascular diseases such as scleroderma may be evident.
- Skin exam may also reveal jaundice indicative of a hepatobiliary disorder, calluses on the dorsum of the hands consistent with self-induced vomiting, or hyperpigmentation associated with primary adrenal failure.
- Loss of dental enamel can indicate recurrent vomiting secondary to bulimia or the consequences of gastroesophageal reflux disease.
- Lymphadenopathy may be related to malignancy or reactive to another underlying process.
- Neurologic examination may show nystagmus, papilledema on funduscopic exam, cranial nerve or other focal deficits, or gait abnormality.
- Psychiatric pathology also may become evident during the history and physical examination.

- **Abdominal exam** may reveal organomegaly, other masses, or the presence of a hernia.
  - Epigastric tenderness may be caused by peptic ulcer disease or pancreatitis.
  - Tenderness in the right upper quadrant suggests cholecystitis or biliary tract pathology.
  - Localization to the right lower quadrant may represent appendicitis or Crohn disease.
  - More diffuse tenderness may suggest small bowel obstruction. Rebound tenderness or involuntary guarding can be seen with peritoneal irritation.
  - Auscultation may reveal decreased or absent bowel sounds in ileus or hyperactive, high-pitched bowel sounds in obstruction.
  - In gastric outlet obstruction or severe gastroparesis, a succession splash may be heard over the epigastrium when the epigastrium is being shaken or rapidly palpated.[1]

Differential Diagnosis

The differential diagnosis is broad. A partial list is shown in Table 13-1.[1,2]

Diagnostic Testing

Laboratories

The history and physical exam may be all that is needed to determine the etiology and will dictate what laboratory and imaging studies are appropriate. Generally, routine blood studies should include

TABLE 13-1 DIFFERENTIAL DIAGNOSIS OF NAUSEA AND VOMITING (PARTIAL LIST)

Medications

Toxins

Infections

Viral gastroenteritis (rotavirus, Norwalk virus, Reovirus, adenovirus)

Bacterial (*Staphylococcus aureus*, *Bacillus cereus*, *Salmonella*, *Clostridium perfringens*)

Other infections (meningitis, acute hepatitis, otitis media)

Gastrointestinal Disorders

Gastroparesis, intestinal obstruction or ischemia, gastric outlet obstruction, pancreatitis, appendicitis, cholecystitis, gastroesophageal reflux disease, peptic ulcer disease, functional motility disorder, cyclical vomiting

Metabolic and Endocrine Disorders

Uremia, diabetic ketoacidosis, hypercalcemia, hyponatremia, adrenal insufficiency, thyroid and parathyroid disease, acute intermittent porphyria

Central Nervous System Disorders

Increased intracranial pressure, vestibular and labyrinthine disorders, migraine, seizure disorders, demyelinating disorders, psychiatric

Other

Pregnancy, postoperative state, cannabinoid hyperemesis syndrome, cardiac disease, collagen vascular disorders, eating disorders, starvation

---

Adapted from Quigley EMM, Hasler WL, Parkman HP. AGA technical review on nausea and vomiting. *Gastroenterology* 2001;120:263–86; Malagelada JR, Malagelada C. Nausea and Vomiting. In: Feldman M, Friedman LS, Brandt LJ, eds. *Sleisenger and Fordtran's Gastrointestinal and Liver Disease*. 10th ed. Philadelphia: Saunders/Elsevier, 2016:207–20.

- Complete blood count (CBC)
  - Leukocytosis may be secondary to infection or reactive to another underlying process.
  - Peripheral eosinophilia may be seen with eosinophilic gastroenteritis or parasitic infection.
- Comprehensive metabolic panel (CMP)
  - Hyponatremia may be secondary to volume depletion or adrenal insufficiency.
  - Hypokalemia and metabolic alkalosis result from the GI loss of hydrochloric acid and potassium.
    - Hypokalemia is exacerbated by the exchange of potassium for sodium as the renal tubule attempts to conserve sodium.
    - Metabolic alkalosis is worsened by the contraction of extracellular fluid and the shifting of hydrogen into cells in exchange for potassium.
  - Renal function may be impaired, depending on volume status.
  - Hyperglycemia, anion gap metabolic acidosis, and serum or urinary ketones will be seen in diabetic ketoacidosis.
  - Abnormal liver function tests may indicate a hepatobiliary cause.
- Thyroid function tests and possibly screening for adrenal disorders may be appropriate.
- Pancreatic enzymes should be obtained if pancreatitis is suspected.
- It may be necessary to obtain an arterial blood gas (ABG) to evaluate acid–base status.
- A urine pregnancy test should be obtained in women of reproductive age.
- Serum drug levels (e.g., of digoxin, theophylline, salicylates, or alcohol) may be helpful.

Imaging
- If obstruction is suspected, an abdominal obstructive series (upright and supine) should be obtained, although plain films may be unrevealing in 22% of those with partial small bowel obstruction.[4]
- If further clarification is required, computed tomography (CT) can localize the intestinal obstruction and identify abdominal masses as well as pancreatic and hepatobiliary pathology.
- Barium contrast studies may also be able to suggest achalasia, gastroparesis, or neoplasm.
- Small bowel follow-through, small bowel enteroclysis, and more recently CT enterography can potentially identify mucosal lesions in the small bowel.
- Ultrasound can identify gallbladder, hepatobiliary, or pancreatic pathology.
- Radioscintigraphy is the most accurate method to assess for delayed gastric emptying as seen in gastroparesis.
- Neurologic imaging should be performed in those with suspicious history or physical exam findings or perhaps in those with severe, unexplained, persistent symptoms. Magnetic resonance imaging is more valuable than CT for visualization of the posterior fossa.

Diagnostic Procedures
- Upper endoscopy is sensitive and specific for mucosal lesions, such as peptic ulcer disease or malignancy, and is one of the tests of choice (along with an upper GI barium study) to evaluate for partial gastric outlet or duodenal obstruction.
- Esophageal manometry to assess esophageal motor activity may be useful in evaluation of suspected achalasia, distal esophageal spasm, or other motor disturbances of the smooth muscle portion of the esophagus.

TREATMENT

- Fluid and electrolyte abnormalities should be corrected.
- If possible, the underlying cause should be eliminated; in the meantime, vomiting should be treated symptomatically.

- For severe symptoms or significant gastric distention, nasogastric tube placement should be considered.
- Literature regarding pharmacological treatment is limited in that most clinical trials have addressed nausea and vomiting associated with chemotherapy, radiation, and surgery, and it may not be appropriate to extrapolate those results to other clinical situations. Pharmacological treatments are discussed below.
- **Dopamine receptor antagonists**
  - Phenothiazines primarily antagonize D2 dopamine receptors in the area postrema of the midbrain and also have M1 muscarinic and H_1 histamine-blocking effects.
    - **Prochlorperazine**, **promethazine**, and **chlorpromazine** are good choices for initial treatment as they are effective for symptoms caused by a wide array of disorders and are generally available in both parenteral and rectal suppository formulations.
    - Limiting side effects include extrapyramidal reactions such as dystonia or tardive dyskinesia, sedation, or orthostatic hypotension.[4]
  - The butyrophenones **droperidol and haloperidol** also block D2 dopamine receptors and muscarinic M1 receptors but are limited by the same safety concerns.
  - The benzamide **metoclopramide** causes central dopamine D2 antagonism at low doses and weak 5-HT_3 blockade at higher doses. It also stimulates peripheral 5-HT_4 receptors on gastric smooth muscle, enhancing acetylcholine release at the neuromuscular junction and therefore creating a prokinetic effect.
    - **Metoclopramide** has a modest antiemetic effect, speeds gastric emptying, and increases lower esophageal sphincter tone.
    - The most common indications for metoclopramide include nausea and vomiting in pregnancy, postoperative state, and that induced by radiation or chemotherapy. Because of its prokinetic effect, the drug is also used for gastroparesis. Metoclopramide crosses the blood–brain barrier and, therefore, may cause neurologic side effects such as dystonia and tardive dyskinesia.
    - Metoclopramide may also prolong the QT interval.[2]
- **Serotonin antagonists:** Because the highest density of 5-HT_3 receptors is in the area postrema, it is thought that the CTZ is the primary site of action of these drugs. They also block gastric wall receptors that relay afferent emetic signals via the vagus nerve, and they have a modest gastric prokinetic action.
  - **Ondansetron**, **granisetron**, **dolasetron**, **ramosetron**, and **tropisetron** are the available first-generation options, and all are especially useful in treatment of chemotherapy- or radiation-induced and postoperative emesis.
    - **Ondansetron** appears to be safe in pregnancy.
    - Headache is the most frequent side effect, and there is a risk of QT prolongation with high doses of ondansetron and other first-generation agents.[2]
  - **Palonosetron** is a second-generation serotonin receptor antagonist that has a much higher affinity for 5-HT_3 receptors and a longer half-life. No prolongation of the QT interval has been seen with its use.[5] Palonosetron is the preferred serotonin receptor antagonist for use with moderately emetogenic chemotherapy.[6]
- **Antihistamines and anticholinergic agents**
  - Histamine H_1-receptor antagonists such as **meclizine**, **dimenhydrinate**, **hydroxyzine**, and **diphenhydramine** have central antiemetic effects and can be helpful for motion sickness, vertigo, and migraine in which symptoms are of labyrinthine origin. Sedation is a common side effect.
  - **Scopolamine**, an M1 muscarinic receptor antagonist, is mainly used as prophylaxis against motion sickness, can be applied transdermally, and may be associated with visual accommodation disturbances. Anticholinergic effects can be problematic for those with glaucoma, benign prostatic hypertrophy, and asthma.[2]

- **Neurokinin-1 receptor antagonists:** Substance P is found in neurons innervating the brainstem nucleus tractus solitarius and the area postrema and has emetogenic effects mediated through the NK-1 receptor.
  - **Aprepitant** and **fosaprepitant** (the parenteral formulation) are used to prevent acute and delayed chemotherapy-induced emesis and work best in conjunction with serotonin receptor antagonists and dexamethasone; this three-drug combination is recommended for patients receiving highly emetogenic chemotherapy.[6]
  - There can be significant drug interactions because aprepitant moderately inhibits the CYP3A4 pathway.
  - Other NK-1 receptor antagonists that appear to be very effective for prevention of nausea and vomiting in patients receiving emetogenic chemotherapy include NEPA, a combined product of netupitant plus palonosetron, and rolapitant, which has a very long half-life of ~7 days and does not interact with the CYP3A4 pathway.[7,8]
- **Corticosteroids:** The antiemetic mechanism of glucocorticoids is not well understood but may relate to inhibition of central prostaglandin synthesis, release of endorphins, or altered synthesis or release of serotonin.[2]
  - Corticosteroids (usually **dexamethasone**) are used alone or in combination with 5-HT$_3$ receptor antagonists and/or NK-1 receptor antagonists for treatment of chemotherapy- or radiation-induced emesis or postoperative emesis.
  - Side effects are uncommon because treatment is usually limited to a short period of time but can include hyperglycemia, insomnia, increased energy, and mood changes.
- **Cannabinoids: Nabilone and dronabinol** are approved for chemotherapy-induced nausea and vomiting refractory to conventional therapy but are potentially more toxic with unfavorable side effects including hypotension and psychotropic reactions.[2] The paradoxical nausea and vomiting seen in cannabinoid hyperemesis syndrome is not well understood but may be related genetic variations in hepatic metabolism or chronic accumulation of tetrahydrocannabinol (THC) after long-term exposure in sensitive patients.[3]
- **Benzodiazepines:** Given alone, benzodiazepines such as lorazepam and alprazolam are relatively weak antiemetic agents. They are primarily used to potentiate the antiemetic actions of serotonin antagonists and dexamethasone. They are also helpful in the treatment of the anticipatory nausea that occurs with chemotherapy. Sedation is the most common side effect.
- **Prokinetic drugs:** In addition to metoclopramide, another drug in the benzamide class with peripheral 5-HT$_4$ agonist effects is **prucalopride**, a drug intended for treatment of constipation but with some prokinetic effects in the upper GI tract as well. Potential uses for 5-HT$_4$ agonists include gastroparesis, intestinal pseudo-obstruction, and functional dyspepsia. Related drugs such as cisapride and tegaserod were withdrawn from the market secondary to cardiac toxicity but that has not been seen with prucalopride.[9] **Prucalopride is not currently available in the United States.**
- Other drugs with prokinetic effects include **erythromycin**, a motilin receptor agonist, and **bethanechol**, a muscarinic receptor agonist. **Erythromycin** may be used to treat acute nausea and vomiting secondary to gastroparesis and to clear the stomach prior to upper endoscopy. However, its symptom-relieving effects are questionable, higher doses often induce abdominal cramping and diarrhea, and it is not useful for prolonged treatment due to prompt tachyphylaxis, uncertain efficacy via the oral route, and risks of pseudomembranous colitis and QT prolongation.[2]
- Ghrelin (a peptide related to motilin) has been identified as a potential treatment for impaired gastric emptying due to its actions on GI motility and food intake. After promising results in initial clinical trials, relamorelin, a ghrelin receptor agonist, is currently in phase II studies in patients with diabetic gastroparesis.[10]

REFERENCES

1. Quigley EMM, Hasler WL, Parkman HP. AGA technical review on nausea and vomiting. *Gastroenterology* 2001;120:263–86.
2. Malagelada JR, Malagelada C. Nausea and Vomiting. In: Feldman M, Friedman LS, Brandt LJ, eds. *Sleisenger and Fordtran's Gastrointestinal and Liver Disease*. 10th ed. Philadelphia: Saunders/Elsevier, 2016:207–20.
3. Soriano-Co M, Batke M, Cappell MS. The cannabis hyperemesis syndrome characterized by persistent nausea and vomiting, abdominal pain, and compulsive bathing associated with chronic marijuana use: a report of eight cases in the United States. *Dig Dis Sci* 2010;55:3113–9.
4. Hasler WL, Chey WD. Nausea and vomiting. *Gastroenterology* 2003;125:1860–7.
5. Gonullu G, Demircan S, Demirag MK, et al. Electrocardiographic findings of palonosetron in cancer patients. *Support Care Cancer* 2012;20:1435–9.
6. Basch E, Prestrud AA, Hesketh PJ. Antiemetics: American Society of Clinical Oncology clinical practice guideline update. *J Clin Oncol* 2011;29:4189–98.
7. Gralla RJ, Bosnjak SM, Hontsa A. A phase III study evaluating the safety and efficacy of NEPA, a fixed-dose combination of netupitant and palonosetron, for prevention of chemotherapy-induced nausea and vomiting over repeated cycles of chemotherapy. *Ann Oncol* 2014;25:1333–9.
8. Rapoport BL, Chasen MR, Gridelli C. Safety and efficacy of rolapitant for prevention of chemotherapy-induced nausea and vomiting after administration of cisplatin-based highly emetogenic chemotherapy in patients with cancer: two randomised active-controlled, double-blind, phase 3 trials. *Lancet Oncol* 2015;16:1079–89.
9. Quigley E. Prucalopride: safety, efficacy and potential applications. *Therap Adv Gastroenterol* 2012;5:23–30.
10. Shin A, Wo J. Therapeutic applications of ghrelin agonists in the treatment of gastroparesis. *Curr Gastroenterol Rep* 2015;17:430.

Approach to Gastrointestinal Bleeding

14

Cheryl R. McDonough

GENERAL PRINCIPLES

- Gastrointestinal (GI) bleeding leads to over 1,000,000 hospitalizations yearly in the United States.
- Fifty percent of GI bleeding admissions are for upper GI bleeding, which originates proximal to the ligament of Treitz; 40% are for lower GI bleeding that arises in the colon and anorectum; and 10% are for mid bleeding from the small intestine.
- GI bleeding may be overt, occult (a positive stool guaiac test [hemoccult] or iron deficiency anemia), or obscure (of unclear etiology despite upper and lower endoscopic evaluation and possibly small bowel radiography).[1]

DIAGNOSIS

Clinical Presentation

History

Important aspects of the history to focus on when seeing a patient with suspected GI bleed include the following:

- Character of the bleeding
  - Vomiting of bright red blood usually indicates significant upper GI bleeding.
  - Coffee-ground emesis usually indicates the patient is not actively bleeding.
  - Hematochezia can indicate upper GI bleeding if it is a very brisk bleed; this is usually associated with signs of hemodynamic compromise.
  - Epistaxis may point to a non-GI source of blood loss.
- Symptoms of anemia or hypovolemia
  - Light-headedness or syncope
  - Dyspnea
  - Angina
- Associated symptoms
  - Retching and vomiting may lead to a Mallory-Weiss tear.
  - Heartburn or dyspepsia may be associated with peptic ulcer disease (PUD), gastritis, or esophagitis.
  - Weight loss, early satiety, night sweats, anorexia, and/or a change in bowel habits or stool caliber are concerning for malignancy.
  - PUD, mesenteric ischemia, and ischemic colitis may be associated with abdominal pain.
  - Bleeding from hemorrhoids is generally painless, while anal fissures are associated with anal pain.
  - Diverticular bleeding is usually painless.
- Medication use
  - Aspirin or other nonsteroidal anti-inflammatory drugs (NSAIDs)
  - Anticoagulants
  - Bismuth or iron

- Medications associated with pill esophagitis
  - Tetracycline, doxycycline, clindamycin
  - Bisphosphonates
- Social habits
  - Alcohol use is associated with gastritis, PUD, and GI malignancy and raises the possibility of variceal bleeding.
  - Tobacco use is associated with GI malignancy and recurrent PUD.
- Medical and surgical history
  - The source of GI bleeding is the same as previous bleeds up to 60% of the time.[2]
  - History of liver disease increases the likelihood of esophageal or gastric varices or portal hypertensive gastropathy.
  - Prior surgery such as an abdominal aortic vascular graft or a known abdominal aortic aneurysm increases the concern for an aortoenteric fistula.
  - Prior intestinal surgical anastomosis raises the possibility of an anastomotic ulceration.
  - Prior radiation therapy may point to radiation-induced telangiectasia or radiation proctosigmoiditis.
  - Patients who have had a recent polypectomy may have postpolypectomy bleeding.

Physical Examination

Important aspects of the physical examination to focus on when examining a patient with suspected GI bleed include the following:

- Assessment of hemodynamic stability, including orthostatic heart rate and blood pressure
- Careful abdominal examination
  - Epigastric tenderness may be present with PUD or gastritis.
  - Abdominal tenderness may be more diffuse with infectious, inflammatory, or ischemic causes of bleeding.
  - Ascites or splenomegaly may be present in chronic liver disease.
  - Hyperactive bowel sounds may be heard with an upper bleed.
- Cutaneous manifestations of systemic diseases
  - Stigmata of chronic liver disease such as jaundice, caput medusa, spider angiomata, telangiectasias, or palmar erythema should heighten the suspicion for variceal bleeding.
  - Skin or mucous membrane telangiectasias could indicate hereditary hemorrhagic telangiectasia (Osler-Weber-Rendu syndrome).
  - Pigmented lip lesions are seen with Peutz-Jeghers syndrome.
  - Cutaneous tumors suggest neurofibromatosis.
  - Purpura is seen with vascular disease such as Henoch-Schonlein purpura or polyarteritis nodosa.
  - Purpura and/or petechiae may be seen with other bleeding disorders.
  - Acanthosis nigricans may reflect underlying malignancy.
- Evaluation of the patient's stool
  - Patients with brown stool are unlikely to have aggressive bleeding.
  - Those who are actively passing stools with red blood, maroon blood, or melena are likely to still have active bleeding.
  - Patients with infrequent stools are unlikely to be actively bleeding.
  - Those with a history of coffee-ground emesis but normal-appearing stools (possibly positive for occult blood) usually have had a trivial bleed.

Differential Diagnosis

- Key to the formulation of a differential diagnosis is classifying a bleed as to whether it arises from an upper or a lower source.
- Upper GI bleeding presents with hematemesis (vomiting of bright red blood or coffee grounds) as well as melena (black, tarry, and foul-smelling stool). As little as 50–100 mL

TABLE 14-1 CAUSES OF ACUTE UPPER GASTROINTESTINAL BLEEDING

Major	Minor
Peptic ulcer disease	Cameron lesion
Esophageal and gastric varices	Gastric antral vascular ectasia (watermelon stomach)
Hemorrhagic gastritis	Portal hypertensive gastropathy
Esophagitis	Past chemotherapy or radiation sequelae
Duodenitis	Gastric polyps
Mallory-Weiss tear	Aortoenteric fistula
Angiodysplasia	Submucosal lesion/mass
Upper GI malignancy	Connective tissue disease
Anastomotic ulcers	Hemobilia
Dieulafoy lesion	Hemosuccus pancreaticus
	Kaposi sarcoma
	Foreign body
	Postprocedural

Adapted from Cappell MS, Friedel D. Initial management of acute upper gastrointestinal bleeding: from initial evaluation up to gastrointestinal endoscopy. *Med Clin North Am* 2008;92:491–509.

of blood in the GI tract can result in melena.[1] See Table 14-1 for a differential diagnosis of upper GI bleeding.[2]

- Bleeding from the lower GI tract usually presents as hematochezia (bright red or maroon colored blood or fresh clots per rectum), although hematochezia can be seen with massive upper GI bleeding, and melena can be seen with proximal lower GI bleeding. See Table 14-2 for a differential diagnosis of lower GI bleeding.[3]

TABLE 14-2 CAUSES OF ACUTE LOWER GASTROINTESTINAL BLEEDING

Lesions Seen in Hematochezia	Frequency
Diverticuli	17–40%
Angiodysplasia	2–30%
Colitis (infectious, inflammatory, ischemic, radiation)	9–21%
Colonic neoplasm or postpolypectomy bleeding	11–14%
Anorectal	4–10%
Upper GI source	0–11%
Small bowel source	2–9%

Adapted from Zuccaro G. Management of the adult patient with acute lower gastrointestinal bleeding. *Am J Gastroenterol* 1998;93:1202–8.

Diagnostic Testing

Although the return of bright red blood on nasogastric lavage (NGL) can help identify patients with high-risk lesions, it is somewhat controversial and is performed with decreasing frequency for the following reasons:

- Approximately 15% of actively bleeding patients still have a negative lavage.[4]
- Those patients who have a bloody NGL tend to have endoscopy performed more promptly, but it makes no difference in clinical outcomes or length of hospitalization.[5]
- A study of bedside procedures performed in the emergency department showed that patients rank NG intubation as the most painful.[6]

Laboratories
- Complete blood count
    - Hematocrit checked soon after the onset of acute bleeding does not accurately reflect the degree of blood loss. Equilibration can take several hours.
    - A low mean corpuscular volume may indicate chronic blood loss and iron deficiency.
- Type and screen or cross-match
- Coagulation studies
- Complete metabolic panel
    - An elevated blood urea nitrogen (BUN) to creatinine ratio is often seen in upper GI bleeding.
    - Abnormal liver function tests in combination with low albumin, low platelets, and elevated international normalized ratio (INR) may indicate cirrhosis and risk for variceal bleeding.
    - Cardiac enzymes and an electrocardiogram should be performed in those with symptoms or risk of cardiac ischemia.

Imaging
If there is suspicion for bowel perforation, upright and supine abdominal x-rays and potentially a CT of the abdomen and pelvis should be performed. Of note, barium radiography is contraindicated in acute upper GI bleeding because of its interference with subsequent endoscopy, angiography, or surgery. Discussion of other imaging tests for GI bleeding occurs in the treatment section.

Diagnostic Procedures
Diagnostic procedures for upper and lower GI bleeding will be discussed under treatment.

TREATMENT

- Initial treatment is aimed at **volume resuscitation**.
    - Volume should be replaced with isotonic fluids.
    - Administration of blood products (O-negative if necessary prior to cross-matching) should be based on the patients clinical condition.
    - In general, transfusion to goal hemoglobin of 7 g/dL is adequate.[7]
- Coagulopathy (INR > 1.5) should be corrected with fresh frozen plasma (FPP) and vitamin K.
- Thrombocytopenia (platelets < 50,000) should be corrected with platelet transfusion.
- Patients whose vital signs do not stabilize with initial resuscitation, who have ongoing transfusion requirements, or who have significant comorbid illness should be considered for intensive care unit admission. Endotracheal intubation should be considered in patients with ongoing hematemesis or in those patients with altered respiratory or mental status.

Treatment of Upper GI Bleeding

- After hemodynamic stabilization and reasonable correction of any coagulopathy, upper endoscopy is the diagnostic study of choice in suspected upper GI bleeding. Endoscopy is ideally performed within 24 hours of presentation but should be performed more urgently after medical resuscitation of those with active hemorrhage. Nearly 80% of patients with upper GI bleeding will stop bleeding spontaneously and not have recurrence; however, the remaining 20% of patients have a high mortality rate of 30–40%.
- Therapeutic endoscopic maneuvers such as injection, thermal coagulation, banding, and/or clipping are often able to achieve hemostasis. In addition, prompt endoscopy can identify low-risk patients who may be appropriate for outpatient treatment as well as triage those particularly high-risk patients to more intensive monitoring.
- Clinical predictors of rebleeding and mortality in upper GI bleeds include the following:
  - Age > 65
  - Syncope or hemodynamic instability
  - Poor overall health status
  - Comorbid illnesses
  - Low initial hemoglobin
  - Melena
  - Transfusion requirement
  - Fresh red blood on rectal exam, emesis, or nasogastric aspirate
  - Sepsis
  - Elevated BUN, creatinine, or serum aminotransferases[7]
  - Endoscopic predictors of risk include peptic ulcer appearance (Table 14-3),[1,8,9] ulcer size >2 cm, ulcer location on the posterior lesser gastric curvature or posterior duodenal wall, and lesion type[7]
- Peptic ulcers with:
  - **High-risk stigmata** (active bleeding and nonbleeding visible vessel) require endoscopic intervention, which can reduce their risk of rebleeding to 15–30%; adjunctive high-dose proton pump inhibitor (PPI) reduces the risk even further to <10%.[1]

TABLE 14-3 MORTALITY, FREQUENCY, AND REBLEEDING RISK BASED ON ENDOSCOPIC APPEARANCE OF ULCER

Endoscopic Appearance	Frequency	Risk of Rebleeding without Intervention	Mortality
Active bleeding	12%	Approaches 100%	11%
Nonbleeding visible vessel	8%	Up to 50%	11%
Adherent clot	8%	8–35%	7%
Flat spot	16%	<8%	3%
Clean ulcer base	55%	<3%	2%

Adapted from Savides TJ, Jensen DM. Gastrointestinal Bleeding. In: Feldman M, Friedman LS, Brandt LJ, eds. *Sleisenger and Fordtran's Gastrointestinal and Liver Disease*. 10th ed. Philadelphia: Saunders/Elsevier, 2016:297–335; Laine L, Jensen DM. Management of patients with ulcer bleeding. *Am J Gastroenterol* 2012;107:345–60; Hwang JH, Fisher DA, Ben-Menachem T, et al. The role of endoscopy in the management of acute non-variceal upper GI bleeding. *Gastrointest Endosc* 2012;75:1132–8.

- An ulcer with oozing or an adherent clot also benefit from endoscopic treatment. Oozing is of intermediate risk, and those patients are generally observed in the hospital for 24–28 hours after endoscopy.[1]
- Patients with clean-based ulcers have a low rebleeding rate of <5%, do not require endoscopic therapy, can be fed after endoscopy, treated with oral acid suppression once daily, and can often be safely discharged home within <24 hours.[1]
- High-dose **proton pump inhibitor** infusion decreases rebleeding in patients with high-risk stigmata on endoscopy.
  - Pre-endoscopic administration of a PPI is cost-effective and decreases the proportion of patients that will have high-risk stigmata on endoscopy.
  - The optimal route of administration and dose are not clearly established, but it is reasonable to use high-dose intravenous PPI (80 mg bolus followed by 8 mg/h) for clinically high-risk patients.[1]
  - Approximately 80% of rebleeding from high-risk peptic ulcers occurs in the first 72 hours after endoscopic hemostasis, and high-risk ulcers generally evolve into a low-risk appearance over the first 72 hours. **Therefore, it is recommended that patients with high-risk stigmata remain hospitalized and be treated with high-dose intravenous PPI for a full 72 hours after endoscopic hemostasis.**[10]
  - Of note, histamine type-2 receptor antagonists are not recommended for the acute management of upper GI bleeding due to a lack of benefit.
- **Eradication of *Helicobacter pylori*** (either immediately or during follow-up) decreases the rate of rebleeding in patients with PUD. Acute bleeding increases the rate of false-negative rapid urease testing, and a negative result requires later confirmation or an alternative method of testing. Eradication should be confirmed after treatment.[2]
- Aspirin or other NSAID use should be stopped if possible after an NSAID-induced bleeding ulcer.
  - Switching an NSAID to a selective cycloxygenase-2 (COX-2) inhibitor (with concurrent PPI) is of lower rebleeding risk as long as there is no cardiovascular contraindication.[1]
  - In patients who require aspirin for cardiovascular protection, the risk of a cardiovascular complication begins to significantly increase within 7–10 days off aspirin; therefore, aspirin should be resumed as soon as possible after hemostasis, certainly within 7 days.[7,8] Concurrent use of a PPI reduces the risk of recurrent GI hemorrhage.[1]
  - Clopidogrel is associated with a high risk for rebleeding, significantly higher than that seen with low-dose aspirin (81 mg) plus a PPI.[1,7] Use of clopidogrel plus a PPI may decrease the antiplatelet effect of clopidogrel; however, for patients who require continuation of clopidogrel, the risk of recurrent bleeding without a PPI is felt to outweigh the potential increase in cardiovascular events.[10]
- If rebleeding after endoscopic treatment occurs, an urgent repeat endoscopy should be performed, as sustained hemostasis will be achieved in 73% of patients who will therefore avoid the need for surgery or other invasive interventions.[1]
  - Next, patients should be considered for angiography with embolization or for surgery.
  - Immediate surgical intervention is required for patients with exsanguinating bleeding or potentially for those with a high-risk lesion that the endoscopist does not feel comfortable treating.
- **Variceal hemorrhage** is the most common nonulcer cause of upper GI hemorrhage, accounting for 10–25% of upper GI bleeding.[2] In patients with cirrhosis, around 60% of initial upper GI bleeds are secondary to esophageal varices, which will stop bleeding spontaneously in over 50% due to the decreased portal pressure created by hypovolemia and splanchnic vasoconstriction.[2,11] In fact, excessive blood transfusion appears to increase the chance of rebleeding due to the negation of this effect.[12]

- **Endoscopic variceal ligation** (EVL) and **endoscopic sclerotherapy** (EST) are both effective for controlling esophageal variceal hemorrhage with cessation of bleeding after initial treatment in 80–90% of patients[11]; however, trials have shown that EVL is superior with regard to less recurrent bleeding, fewer local adverse reactions, and better survival.[13] Mortality with an acute variceal hemorrhage is 5–8% at 1 week and about 20% at 6 weeks, with up to one-third of treated patients rebleeding within 6 weeks.[11]
- A **transjugular intrahepatic portosystemic shunt** (TIPS) is placed for refractory bleeding uncontrolled by two sessions of endoscopic therapy within 24 hours.[11]
- If necessary, balloon tamponade using a Sengstaken-Blakemore tube, a Minnesota tube, or a Linton-Nachlas tube can be used as a temporizing measure until TIPS can be performed.
- **Somatostatin** and its long-acting analog **octreotide** cause splanchnic vasoconstriction and decreased portal inflow; these can be used in acute variceal hemorrhage to decrease portal and intravariceal pressure. Octreotide (50 mcg IV bolus followed by 50 mcg/h IV infusion for up to 5 days) is the usual choice because of its easy availability and should be started as soon as possible when a variceal bleed is suspected.[1,11]
- Endoscopic treatment of gastric variceal hemorrhage is somewhat less well defined; however, **gastric variceal obturation** (GVO) using adhesives or fibrin glue appears to be more effective than EST or EVL.[13] TIPS or **balloon-occluded retrograde transvenous obliteration** (BRTO) should be performed for uncontrollable hemorrhage.[13]
- Cirrhotic patients with upper GI bleeding (including nonvariceal) should be treated with
  - **Prophylactic antibiotics**, preferably prior to endoscopy, to prevent bacteremia and spontaneous bacterial peritonitis. In a patient who is tolerating oral intake, the preferred choice is norfloxacin 400 mg daily for 7 days; intravenous options include ceftriaxone 1000 mg daily for 7 days, ciprofloxacin 400 mg twice daily for 7 days, or levofloxacin 500 mg daily for 7 days.[11]
  - Addition of a **nonselective β-blocker** such as propranolol or nadolol can decrease the risk of rebleeding.[11]
  - An oral **PPI** is also recommended to decrease the risk for postbanding ulceration.[13]
  - **Liver transplant** is the only treatment that significantly improves long-term prognosis.

Treatment of Lower GI Bleeding

- Twenty to thirty percent of patients presenting with a major GI bleed will be found to have lower GI bleeding, the incidence of which increases with age.[14]
- Those with lower GI bleeding are more likely to present with normal hemoglobin, less likely to develop shock or require blood transfusion, and have a mortality ranging from 2% to 4%.[14]
- Clinical predictors of outcome are not as well defined for lower GI bleeding as compared with upper, but high-risk characteristics have been shown to include tachycardia, hypotension, syncope, a nontender abdomen, rectal bleeding on presentation, aspirin use, and more than two comorbid illnesses.[1]
- Causes of lower GI bleeding
  - **Diverticulosis** is the most common cause of lower GI bleeding; about 70–80% of these cases (including virtually all those requiring <4 units of packed RBC transfusion in a 24-hour period) stop spontaneously.[3]
  - **Angiodysplasia** is also a common cause of lower GI bleeding, especially in those patients >65 years of age.
  - **Ischemic colitis** generally affects the watershed areas of the colon (splenic flexure and rectosigmoid junction), and patients usually have underlying cardiovascular disease; most improve with conservative management.
- Occasionally, upper endoscopy may be required to evaluate for an upper GI source of bleeding, as 10–15% of patients with severe hematochezia (usually associated with hemodynamic compromise) will have an upper source.[1] After an upper GI source has

been ruled out, **colonoscopy** has a diagnostic yield ranging from 45 to 90% and offers the potential for therapeutic interventions such as thermal coagulation, epinephrine injection, and/or endoscopic clip placement, which can achieve hemostasis in 50–100% of patients undergoing early colonoscopy.[1,14]

- Appropriate timing for colonoscopy in acute lower GI bleeding is somewhat unclear, but most recommend urgent colonoscopy within 8–24 hours of presentation with severe hematochezia.[14] Colon preparation is recommended, usually with a polyethylene glycol–based solution; there is no evidence that rapid bowel preparation reactivates or increases the rate of bleeding.
- **Radionuclide imaging** (tagged RBC study) is a noninvasive option that can detect active bleeding at a rate as low as 0.04 mL/min.[1] Bleeding is localized only to an area of the abdomen rather than to an anatomic part of the bowel. False-positive results can occur with rapid transit of intraluminal blood when radiolabeled blood is detected in the colon even though it originated in the upper GI tract.
- **CT angiography** can detect bleeding of 0.3–0.5 mL/min with 85% sensitivity. This modality is widely available, fast, and minimally invasive, but it requires intravenous contrast and has no therapeutic capacity. Its role in evaluation of acute GI bleeding is still being determined, but it has replaced the nuclear tagged red blood cell scan at some centers.[14]
- **Mesenteric angiography** is most likely to detect a bleeding site when the rate of active bleeding is at least 0.5 mL/min.[1] Anatomic localization of the bleed is very accurate, but sensitivity is variable. Often radionuclide imaging is obtained prior to angiography to localize the bleed, but this delay can also prevent obtaining a positive angiogram if the bleeding stops. Angiography does not require bowel prep and can allow therapeutic intervention via superselective transcatheter embolization. Colonoscopy has a higher diagnostic yield and lower rate of complications. **Angiography is reserved for patients with massive, ongoing bleeding where endoscopy is not feasible or for those with persistent and/or recurrent hematochezia with a source not apparent on endoscopy.**
- Despite lower GI evaluation, a bleeding site may not be identified. An upper **endoscopy with push enteroscopy**, which allows visualization of the proximal jejunum approximately 50–150 cm beyond the ligament of Treitz, can be considered and identifies a potential bleeding site in about 50% of patients.[1] Up to 15% of these patients with an initially suspected lower GI bleed will prove to have a bleeding site in the upper GI tract.[1]
- **Capsule endoscopy** is more sensitive than other methods for the diagnosis of a small bowel source of bleeding and is generally the next step following nondiagnostic upper and lower endoscopies. It is a noninvasive test and allows examination of the entire small bowel, but no tissue sampling or therapeutic intervention is possible. If a lesion is seen in the proximal jejunum, push enteroscopy can then be performed.
- **Small bowel follow-through** may detect intraluminal lesions. **Small bowel enteroclysis** may have an increased diagnostic yield over standard small bowel follow-through and can be performed in conjunction with computed tomography and magnetic resonance imaging. Its role may be in settings where capsule endoscopy and enteroscopy are unavailable or contraindicated. However, barium studies are not recommended in acute bleeding because residual barium in the GI tract makes subsequent endoscopy or angiography difficult to perform.
- Nuclear scanning for Meckel diverticulum should be considered in younger patients. Deep enteroscopy of the jejunum or ileum can be performed via the oral or rectal route with a double-balloon endoscope, single-balloon system, or a spiral overtube using no balloon. Interventions are also possible using this method, but risk of major complications is approximately 1%.[1]
- Intractable bleeding may require surgical intervention. Morbidity and mortality are reduced if the site of blood loss has been identified preoperatively. It is helpful to consult surgical colleagues early on if this is a possibility.

REFERENCES

1. Savides TJ, Jensen DM. Gastrointestinal Bleeding. In: Feldman M, Friedman LS, Brandt LJ, eds. *Sleisenger and Fordtran's Gastrointestinal and Liver Disease*. 10th ed. Philadelphia: Saunders/Elsevier, 2016:297–335.
2. Cappell MS, Friedel D. Initial management of acute upper gastrointestinal bleeding: from initial evaluation up to gastrointestinal endoscopy. *Med Clin North Am* 2008;92:491–509.
3. Zuccaro G. Management of the adult patient with acute lower gastrointestinal bleeding. *Am J Gastroenterol* 2008;93:1202–8.
4. Alijebreen AM, Fallone CA, Barkun AN. Nasogastric aspirate predicts high-risk endoscopic lesions in patients with acute upper-GI bleeding. *Gastrointest Endosc* 2004;59:172–8.
5. Huang ES, Karsan S, Kanwal F, et al. Impact of nasogastric lavage on outcomes in acute GI bleeding. *Gastrointest Endosc* 2011;74:971–80.
6. Singer AJ, Richman PB, Kowalska A, Thode HC Jr. Comparison of patient and practitioner assessments of pain from commonly performed emergency department procedures. *Ann Emerg Med* 1999;33:652–8.
7. Barkun AN, Bardou M, Kuipers EJ, et al. International consensus recommendations on the management of patients with nonvariceal upper gastrointestinal bleeding. *Ann Intern Med* 2010;152:101–13.
8. Laine L, Jensen DM. Management of patients with ulcer bleeding. *Am J Gastroenterol* 2012;107:345–60.
9. Hwang JH, Fisher DA, Ben-Menachem T, et al. The role of endoscopy in the management of acute non-variceal upper GI bleeding. *Gastrointest Endosc* 2012;75:1132–8.
10. Greenspoon J, Barkun A, Bardou M. Management of patients with nonvariceal upper gastrointestinal bleeding. *Clin Gastroenterol Hepatol* 2012;10:234–9.
11. Shah VH, Kamath PS. Portal Hypertension and Variceal Bleeding. Gastrointestinal Bleeding. In: Feldman M, Friedman LS, Brandt LJ, eds. *Sleisenger and Fordtran's Gastrointestinal and Liver Disease*. 10th ed. Philadelphia: Saunders/Elsevier, 2016:1524–52.
12. Villanueva C, Colomo A, Bosch A, et al. Transfusion strategies for acute upper gastrointestinal bleeding. *N Engl J Med* 2013;368:11–21.
13. Hwang JH, Shergill AK, Acosta RD, et al. The role of endoscopy in the management of variceal hemorrhage. *Gastrointest Endosc* 2014;80:221–7.
14. Pasha SF, Shergill A, Acosta RD, et al. The role of endoscopy in the patient with lower GI bleeding. *Gastrointest Endosc* 2014;79(6):875–85.

Approach to Abdominal Pain

15

Surachai Amornsawadwattana

GENERAL PRINCIPLES

- Abdominal pain is one of the most common complaints and is the most common GI symptom for outpatient clinic visits in the United States in 2009.[1]
- It presents in many settings and to most clinical specialists. General internists are often called upon to evaluate patients with abdominal pain and determine the seriousness of the problem—in particular, whether or not the situation is emergent and/or if a surgical consultation is required.
- Diagnosis may be especially challenging in children, immunocompromised hosts, the elderly, those who are pregnant or obese, and patients with a history of chronic abdominal pain.
- Because there are literally hundreds of disorders that can result in the perception of pain in the abdomen, an orderly approach is critical to avoid unnecessary testing and potentially harmful delays in diagnosis.
- Possible diagnoses range from trivial to life threatening. The latter conditions add to the complexity and the possibility of bad outcomes with misdiagnosis. Many organ systems and disease mechanisms can be involved.
- The time-honored approach to the differential relies on location (Fig. 15-1; Table 15-1).
- While effective, this approach may overlook some anatomic structures such as the skin/abdominal wall (e.g., herpes zoster, rectus sheath hematoma), vasculature (e.g., aortic aneurysm/dissection), and the retroperitoneal area (e.g., retroperitoneal fibrosis, psoas abscess).
- Additionally, certain mechanisms of disease, especially those that are more diffuse or systemic in nature, may be missed, including toxic, metabolic, allergic, autoimmune, and psychiatric. Any approach may neglect pain originating outside of but referred to the abdomen (e.g., myocardial ischemia/infarction, pneumonia, pulmonary embolism).
- No single approach will be clearly the most effective in every patient; therefore, **systematic thoroughness and identification of the surgical abdomen** are ultimately the keys to diagnostic management.
- Table 15-2 lists some important items on the differential diagnosis of abdominal pain.

DIAGNOSIS

Clinical Presentation

History

The two most important mechanisms of pain are parietal pain and visceral pain (Table 15-3).

- **Parietal (somatic) pain** is caused by irritation of the parietal peritoneum, which may be produced by inflammation of an adjacent organ. The presence of blood, stool, or gastric contents against the peritoneum also causes parietal pain. It is aching to sharp in character, often steady, and well localized directly over the inflamed area.

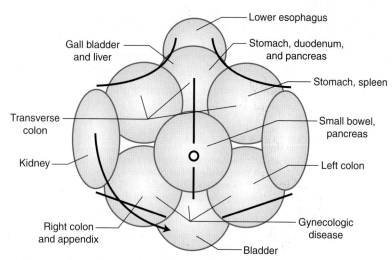

FIGURE 15-1 Anatomic approach to abdominal pain.

- **Visceral pain** is due to noxious stimuli to the visceral organs and has such causes as traction on the peritoneum, distention of a hollow viscus, or muscular contraction, often against an obstructed lumen. It is usually dull in nature, vaguely localized, and intermittent (colicky), but it may also be steady (e.g., biliary "colic"). Seemingly odd localization/referral of pain is readily explained by the particular spinal nerve involved.

TABLE 15-1	ORGAN INVOLVEMENT AND PERCEIVED LOCATION OF PAIN
Organ	**Perceived Location of Pain**
Esophagus	Chest, epigastrium
Stomach	Epigastrium, chest, left upper quadrant
Small intestine	Periumbilical region
Colon	Lower abdomen
Gallbladder	Right upper quadrant or epigastric, radiation to right scapula or shoulder
Liver	Right upper quadrant
Kidney or ureter	Costovertebral angle, flank, radiation to groin
Bladder	Suprapubic region
Aorta	Midback region
Spleen	Left upper quadrant or epigastric, radiation to left shoulder
Pancreas	Epigastric, radiation to the back
Colonic diverticula	Typically left lower quadrant
Ovaries	Lower quadrants

TABLE 15-2 ABBREVIATED DIFFERENTIAL DIAGNOSIS OF ABDOMINAL PAIN

Vascular/Ischemic
Ruptured aortic aneurysm/dissection
Ruptured ectopic pregnancy
Mesenteric ischemia
Splenic infarction
Sickle cell disease

Inflammatory/Infectious
Peptic ulcer disease
Gastroesophageal reflux disease
Hepatitis
Cholecystitis/gallstones
Acute cholangitis
Pancreatitis/psuedocyst
Appendicitis
Acute gastroenteritis
Acute colitis
Chronic parasitic infections
Whipple disease
Diverticulitis
Inflammatory bowel disease
Spontaneous bacterial peritonitis
Cystitis
Pyelonephritis
Pelvic inflammatory disease

Traumatic/Toxic
Abdominal organ rupture/hemorrhage
Abdominal wall muscular strain/tear/hematoma
Lead and arsenic poisoning
Spider and scorpion envenomation
Ethanol
Narcotic withdrawal

Allergic/Autoimmune
Sprue
Eosinophilic gastroenteritis
C1 esterase inhibitor deficiency
Food allergies
Systemic lupus erythematosus
Vasculitis

Metabolic
Diabetic ketoacidosis
Uremia
Porphyria
Lactose intolerance

Idiopathic/Iatrogenic
Irritable bowel syndrome
Other GI functional disorders
Amyloidosis
Sarcoidosis
Endometriosis
Retroperitoneal fibrosis
Perforation secondary to endoscopic procedures

Neoplastic
Gastric cancer
Colon cancer
Hepatocellular carcinoma
Pancreatic cancer
Renal cell carcinoma
Biliary cancer
Gynecologic cancer
Uterine fibroids
Prostate cancer
Lymphoma

Congenital/Genetic
Familial Mediterranean fever
Porphyria
Sickle cell disease

Drugs/Degenerative
Nonsteroidal anti-inflammatory drugs
Antibiotics
Iron

Endocrinologic
Diabetic ketoacidosis
Addison disease

Psychiatric/Psychosocial
Somatization disorders
Domestic violence
Sexual abuse

Mechanical
Small or large bowel obstruction
Intestinal hernia
Volvulus
Biliary obstruction
Ureteral obstruction/nephrolithiasis
Intussusception

Neurologic
Herpes zoster
Tabes dorsalis

Other
Thoracic disorders (referred)
Testicular torsion (referred)
Radiculopathy
Constipation
Menstrual cramps
Mittelschmerz
Ovarian cyst

TABLE 15-3 CHARACTERISTICS OF PARIETAL AND VISCERAL PAIN

	Parietal Pain	Visceral Pain
Localization	Well localized and lateralizing	Often midline or diffuse
Character	Constant, worse with movement or coughing	Often dull, colicky, or intermittent but may be constant
Associated symptoms	Pain with bed shaking	Autonomic symptoms such as nausea, vomiting, diaphoresis, pallor
Exam findings	Involuntary and voluntary guarding; abdominal rigidity	Voluntary guarding, soft abdomen

- Referred pain is characterized by pain that is felt distant to affected organs. For example, pathologies irritating right hemidiaphram may produce referred pain to the right shoulder. Therefore, obtaining information in regard to referred pain would help to localize the diseased organ.
- In addition, the onset of pain can usually indicate the severity of diseases and determine the urgency/emergency of evaluation.
  - Pain that begins abruptly suggests possible intra-abdominal catastrophe, including ruptured abdominal vasculature, acute mesenteric ischemia/infarction, or perforated viscus.
  - Pain that develops rapidly over minutes suggests inflammation or obstruction of a viscus. Gradual onset over a few hours also suggests inflammation.
  - Pain from duodenal ulcer often improves with eating or antacids. On the other hand, pain from gastric ulcer may worsen after eating.
- Hematemesis, hematochezia, melena, obstipation, hematuria, and fever may further focus the diagnostic evaluation.
- Always take a menstrual history in women of childbearing age. **Do not miss an ectopic pregnancy or other obstetric emergency.**

Physical Examination
- The presence of tachycardia or orthostatic hypotension suggests significant volume depletion and should prompt an immediate resuscitation and search for the underlying cause (hemorrhage, vomiting, diarrhea, and/or third spacing). Tachycardia may be the only sign of impending hemodynamic collapse in a patient with a vascular catastrophe. Fever suggests an inflammatory process, often infectious.
- Patients with peritonitis will often lie very still, whereas those with renal colic will often writhe in bed.
- Jaundice usually indicates pathologies of hepatobiliary tract.
- Skin lesions can sometimes be crucial clues to diagnose certain diseases such as inflammatory bowel disease, Henoch-Schönlein purpura, porphyria, or autoimmune disorders.
- Palpable lymph node(s) may suggest underlying malignancies.
- **Inspect** the abdomen for surgical scars, distention, bulging flanks, hernias, or other obvious abnormalities. The entire abdomen should be visualized, from just above the lower costal margins to thighs.
- **Auscultate** for the presence and quality of bowel sounds.
  - Listen for at least several minutes before presuming that bowel sounds are **absent**, which suggests ileus or peritonitis.

- High-pitched **tinkling** bowel sounds are said to be indicative of intestinal fluid and air under tension in a dilated bowel.
- High-pitched **rushing** bowel sounds with abdominal cramps are reportedly due to intestinal obstruction.
- The sensitivity and specificity of these findings for intra-abdominal pathology is probably quite low. Serious abdominal problems may exist in spite of the presence "normal active bowel sounds."
- Arterial bruits may be heard. Gentle pressure with the stethoscope during auscultation may allow for assessment of tenderness without alarming the patient.
- **Percussion and palpation** should begin furthest from the area of reported pain.
  - **Peritoneal inflammation** may be determined by light percussion on the abdomen, gently shaking the bed, or asking the patient to cough. It may be helpful to ask the patient to point to where the pain is worst.
  - Lightly percuss all four quadrants. If the patient can tolerate it, tap out the size of the liver. If indicated, percuss for shifting dullness.
  - Palpation should be very gentle at first and then increased as the patient tolerates. Observe the patient closely while doing so. It may be necessary to help the patient to relax and thereby decrease voluntary guarding. If true **involuntary guarding** is present, the abdominal musculature will stay in spasm throughout deep breathing with gentle palpation.
  - **Rebound tenderness** is less specific for peritoneal inflammation, whereas involuntary guarding and rigidity are more specific. The traditional assessment of rebound tenderness may also be very painful (and generally unnecessary) for patients with peritonitis.
  - Masses, organomegaly, and aortic pulsations/size should be noted.
  - **Ruptured abdominal aortic aneurysm** must be immediately considered in patients with **abdominal/back pain, a pulsatile abdominal mass, and hypotension**.
  - If ascites is suspected, assess for a fluid wave as well.
- Be sure to examine for the presence of hernias.
- All patients with acute abdominal pain must have a **rectal and pelvic** (women) exam performed.
- Severe pain out of proportion to abdominal findings suggests mesenteric ischemia.
- A recent systematic review concluded that findings of abdominal pain, fever, rebound tenderness, and midabdominal pain migrating to the right lower quadrant in children are associated with appendicitis.[2] A lack of leukocytosis is associated with its absence. These findings seem to be most useful in combination but are insufficient to establish the diagnosis with certainty. They do, however, suggest when further evaluation is indicated.
- Similarly in adults, individual clinical features are not particularly discriminatory but may be very useful in combination, particularly laboratory markers of inflammation (neutrophil count and CRP level), findings of peritonitis (rigidity and percussion/rebound tenderness), and a history of pain migration.[3]

Diagnostic Testing

Laboratories

As most patients with acute abdominal pain can be diagnosed with a careful history and physical exam, further diagnostic evaluation should be targeted to the specific clinical scenario. **Always obtain a urine β-hCG in women of childbearing age**. Excessive undirected testing increases the costs and may cause unnecessary delays in diagnosis and treatment. Some basic tests to consider include

- Complete blood count
- Basic metabolic panel

- Hepatic function panel
- Amylase/lipase
- Urinalysis

Imaging
- Not all patients with acute abdominal pain require plain or upright films of the abdomen. However, abdominal radiographs are useful for diagnosing a perforated viscus (identified as free air), foreign bodies, ileus, or bowel obstruction. If there is no real suspicion, then plain films will generally be of no diagnostic value.
- Transabdominal US is useful for patients with suspected biliary tract disease, including acute cholecystitis, biliary pain, and choledocholithiasis. It is the initial test of choice for right-upper-quadrant pain. US also allows rapid diagnosis of abdominal aortic aneurysms. However, its diagnostic yield also depends on the experience of the ultrasonographers. Recently, a study supported the use of ultrasound as an initial imaging in patients with suspected nephrolithiasis without increasing risks of adverse events.[4]
- Abdominal CT is a powerful imaging tool and is very sensitive for identifying a perforated viscus, bowel obstruction, intra-abdominal abscess, appendicitis, ruptured aortic aneurysm, pancreatitis, and diverticulitis. It also can alter intial diagnosis and influence management decisions.[5] However, care must be used in selecting patients for abdominal CT. The test is time consuming and costly and may unnecessarily delay diagnosis and treatment, especially in patients who require urgent surgery. In addition, CT requires higher doses of radiation and may increase cancer risks in the future.[6] So, it should be used judiciously.
- MRI can be used safely to evaluate abdominal pain in pregnant patients since there is no radiation exposure to a fetus. It also has high accuracy to diagnose acute appendicitis and other conditions.[7] Still, it may be challenging to obtain MRI during urgent/emergent evaluation.

TREATMENT

The appropriate treatment of the many causes of abdominal pain is well beyond the scope of this chapter. Although there are growing evidences that patients with uncomplicated acute appendicitis can be treated with only antibiotic therapy, this treatment should be carefully evaluated and offered to the appropriate patients.[8] Keep in mind that appendectomy is still the gold standard. Most patients will very frequently want symptomatic treatment of their pain. Historically, this has been strongly discouraged on the grounds that opiates may mask important symptoms and signs and thereby inhibit a rapid and accurate diagnosis. There is no convincing objective evidence for this assumption, and opioid analgesics are probably indicated for patient comfort once an initial history and physical exam have been done.[9]

REFERENCES

1. Peery AF, Dellon ES, Lund J, et al. Burden of gastrointestinal disease in the United States: 2012 update. *Gastroenterology* 2012;143:1179–87, e1–3.
2. Bundy DG, Byerley JS, Liles EA, et al. Does this child have appendicitis? *JAMA* 2007;298:438–51.
3. Andersson RE. Meta-analysis of the clinical and laboratory diagnosis of appendicitis. *Br J Surg* 2004;91:28–37.
4. Smith-Bindman R, Aubin C, Bailitz J, et al. Ultrasonography versus computed tomography for suspected nephrolithiasis. *New Engl J Med* 2014;371:1100–10.
5. Abujudeh HH, Kaewlai R, McMahon PM, et al. Abdominopelvic CT increases diagnostic certainty and guides management decisions: a prospective investigation of 584 patients in a large academic medical center. *AJR Am J Roentgenol* 2011;196:238–43.

6. Brenner DJ, Hall EJ. Computed tomography—an increasing source of radiation exposure. *New Engl J Med* 2007;357:2277–84.
7. Spalluto LB, Woodfield CA, DeBenedectis CM, Lazarus E. MR imaging evaluation of abdominal pain during pregnancy: appendicitis and other nonobstetric causes. *Radiographics* 2012;32:317–34.
8. Varadhan KK, Neal KR, Lobo DN. Safety and efficacy of antibiotics compared with appendicectomy for treatment of uncomplicated acute appendicitis: meta-analysis of randomised controlled trials. *BMJ* 2012;344:e2156.
9. Ranji SR, Goldman LE, Simel DL, Shojania KG. Do opiates affect the clinical evaluation of patients with acute abdominal pain? *JAMA* 2006;296:1764–74.

Approach to Abnormal Liver Enzymes

James Matthew Freer

GENERAL PRINCIPLES

- Alkaline phosphatase and the transaminases aspartate aminotransferase (AST) and alanine aminotransferase (ALT) are commonly called liver function tests (LFTs), although the AST and ALT are actually indicators more of inflammation than of dysfunction. ALT is more specific than AST for liver damage.
- Albumin, bilirubin, and the prothrombin time (PT) are better tests for the synthetic function of the liver and are often included in panels of "liver function tests"; however, these tests are not specific to liver disease. Abnormalities in LFTs can be classified as being reflective of either of the following:
  - **Hepatocellular injury**, which is characterized by a predominant elevation in AST, ALT and, to a lesser extent, bilirubin. Tests of liver synthetic function may be normal or abnormal.
  - **Cholestatic disorders**: characterized by a predominant elevation in alkaline phosphatase and possibly bilirubin, with lesser elevations in the transaminases.
  - This distinction is useful in the workup of patients with abnormalities in LFTs, though significant overlap occurs between the two patterns.
- **Nonhepatic causes** may result in elevations of many of the hepatic enzymes.
  - Alkaline phosphatase may be elevated in diseases of the bone (fractures, metastatic lesions, Paget disease, hyperparathyroidism), from intestinal disorders, or from the placenta (pregnancy, uterine disease). Alkaline phosphatase is also appropriately elevated in times of growth and increased bone turnover (i.e., adolescence). Finally, patients with blood types O or B may have elevated alkaline phosphatase after a fatty meal due to an influx of intestinal alkaline phosphatase, and there are rare reports of familial elevation of alkaline phosphatase due to a similar mechanism.[1]
  - AST may be elevated in myocardial infarction or other disorders involving muscle damage (where creatine kinase and aldolase may also be elevated), thyroidal illness, Addison disease, anorexia, and celiac sprue.
  - Isolated hyperbilirubinemia should be classified as either predominantly direct or predominantly indirect hyperbilirubinemia.
    - Direct hyperbilirubinemia can be caused by an obstruction in the biliary tree as well as Dubin-Johnson and Rotor syndromes.
    - Indirect hyperbilirubinemia is caused by hemolysis, ineffective hematopoiesis, resorption of hematomas, Gilbert disease, and Crigler-Najjar syndrome.
  - An elevation in the PT and international normalized ratio (INR) can be seen in liver disease, nutritional deficiency or malabsorption of vitamin K, warfarin administration, or factor VII deficiency or inhibitor.
- A variety of **hepatic** and **biliary** disorders (Tables 16-1 and 16-2) cause elevation of one or more liver enzymes. These are discussed further below. Other **distinctive patterns** of liver enzyme elevation are noted below:

TABLE 16-1 DIFFERENTIAL DIAGNOSIS OF HEPATOCELLULAR PATTERNS OF INJURY

Viral hepatitis	Muscle disorders
Medication induced (especially acetaminophen)	Celiac sprue
Toxins (e.g., alcohol)	Congestive hepatopathy
Wilson disease	Autoimmune hepatitis
Hemochromatosis	Various bacterial infections
α_1-Antitrypsin deficiency	Thyroid disease
Nonalcoholic steatohepatitis	Adrenal insufficiency
Ischemia (i.e., "shock liver")	Venoocclusive disease
Anorexia	

- AST:ALT >2 is typical of alcoholic injury, whereas ALT > AST is typical of viral injury and nonalcoholic steatohepatitis (NASH). In one study, >90% of patients with AST:ALT >2 had alcoholic liver disease, and this increased to 96% when the ratio was >3:1.[2]
- Transaminases in the thousands are generally seen with toxic, ischemic, or viral causes. Alcoholic hepatitis rarely causes transaminase elevations greater than several hundred.[2]

DIAGNOSIS

Clinical Presentation

History
- Symptoms of malaise, jaundice, nausea, vomiting, abdominal pain, and weight loss are nonspecific but may aid in estimating the onset of disease.
- **Hemochromatosis** may be associated with diabetes, skin bronzing, congestive heart failure, arthritis, and hypogonadism.
- **Wilson disease** may present with movement disorders and psychiatric symptoms.
- **α_1-Antitrypsin deficiency** is associated with early emphysema (emphysema in nonsmokers should raise suspicion).

TABLE 16-2 DIFFERENTIAL DIAGNOSIS OF CHOLESTATIC PATTERNS OF INJURY

Primary biliary cirrhosis	Bone disorders
Primary sclerosing cholangitis	Various intestinal disorders
Total parenteral nutrition (TPN)	Pregnancy
Sepsis and postoperative states	Disorders of the placenta
Infiltrating malignancy (e.g., lymphoma)	Granulomatous hepatitis (e.g., sarcoidosis)
Extrahepatic obstruction (e.g., choledocholithiasis, malignancy, stricture)	Medication induced
	Other infiltrative disorders (e.g., amyloidosis)

- **Venoocclusive disease** of the liver is associated with several hematologic disorders and the use of oral contraceptives.
- Exposure to blood products (especially remote), IV drug abuse, tattoos, or close family members with hepatitis should raise suspicion of **viral hepatitis**. Raw oysters and other contaminated foods may spread hepatitis A. The travel history may be revealing.
- **Autoimmune hepatitis (AIH)** is most common in women <40 years of age and may be associated with thyroid disease, rheumatoid arthritis, and other autoimmune disorders.
- **Primary biliary cirrhosis** (PBC) affects mostly middle-aged women and may be associated with several autoimmune disorders. **Primary sclerosing cholangitis** is seen more commonly in men and is strongly associated with ulcerative colitis. Both disorders present with a cholestatic picture.
- **Ischemic hepatitis** is usually seen in the setting of a critical illness such as respiratory or heart failure. The vast majority will also have some degree of acute kidney injury. Transaminases are usually elevated in the thousands, and the INR can also be markedly elevated.[3]
- **Nonalcoholic steatohepatitis** is commonly seen in obese patients, diabetics, and patients with hypertriglyceridemia.
- **Medication use and toxins** are important causes of liver enzyme abnormalities (Table 16-3). Perform a thorough history of alcohol and medication use (including herbal preparations) and work and environmental exposures. Always consider acetaminophen toxicity, especially in alcoholics, who may suffer toxicity at levels that would otherwise be tolerable. Do not assume that liver disease in an alcoholic is due to alcohol alone.
- **Family history** should include inquiries into Wilson disease, α_1-antitrypsin deficiency, and hemochromatosis.

Physical Examination
- Look for **stigmata of chronic liver disease** such as spider telangiectasias, palmar erythema, testicular atrophy, and gynecomastia. Jaundice and ascites may be seen in acute or chronic liver disease.
- Extrahepatic manifestations of viral hepatitis may include **arthritis** or a **skin rash**.
- Assess for the copper discoloration of Descemet membrane from Wilson disease (**Kayser-Fleischer rings**) and the **bronze discoloration of the skin** from hemochromatosis.
- Volume overload and severe congestive heart failure, especially with severe tricuspid regurgitation, may result in a **congestive hepatopathy**. Elevated jugular venous pressure and a pulsatile and markedly enlarged liver are suggestive findings.
- Confusion, hyperreflexia, and asterixis can be seen in patients with **portosystemic encephalopathy**.

Diagnostic Testing
Diagnostic workup of abnormal liver enzymes will be discussed in the context of predominately hepatocellular pattern followed by predominately cholestatic pattern.

Predominantly Hepatocellular Pattern
- First, repeat the transaminases to confirm elevation. If the repeat assay is normal, no further evaluation is indicated. Controversy exists over the true upper limit of normal (ULN) for ALT, as various laboratories report different reference ranges. One paper concluded that using a lower cutoff for the ALT ULN would classify approximately 30% of the US population as having an abnormal value, resulting in unnecessary testing and increased cost as the majority of these patients either would have a negative workup for causes of chronic liver disease or would have NASH.[4]
- If only AST is elevated, alcohol abuse or a nonhepatic cause of the AST elevation should be considered. If a medication is suspected as the culprit, weigh the benefits of continuing the drug against the risks of liver injury (Table 16-3). In either case, serial lab monitoring should ensue.

TABLE 16-3 CAUSES OF MEDICATION-INDUCED HEPATOTOXICITY (PARTIAL LIST)

Acetaminophen

Angiotensin-converting enzyme inhibitors

Allopurinol

Amiodarone

Amoxicillin–clavulanic acid (cholestatic picture)

Anabolic steroids (cholestatic picture)

Angiotensin receptor blockers

Anticonvulsants (e.g., valproic acid, carbamazepine, phenytoin, phenobarbital)

Antituberculosis drugs (especially isoniazid and rifampin)

Azathioprine

Ceftriaxone (cholestatic picture)

Chlorpromazine (cholestatic picture)

Clindamycin

Clopidogrel (cholestatic picture)

Erythromycins (cholestatic picture)

Highly active antiretroviral therapy (HAART)

Herbal preparations (e.g., kava kava, germander, chaparral)

HMG-CoA reductase inhibitors (i.e., statins)

Ketoconazole

Methimazole

Methotrexate

Nitrofurantion

Nonsteroidal anti-inflammatory drugs (NSAIDs)

Oral contraceptives (cholestatic picture)

Other antidepressants (e.g., bupropion, mirtazapine, trazodone)

Phenothiazines (cholestatic picture)

Selective serotonin reuptake inhibitors (SSRIs)

Terbinafine (cholestatic picture)

Tetracyclines

Tricyclic antidepressants (cholestatic picture)

Trimethoprim–sulfamethoxazole

Verapamil

- If history and physical exam do not point to an obvious cause, then a cost-effective stepwise approach to laboratory testing and imaging may be undertaken. Alternatively, a broader battery of tests may be ordered initially if a quick diagnosis is essential. An acetaminophen level should be obtained if appropriate.

- Initial laboratory evaluation should include an acute hepatitis panel (hepatitis A IgM virus antibody [Ab], hepatitis C virus Ab, hepatitis B virus surface antigen [Ag], hepatitis B surface Ab, and hepatitis B core Ab).
  - A combination of hepatitis B surface Ag and core Ab positivity suggests chronic infection; additional testing can be undertaken to determine the degree of viral activity and replication.
  - The combination of hepatitis B surface Ab and core Ab positivity represents immunity. An isolated positive hepatitis B surface Ab indicates past immunization.
  - A positive hepatitis C Ab should prompt further testing including a viral load, viral genotyping, and possibly a liver biopsy to assess the need for antiviral therapy.
- A right-upper-quadrant ultrasound should be obtained to identify fatty liver, a biliary obstruction, or mass lesion.
- Iron and total iron-binding capacity (TIBC) should be checked as a screen for hemochromatosis. A ferritin can also be obtained but is a less specific test for hemochromatosis. The iron/TIBC equals the transferrin saturation, and a value of >45% should trigger further genetic testing and/or a liver biopsy.

• If the initial workup outlined above is unrevealing, additional tests to search for other causes may be ordered. These include the following:
  - Antitissue transglutaminase antibodies and IgA levels, or upper endoscopy (to evaluate for celiac disease)
  - Thyroid-stimulating hormone
  - Cortisol or cosyntropin stimulation test (to evaluate for adrenal insufficiency)
  - Ceruloplasmin (to assess for Wilson disease)
  - Serum protein electrophoresis or immunoglobulin (Ig) levels (nearly all patients with autoimmune hepatitis have some degree of IgG elevation; also helpful in α1-antitrypsin deficiency)[5]
  - Antinuclear antibody (ANA) titer (fairly sensitive for autoimmune hepatitis but not specific)
  - Anti–smooth muscle antibodies (less sensitive than ANA for autoimmune hepatitis though positive titers of both antibodies have a high specificity)[5]
  - α_1-antitrypsin levels
  - Additional viral serologies may be indicated as well, as Epstein-Barr virus, cytomegalovirus, and others can also cause acute viral hepatitis.
• If the above tests are unrevealing, then one may consider a liver biopsy. Note that a liver biopsy may also be indicated to confirm a specific diagnosis or to assess for disease severity in patients with one or more abnormal laboratory values listed above. For those with a negative laboratory and imaging workup, the utility of a liver biopsy may be limited, especially for asymptomatic patients with transaminase elevations <2 times the ULN. The vast majority of these patients will have biopsies that reveal steatosis or steatohepatitis, resulting in no new monitoring or management recommendations.[6,7]

Predominately Cholestatic Pattern
- This is an isolated elevation in alkaline phosphatase with or without hyperbilirubinemia.
- Obtain a β-hCG in the appropriate clinical setting to exclude **pregnancy** as a cause.
- The patient's medication list should be reviewed, as a number of drugs may cause cholestasis (Table 16-3).
- Confirm a hepatic source using γ-glutamyl transferase levels and/or 5′ nucleotidase (concomitant elevation suggests a hepatic source). Alkaline phosphatase isoenzymes may also be checked but are less readily available. If the elevation of the alkaline phosphatase is found to be from a bone source, subsequent evaluation for primary bone disorders should follow.

- If the elevation is found to be from a liver source, evaluation should include the following:
  - A right-upper-quadrant ultrasound or abdominal computed tomography to assess for liver parenchymal disease or dilated ducts. Further testing with magnetic resonance cholangiopancreatography (MRCP) or with endoscopic retrograde cholangiopancreatography (ERCP) may be necessary.
  - Antimitochondrial antibodies (AMA) to assess for PBC. AMA have a sensitivity and specificity of ~95%.[8] As many as 10% of patients may have an overlap AIH/PBC syndrome.[9]
  - Primary sclerosing cholangitis is suspected in a patient with inflammatory bowel disease and is best diagnosed by MRCP or ERCP. AMA are generally negative, though ANA and antineutrophil cytoplasmic antibodies may be present.
- If the above workup is unrevealing, a liver biopsy may be indicated, especially if the alkaline phosphatase is consistently 50% more than the ULN.

REFERENCES

1. Pratt DS, Kaplan MM. Evaluation of abnormal liver-enzyme results in asymptomatic patients. *N Engl J Med* 2000;342:1266–71.
2. Fuchs S, Bogomolski-Yahalom V, Paltiel O, Ackerman Z. Ischemic hepatitis: clinical and laboratory observations of 34 patients. *J Clin Gastroenterol* 1998;26:183–6.
3. Ruhl CE, Everhart JE. Upper limits of normal for alanine aminotransferase activity in the United States population. *Hepatology* 2012;55:447–54.
4. Czaja AJ. Diagnosis and management of autoimmune hepatitis. *Clin Liver Dis* 2015;19:57–79.
5. Sorbi D, McGill DB, Thistle JL, et al. An assessment of the role of liver biopsies in asymptomatic patients with chronic liver test abnormalities. *Am J Gastroenterol* 2000;95:3206–10.
6. Daniel S, Ben-Menachem T, Vasudevan G, et al. Prospective evaluation of unexplained chronic liver transaminase abnormalities in asymptomatic and symptomatic patients. *Am J Gastroenterol* 1999;94:3010–4.
7. Invernizzi P, Lleo A, Podda M. Interpreting serological tests in diagnosing autoimmune liver diseases. *Semin Liver Dis* 2007;27:161–72.
8. Heathcote EJ. Overlap of autoimmune hepatitis and primary biliary cirrhosis: an evaluation of a modified scoring system. *Am J Gastroenterol* 2002;97:1090–2.

V Nephrology

Approach to Acute Kidney Injury

Joshua M. Saef and Melvin Blanchard

GENERAL PRINCIPLES

- Acute kidney injury (AKI) refers to a rapid decline in glomerular filtration rate (GFR) that occurs over hours to days. It is associated with a reduced ability to excrete nitrogenous metabolic waste such as blood urea nitrogen (BUN) and creatinine.
- AKI replaces the historic term acute renal failure to highlight the concept that acute changes in renal function can have a profound impact on the patient even in the absence of overt renal failure.

Definition

The Acute Kidney Injury Network (AKIN) defines AKI as an abrupt (within 48 hours) reduction in kidney function: rise in serum creatinine (S_{Cr}) by ≥ 0.3 mg/dL, a percentage increase in S_{Cr} of $\geq 50\%$ from baseline, or documented oliguria of < 0.5 mL/kg/h for more than 6 hours.[1]

Classification

The AKIN group has also published a classification or staging system for AKI (Table 17-1).[1]

Etiology

The causes of AKI can be divided into three broad categories:

- **Prerenal azotemia**, the most common cause of renal failure in the hospital, results from the kidney's normal physiologic response to a decrease in effective perfusion of its vasculature. The causes include the following:
  - Hypovolemia
  - Heart failure
  - Decompensated cirrhosis
  - Hypotension
  - Medications such as angiotensin-converting enzyme (ACE) inhibitors, angiotensin receptor blockers, and nonsteroidal anti-inflammatory drugs (NSAIDs), through alteration of intrarenal blood flow, also contribute to prerenal azotemia.
- **Postrenal azotemia** is due to obstruction (intrinsic or extrinsic) of the urinary tract. AKI due to postrenal causes must involve both kidneys (unless the patient has only a solitary kidney or baseline poor renal function). The most common causes include the following:
  - The prostate (benign prostatic hyperplasia and prostatic carcinoma)
  - The cervix (cervical carcinoma)
  - Catheters
  - Bilateral stones
  - Retroperitoneal fibrosis
  - Neurogenic bladder

TABLE 17-1 CLASSIFICATION/STAGING OF ACUTE KIDNEY INJURY

Stage[a]	Serum Creatinine Criteria	Urine Output Criteria
1	Rise in S_{Cr} ≥0.3 mg/dL or ≥150–200% from baseline	<0.5 mL/kg/h for >6 h
2	Rise in S_{Cr} >200–300% from baseline	<0.5 mL/kg/h for >12 h
3[b]	Rise in S_{Cr} >300% from baseline or S_{Cr} ≥4 mg/dL with an acute increase of at least 0.5 mg/dL	<0.3 mL/kg/h for >24 h or anuria >12 h

[a]Only one criterion has to be fulfilled to qualify for a stage.
[b]Individuals who receive renal replacement therapy are considered to have met the criteria for stage 3 irrespective of the other criteria.
S_{Cr}, serum creatinine.
Adapted from Mehta RL, Kellum JA, Shah SV, et al. Acute Kidney Injury Network: report of an initiative to improve outcomes in acute kidney injury. *Crit Care* 2007;11:R31.

- **Intrinsic azotemia** is characterized by disease affecting the renal parenchyma itself, the causes of which can be divided into the portion of the kidney affected.
  - **Vasculature:** Vessel at all levels of the renal vascular system may cause AKI. Large vessels (atheroembolic disease, renal artery stenosis, renal artery dissection, aortic diseases), small vessels (vasculitides, thrombotic angiopathies), and veins (renal vein thrombosis) may all cause AKI.
  - **Tubules:** Tubular injury may be due to ischemia or toxins. Renal hypoperfusion may cause prerenal azotemia; when prolonged or severe, it can cause acute tubular necrosis (ATN). ATN may also result from medications (e.g., aminoglycosides, radiographic contrast), or it may be due to endogenous (e.g., crystals, myoglobin, hemoglobin) or exogenous (radiographic contrast) toxins. Urinary sediment will contain coarse granular casts or large muddy-brown casts.
  - **Interstitium:** Acute interstitial nephritis (AIN) is seen most commonly in the setting of an allergic reaction to medications, but it can also result from autoimmune disease and infection. Common drug causes include the semisynthetic penicillins (methicillin and nafcillin) and sulfa drugs, but any medication can be a culprit. Onset may occur days after drug initiation or after months of use. This condition is often associated with a skin rash, peripheral eosinophilia, and eosinophiluria.
  - **Glomeruli:** Acute glomerulonephritis is relatively uncommon but is characterized by hematuria, oliguria, and hypertension (HTN). Examination of the urine sediment will usually reveal red blood cell (RBC) casts and dysmorphic RBCs.[2]

DIAGNOSIS

Clinical Presentation

It is important to determine whether a patient with an abnormal creatinine truly has AKI or whether the abnormality is longer standing (i.e., chronic). Some clues to differentiating acute from chronic kidney disease include the following:

- **Previous creatinine:** If prior serum creatinine measurements are similar, then the patient likely has chronic rather than acute kidney disease.

- **Renal size:** Patients with chronic renal failure tend to have bilaterally shrunken kidneys, whereas renal size is usually normal in acute failure. Some exceptions are diabetic nephropathy, polycystic kidney disease, myeloma kidney, amyloidosis, and nephropathy due to human immunodeficiency virus (HIV), in which renal size is normal or increased.
- **Anemia:** Patients with a GFR <30 mL/min and chronic kidney disease tend to be anemic secondary to decreased erythropoietin production. One exception is chronic renal failure from autosomal dominant polycystic kidney disease, in which patients are typically **not** anemic.
- **Renal osteodystrophy:** Patients with prolonged chronic renal failure may have evidence of renal osteodystrophy. The clavicles and wrists are common sites at which changes are seen.

History

The history can also provide important clues to the likely cause of AKI. Key elements of the history include the following:

- Fluid balance: dehydration from vomiting, diarrhea, or poor oral intake. A chart review to assess for hypotension, inputs (e.g., oral or IV fluids) and outputs (e.g., gastrointestinal, urinary), as well as weight change can be helpful.
- Symptoms of volume depletion: orthostasis
- Poorly controlled diabetes mellitus, especially those who are insulin dependent, may have glycosuria and osmotic diuresis.
- Recent trauma: crush injuries (rhabdomyolysis)
- Recent infections: pharyngitis (poststreptococcal glomerulonephritis), upper respiratory infection (IgA nephropathy), sinusitis (Granulomatosis with polyangiitis), and bloody diarrhea (hemolytic uremic syndrome)
- Hemoptysis: lupus, granulomatosis with polyangiitis, Goodpasture's, and endocarditis
- Urine appearance: hematuria (glomerulonephritis or nephrolithiasis)
- Rashes: allergic, interstitial nephritis, vasculitis, or autoimmune
- Medication history: allergic interstitial nephritis, NSAID nephropathy, and nephrotoxins. Anticholinergics (e.g., tricyclic antidepressants [TCAs]) may cause urinary retention and postrenal failure.
- Toxic ingestions (e.g., polyethylene glycol)
- Recent procedure involving the aorta or other large vessels (atheroembolic disease, ischemia)
- Recent IV contrast administration
- Social history: IV drug abuse (HIV, hepatitis, endocarditis)
- Medical history: chronic kidney disease and AKI are closely interconnected. Patients with chronic kidney disease are more prone to AKI than the general population.[3]

Physical Examination

- Determine whether the patient is oliguric (0.5 mL/kg/h for more than 6 hours) or anuric (<100 mL/d). Anuria should raise the possibility of obstructive uropathy, occlusion of the renal arteries, or severe ATN/cortical necrosis.
- Volume status is critical for both diagnosis (to identify a prerenal state) and fluid management. Assess volume status with orthostatic vital signs, examination of jugular venous pressure, skin turgor, moistness of mucous membranes, and axillary sweat.
- Examine the fundi in diabetics with chronic renal insufficiency. It is unusual to develop diabetic nephropathy without retinopathy. Retinal exam may also reveal the bright-orange arteriolar changes of atheroembolic disease (Hollenhorst plaque).
- The cardiac examination may reveal a pericardial rub, indicative of uremic pericarditis. It is important to look for signs of congestive heart failure or cirrhosis as a cause of

decreased renal perfusion. Listen for systolic–diastolic abdominal bruits, which may be audible with renal artery stenosis.
- Palpate and percuss the suprapubic region for an enlarged bladder (from prostatic obstructive uropathy) and the abdomen for enlarged kidneys.
- Evaluate for musculoskeletal trauma or signs of myopathy that could be culprit in rhabdomyolysis.
- Skin exam may reveal evidence of vasculitis, lupus, livedo reticularis (from cholesterol emboli), drug rash, or peripheral stigmata of endocarditis.
- A pelvic and prostate exam may identify a source of urinary tract obstruction.
- In the neurologic examination, it is important to look for evidence of uremic encephalopathy with confusion and sometimes asterixis.

Diagnostic Testing

Laboratories
- The urinalysis (UA), including a microscopic examination of urinary sediment, is the single most important test in evaluating AKI.
  ○ The sediment in prerenal AKI tends to be acellular but may consist of hyaline casts, which are found in normal concentrated urine.
  ○ Pigmented granular and tubular cell casts are found in ATN.
  ○ Red cell casts are found in glomerular disease.
  ○ White cell casts are found in interstitial AKI.
  ○ The finding of eosinophils in urine suggests allergic interstitial or atheroembolic disease. Eosinophils are better visualized with the Hansel stain than with the Wright stain.
  ○ Urinary crystals are found with certain exposures (e.g., acyclovir, ethylene glycol) and acute uric acid nephropathy.
- Laboratory data should also include electrolytes, a complete blood count (CBC), urine electrolytes, and creatine kinase. Peripheral eosinophilia should raise the possibility of allergic interstitial nephritis or atheroembolic disease.
- Figure 17-1 is a simple algorithm that may be followed in assessing someone with AKI. This algorithm assumes that patients are not on diuretics.
  ○ The fractional excretion of sodium (FE_{Na}) is most useful in patients who have acute **oliguric** (0.5 mL/kg/h for more than 6 hours) renal failure. A FE_{Na} <1% is consistent with a prerenal state.
  ○ % FE_{Na} = [(urine Na/plasma Na)/(urine creatinine/plasma creatinine)] × 100.
  ○ If the patient is on a diuretic, the fractional excretion of urea may be substituted. A FE_{urea} <35% is indicative of prerenal azotemia.
  ○ % FE_{urea} = [(urine urea nitrogen/blood urea nitrogen)/(urine creatinine/plasma creatinine)] × 100.[4]
  ○ The serum creatinine is not a useful surrogate marker of GFR in AKI, and Cockgraft-Gault or other equations used to calculate creatinine clearance should be avoided. The creatinine in acute rapid-onset renal failure may lag far behind its estimation of renal function.[5] A creatinine that increases by 1 mg/dL/d is called an anephric rise, or roughly the amount that an average person's creatinine would increase in a noncatabolic state with a GFR of 0 mL/min. Therefore, a patient whose creatinine rises from 2 to 3 mg/dL may have a creatinine clearance of 0 mL/min.[6]

Imaging
A renal ultrasound is helpful in assessing kidney size and excluding obstruction of the urinary tract.

Diagnostic Procedures
It is important to assess for obstruction at the bladder outlet in men by placing a Foley catheter. A normal urine output does **not** exclude obstruction.

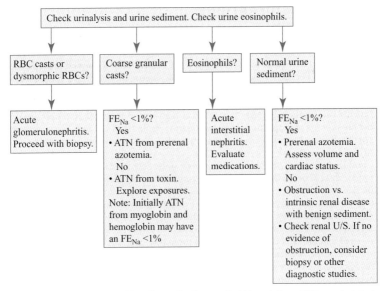

FIGURE 17-1 A simple algorithm for evaluating acute kidney injury. ATN, acute tubular necrosis.

TREATMENT

- The treatment of AKI is determined by its etiology.
- Important aspects in the management of AKI include avoidance of nephrotoxic agents; the acute treatment of hyperphosphatemia, hyperkalemia, and metabolic acidosis; and maintaining a euvolemic state.
- Furosemide to convert a patient to nonoliguric renal failure has not been shown to affect prognosis but may help with fluid management.
- Except in cases of hypotension or cardiogenic shock, dopamine has also not been shown to affect outcomes of renal function and may hold an increased risk of arrhythmias compared to other vasopressor medications.[7]
- Whenever possible, avoid administration of intravenous contrast to patients with AKI.
- One should strive to **maximize renal perfusion** as well. Avoid hypotension, and keep the patient well hydrated. Correct intravascular volume loss with preference to isotonic crystalloid intravenous fluids rather than colloids.[8] Loop diuretics are useful for management of volume overload but otherwise are not considered a treatment for AKI.[9] Remember to adjust medication doses for changing renal function.
- Since many of the causes of AKI are readily reversible, it is important to establish a prompt diagnosis and treat the previously mentioned acute complications. Renal replacement therapy (e.g., hemodialysis) is indicated in the following situations:
  ○ Hyperkalemia or acidosis is refractory to medical management.
  ○ There is evidence of volume overload (pulmonary edema).
  ○ There are symptoms of uremia (encephalopathy, pericarditis, etc.).[10]
- Renal failure from ATN is classically associated with a peak creatinine at 8–14 days, although there is wide variation. Most patients will recover adequate renal function within 6 weeks. Patients may experience a rebound, polyuric phase with the relief of an obstructive process or recovery of renal function following ATN. Close attention to electrolyte levels and fluid balance is imperative.[11]

SPECIAL CONSIDERATIONS

Additional considerations in postoperative renal failure include the following:

- Examine the intraoperative flow sheet carefully for episodes of hypotension during surgery. **Intraoperative renal hypoperfusion is the most common cause of postoperative renal failure.** Because of high vasopressin levels due to anesthesia and surgical stress, most patients will have a decreased urine output with concentrated urine for a few hours after surgery despite adequate renal blood flow and renal function.[12]
- Patients with cardiopulmonary bypass are at high risk of renal failure proportional to the duration of cardiopulmonary bypass or cross clamping of the aorta above the renal arteries. Preoperative placement of an intra-aortic balloon pump increases likelihood of AKI postoperatively.[13]
- Consider mechanical obstruction of the ureter or bladder by inadvertent ligation, hematomas, abscess, or (in the case of urologic surgery) ureteral edema.
- In patients who are immobilized in awkward positions during surgery (e.g., urologic surgery, hip arthroplasty), consider rhabdomyolysis and myoglobinuric renal failure. Approximately one-third of patients with rhabdomyolysis develop ATN. Hyperphosphatemia, hyperkalemia, hyperuricemia, and hypocalcemia out of proportion to renal failure may be clues. Tea-colored urine that is dipstick positive for blood but without RBCs on microscopy is highly suggestive of the diagnosis. Evaluate with serum myoglobin or creatine kinase. Copious IV fluids are paramount. Mannitol and urinary alkalinization have been recommended in the past but have not clearly demonstrated benefit.[14]
- Identify any history of IV dye administration in patients at high risk for dye-induced renal failure, who are those with poor renal perfusion (congestive heart failure, volume depletion), diabetes mellitus, chronic renal insufficiency, or multiple myeloma. **Contrast-induced nephropathy** will have UA and urine electrolyte changes that are usually indistinguishable from prerenal failure. Rarely, there may be a concomitant mild ATN. Initial rise in creatinine is within 48 hours of dye administration, peaking at about 3–4 days and then normalizing in 1 week. The best "treatment" is prevention by ensuring that patients at risk are well hydrated before contrast administration.[15] The role of oral *N*-acetylcysteine in preventing dye nephropathy is not well established,[16] though it may be used in patients at increased risk.[8] There is no indication for prophylactic hemodialysis in patients at risk for contrast-induced nephropathy.[17]
- Patients who have had intravascular manipulation (e.g., aortic surgeries, cardiac catheterizations) may suffer from renal failure due to cholesterol emboli or atheroembolus. Cholesterol emboli may also occur spontaneously or with anticoagulation in patients with aortic atherosclerosis. Livedo reticularis, blue toes, and bright-orange retinal arterioles may be evident. Blood eosinophil counts are often high, complements are usually low, and UA may resemble prerenal failure. Biopsy of skin lesions may be diagnostic. Classically, the loss of renal function is stepwise. Prognosis for renal recovery is dismal.[18]
- Recognize the abdominal compartment syndrome. This presents in patients with severe pelvic or abdominal trauma and in those who develop large intra-abdominal fluid collections (ruptured abdominal aortic aneurysm, retroperitoneal bleed, pancreatitis, following the reduction of a large hernia, massive ascites, etc.). Clinically, they develop distended, usually tense abdomens. Renal failure develops owing to decreased cardiac output (from decreased blood return) and increased pressure on the renal parenchyma and vasculature. Respiratory compromise may also develop. Diagnosis is suggested by elevated intra-abdominal pressures, usually measured through a Foley catheter. Normal intra-abdominal pressure is <5 mm Hg (oliguria develops at >15 mm Hg, anuria at >30 mm Hg). Treatment involves surgical decompression.[19]

REFERENCES

1. Mehta RL, Kellum JA, Shah SV, et al. Acute Kidney Injury Network: report of an initiative to improve outcomes in acute kidney injury. *Crit Care* 2007;11:R31.
2. Thadhani R, Pascual M, Bonventre JV. Acute renal failure. *N Engl J Med* 1996;334:1448–60.
3. Chawla LS, Eggers PW, Star RA, Kimmel PL. Acute kidney injury and chronic kidney disease as interconnected syndromes. *N Engl J Med* 2014;371:58–66.
4. Abuelo JG. Normotensive ischemic acute renal failure. *N Engl J Med* 2007;357:797–805.
5. Bragadottir G, Redfors B, Ricksten SE. Assessing glomerular filtration rate (GFR) in critically ill patients with acute kidney injury—true GFR versus urinary creatinine clearance and estimating equations. *Crit Care* 2013;17:R108.
6. Chen S. Retooling the creatinine clearance equation to estimate kinetic GFR when the plasma creatinine is changing acutely. *J Am Soc Nephrol* 2013;2:877–88.
7. De Backer D, Biston P, Devriendt J, et al. Comparison of dopamine and norepinephrine in the treatment of shock. *N Engl J Med* 2010;362:779–89.
8. Kidney Disease: Improving Global Outcomes (KDIGO) Acute Kidney Injury Work Group. KDIGO Clinical Practice Guideline for Acute Kidney Injury. *Kidney inter., Suppl* 2012;2:1–138.
9. Kellum JA, Lameire N, et al. Diagnosis, evaluation, and management of acute kidney injury: a KDIGO summary (Part 1). *Crit Care* 2013;17:204.
10. Ronco C, Ricci Z, De Backer D, et al. Renal replacement therapy in acute kidney injury: controversy and consensus. *Crit Care* 2015;19:146.
11. Lameire N, Van Biesen W, Vanholder R. Acute renal failure. *Lancet* 2005;365:417–30.
12. Walsh M, Devereaux PJ, Garg AX, et al. Relationship between intraoperative mean arterial pressure and clinical outcomes after noncardiac surgery: toward an empirical definition of hypotension. *Anesthesiology* 2013;119:507–15.
13. Karkouti K, Wijeysundera DN, Yau TM, et al. Acute kidney injury after cardiac surgery: focus on modifiable risk factors. *Circulation* 2009;119:495–502.
14. Bosch X, Poch E, Grau JM. Rhabdomyolysis and acute kidney injury. *N Engl J Med* 2009;361:62–72.
15. Tepel M, Aspelin P, Lameire N. Contrast-induced nephropathy: a clinical and evidence-based approach. *Circulation* 2006;113:1799–806.
16. ACT Investigators. Acetylcysteine for prevention of renal outcomes in patients undergoing coronary and peripheral vascular angiography: main results from the randomized Acetylcysteine for Contrast-induced nephropathy Trial (ACT). *Circulation* 2011;124:1250–9.
17. Lameire N, Kellum JA, et al. Contrast-induced acute kidney injury and renal support for acute kidney injury: a KDIGO summary (Part 2). *Crit Care* 2013;17:205.
18. Scolari F, Ravani P. Atheroembolic renal disease. *Lancet* 2010;375:1650–60.
19. Papavramidis TS, Marinis AD, Pliakos I, et al. Abdominal compartment syndrome—intra-abdominal hypertension: defining, diagnosing, and managing. *J Emerg Trauma Shock* 2011;4:279–91.

Approach to Hyperkalemia and Hypokalemia

Stacy Dai and Melvin Blanchard

Hyperkalemia

GENERAL PRINCIPLES

- Hyperkalemia is a plasma potassium level >5.0 mmol/L. Although this condition is often asymptomatic, neuromuscular weakness and cardiac conduction abnormalities may occur with increasing levels of serum potassium and concomitantly decreased transmembrane potentials.
- The systematic consideration of hyperkalemia includes a review of potassium intake, transcellular shifts, and changes in excretion, particularly from the kidney.
- Causes are often multifactorial, but acute and chronic renal impairment is usually the common underlying etiology due to the kidneys' central role in maintaining potassium homeostasis.
- Medications inhibiting the renal angiotensin aldosterone system (RAAS) are another common etiology; management of these medications in the setting of hyperkalemia can be difficult given their significant long-term benefit in cardiovascular disease, diabetes mellitus, and chronic kidney disease.
- **Differential diagnoses** of hyperkalemia and hypoaldosteronism are addressed in Tables 18-1 and 18-2, respectively.

DIAGNOSIS

Clinical Presentation
History
- **Dietary:** Increased potassium intake may be due to unwitting use of potassium-containing salt substitutes or drinking water softened with potassium salts. Foods such as oranges, bananas, spinach, tomatoes, potatoes, dried fruits, and nuts are high in potassium, and juices from these foods can be especially potassium rich.
- Review of **medications:** Particular attention should be paid to angiotensin-converting enzyme (ACE) inhibitors, angiotensin receptor blockers, and aldosterone antagonists. Other common etiologies include β-blockers, nonsteroidal anti-inflammatory drugs (NSAIDs), potassium supplements, trimethoprim, pentamidine, and heparin. Some drug infusions (penicillins) may also contain potassium.
- Marked cellular injury such as tumor lysis syndrome or large crush injuries can result in significant release of intracellular potassium well as acute kidney injury. Massive **blood transfusions** of unwashed RBCs can also contribute to hyperkalemia especially in the setting of rapid transfusion.[1]
- Past medical history: The presence of **diabetes** may suggest concomitant development of hyporeninemic hypoaldosteronism and type IV renal tubular acidosis. In patients with **sickle cell disease** and those with **obstructive uropathy**, aldosterone resistance may cause hyperkalemia. Underlying kidney disease should be assessed.

TABLE 18-1 CAUSES OF HYPERKALEMIA

Increased potassium intake	PO (massive ingestion required)
	IV (including stored, nonwashed packed red blood cells)
Decreased cellular uptake	Insulin deficiency
	β-blockade (nonselective), digitalis toxicity
Extracellular shift of potassium	Hyperosmolar states
	Metabolic acidosis (nonorganic)
	Tumor lysis, rhabdomyolysis, extreme exercise, trauma
	Familial periodic paralysis, succinylcholine
Decreased renal excretion	Hypoaldosteronism (see Table 18-2)
	Chronic kidney disease
	Congestive heart failure, liver disease
	Hyperkalemic type I renal tubular acidosis
	Chloride shunt
	Selective defect in potassium excretion
Pseudohyperkalemia	Mechanical trauma during blood draw
	Increase in platelets or white blood cells
	Repeated clinching of fist/tourniquet

TABLE 18-2 CAUSES OF HYPOALDOSTERONISM

Decreased renin	Hyporeninemic hypoaldosteronism/type IV renal tubular acidosis
	Medications: NSAIDs, cyclosporine, β-blockers
	HIV/AIDS
Decreased aldosterone	Primary adrenal failure, adrenal enzyme defects
	ACE inhibitors/angiotensin receptor blockers, heparin
	HIV/AIDS
Blockade of aldosterone receptor	Medications: amiloride, triamterene, trimethoprim

ACE, angiotensin-converting enzyme; HIV/AIDS, human immunodeficiency virus/acquired immunodeficiency syndrome; NSAIDs, nonsteroidal anti-inflammatory drugs.

Approach to Hyperkalemia and Hypokalemia

Physical Examination

The physical exam should focus on the **neurologic system** for new-onset generalized muscle weakness; its presence necessitates immediate treatment for hyperkalemia to prevent progression to flaccid paralysis.

Diagnostic Testing

Laboratories

- A rapid confirmation of extracellular K⁺ level can be done on an arterial blood gas (ABG) sample if the diagnosis is in doubt; elevated potassium due to measurement error is called pseudohyperkalemia.
- Serum creatinine should be obtained to evaluate renal function.
- Previously, if the cause of hyperkalemia is not apparent from history and hypoaldosteronism is suspected, an evaluation of urinary potassium excretion through calculating the transtubular potassium gradient (TTKG) was thought to be helpful. However, one of the core assumptions on which the formula was based was shown to be inaccurate, and thus its calculation is no longer routinely recommended.[2]
- Instead, workup in suspected hypoaldosteronism should include plasma renin, aldosterone, and morning cortisol levels (sample should be collected after the patient has been upright for at least 3 hours or after the administration of furosemide the previous evening and again in the morning). The different levels will help differentiate primary adrenal insufficiency from hyporeninemic hypoaldosteronism. A low cortisol level implies adrenal insufficiency. See Table 18-3 for interpretation of renin/aldosterone ratio levels.

Electrocardiography

- ECG evaluation is paramount in determining the urgency of treatment in hyperkalemia. Although there may be marked interpatient variability in the relationship between K⁺ levels and ECG changes, severe hyperkalemia with ECG changes constitutes a clinical emergency.
- EKG findings include the following:
  - Peaked T waves and shortened QT interval (usually at [K⁺] > 6 mmol/L).
  - Prolonged PR interval, loss of P wave, and QRS widening (usually at [K⁺] ≥ 7–8 mmol/L). Bradyarrhythmias can occur.
  - The final stages include a sine wave pattern, which can degenerate rapidly to ventricular fibrillation or asystole if left untreated.
- All patients with K > 6 should be monitored on telemetry. Repeat potassium should be checked within 2 hours of treatment to monitor treatment response.

TABLE 18-3 RENIN AND ALDOSTERONE LEVELS WITH HYPERKALEMIA AND A LOW TTKG

Disorder	Renin	Aldosterone
Primary or secondary hypoaldosteronism	↑	↓
Aldosterone receptor blockade, pseudohypoaldosteronism	↑	↑
Hyporeninemic hypoaldosteronism, chloride shunt	↓	↓

↑, increased; ↓, decreased.

TREATMENT

- Potassium levels >7 mmol/L require close clinical and cardiac monitoring and often indicate the need for acute treatment. The immediate goal is to promote the stabilization of the cell membrane potential, followed by therapy directed at moving potassium intracellularly and restoring the membrane potassium gradient.
- Temporary potassium-lowering therapy includes insulin, β_2-adrenergic agents, and sodium bicarbonate; these agents promote the rapid redistribution of potassium into the intracellular space but do not decrease total body potassium levels. Definitive management requires potassium excretion through the GI tract or kidneys, or removal through dialysis. All patients with severe hyperkalemia should be monitored on telemetry. Dietary elements and any medications that could be contributing to hyperkalemia should be discontinued as appropriate.
- Temporizing medications include the following:
  - **Calcium gluconate** (1 g [10 mL of a 10% solution] given IV over 2 minutes) should be given to stabilize the membrane cell potential in cases of hyperkalemia associated with severe weakness or marked ECG changes. The dose is repeated again in several minutes if there is no clinical improvement.
  - **Insulin** can be given as a dose of 10 U of regular insulin IV, along with 25–50 g of dextrose (1–2 ampules of D_{50}). If the patient is already hyperglycemic (>250 mg/dL), insulin can be given alone. Treatment effects should be seen by 30 minutes–1 hour and lasts for several hours, with an expected decrease of 1–1.5 mmol/L.
  - **β_2-adrenergic agents**, namely albuterol, is classically given in a dose of 10–20 mg in 4 mL by nebulizer over 10 minutes. Onset of action is similar to insulin.
  - **Sodium bicarbonate** is given as one ampule (8.4% solution [100 mmol $NaHCO_3$ in 100 mL] = 4.2 g $NaHCO_3$ = 50 mEq HCO_3^- in 50 mL) IV over several minutes. The onset and duration of effect are approximately the same as with insulin. The utility has come under question and is likely only efficacious in patients with acidemia. In patients with end-stage renal disease, the effect is limited and notably also provides a significant sodium load (~1150 mg).
  - **Loop diuretics** such as furosemide administered as 40 mg IV per dose will cause forced diuresis and salt wasting in those with some intact renal function. Higher doses are likely needed in those who have underlying chronic kidney disease.
  - **Cation-exchange resins** (sodium polystyrene), administered orally or rectally, can be used to eliminate excess potassium by exchanging potassium for sodium in the GI tract. Sorbitol is added to reduce constipation and intestinal blockage. The usual oral dose is 15 g by mouth in 20% sorbitol, given every 6 hours as needed. Notably, sodium polystyrene takes many hours to take effect, and over the years, its efficacy and safety have come under question. There is a significant risk of upper GI ulcers and bowel necrosis, especially in patients with decreased GI motility or perfusion.[3] Sodium polystyrene should therefore be avoided in postoperative patients and in those requiring vasopressors. Each gram will remove up to 1 mmol of potassium.
  - New novel potassium binders are under development and have shown early promise.[4] In October 2015, the FDA approved the use of patiromer to treat hyperkalemia, though it comes with a box warning since it can bind other orally administered drugs. The clinical impact of these medications is currently still unclear.
  - **Hemodialysis** is used when hyperkalemia is not responsive to the usual measures or when an extremely high [K^+] associated with significant ECG changes or severe weakness is present. Predialysis treatment should be limited to a dose of calcium gluconate and a single agent, such as insulin, since further intracellular shift can limit the amount of potassium removed during dialysis.

- For chronic management of aldosterone deficiency, fludrocortisone given as a starting dose of 0.1 mg daily can be considered. Side effects include hypertension and sodium retention.

Hypokalemia

GENERAL PRINCIPLES

- Hypokalemia is defined as a plasma potassium level <3.5 mmol/L. When mild (3–3.5 mmol/L), the diagnosis is usually an incidental finding on routine laboratory testing. Severe hypokalemia (<3 mmol/L), however, is often symptomatic. Since potassium is primarily an intracellular ion, a decrease in serum potassium could represent a significant decrease in whole body potassium.
- Causes of hypokalemia are listed in Table 18-4; they include decreased intake, intracellular shift, increased excretion, and occasionally hypomagnesemia. Table 18-5 lists causes of primary or apparent hyperaldosteronism that can contribute to hypokalemia.

TABLE 18-4 CAUSES OF HYPOKALEMIA

Decreased intake	
Increased cellular uptake	Insulin
	Sympathetic stimulation (β_2-agonists, myocardial infarction, arrhythmias)
	Red or white blood cell production and transfusions
	Hypokalemic periodic paralysis (rare)
	Alkalosis
	Hyperthyroidism
Renal losses	Increased flow to distal tubule and collecting duct
	Nonabsorbed anions (e.g., glucosuria)
	Increased or apparent increased aldosterone (see Table 18-5)
	Type I and type II renal tubular acidosis
	Amphotericin, cisplatin, aminoglycosides
	Diuretics (thiazide, loop, acetazolamide)
	Hypomagnesemia
Nonrenal losses	Gastrointestinal (e.g., diarrhea), sweat

TABLE 18-5 PRIMARY OR APPARENT EXCESS ALDOSTERONE

Primary hyperaldosteronism (low renin–high aldosterone)	Adrenal adenoma, hyperplasia, carcinoma; glucocorticoid-remediable hyperaldosteronism; congenital adrenal hyperplasia
Secondary hyperaldosteronism (high renin–high aldosterone)	Renal artery stenosis, hypertension; renin-secreting tumors, low effective circulating volume
Increased alternate mineralocorticoids (low renin–low aldosterone)	11-β-hydroxysteroid dehydrogenase deficiency (real licorice, chewing tobacco)
	Overwhelmed 11-β-hydroxysteroid dehydrogenase (Cushing syndrome)
Apparent mineralocorticoid excess (low renin–low aldosterone)	Liddle syndrome (pseudohyperaldosteronism)
Apparent mineralocorticoid excess (high renin–high aldosterone)	Gitelman syndrome (pseudothiazide), Bartter syndrome (pseudofurosemide)

DIAGNOSIS

Clinical Presentation

History

The clinical findings may reveal the following:

- Use of **drugs that cause excessive loss of potassium** (overt or covert), such as thiazides, loop diuretics, and laxatives.
- Use of **drugs that shift potassium into cells**: insulin, prolonged bronchodilator use, and phosphodiesterase inhibitors such as theophylline and caffeine.
- **Administration of glucose** in hospitalized patients may increase insulin secretion enough to lower serum potassium.
- **Vomiting or nasogastric suction** since gastric fluid is high in potassium.
- **Insufficient intake**, which may be seen in individuals with poor access to food.
- As in hyperkalemia, the **symptoms** of hypokalemia are usually related to the cardiac, GI, and neuromuscular systems, including the following:
  - Tremor and weakness, due to a significant increase in the intra-to-extracellular ratio of potassium, which can lead to paralysis. In severe hypokalemia, the muscles of respiration can be involved, leading to respiratory failure.
  - An ileus, due to the hypokalemic effects on smooth muscle.
  - Rhabdomyolysis can occur with severe hypokalemia. This elevates the [K^+] and prevents further decrements, although it may also serve to mask the underlying etiology.
  - Increased blood pressure and glucose intolerance may be a manifestation of chronic, mild hypokalemia.
  - Nephrogenic diabetes insipidus.
  - Increased renal ammonia synthesis due to intracellular acidosis. In severe liver disease, this may trigger hepatic encephalopathy.

Physical Examination

Physical findings generally do not become apparent until the degree of hypokalemia is moderate or severe or the fall in potassium occurs rapidly. Hypertension, ascending muscle weakness (eventually affecting respiration), signs of ileus, tetany, and muscle tenderness may be observed.

Diagnostic Testing
Laboratories
- A **24-hour urine collection for potassium** can be useful to distinguish whole body potassium depletion versus intracellular shift, as the total urine excretion per day should be <15–25 mmol of potassium in the presence of total body hypokalemia.
- If hypokalemia-induced rhabdomyolysis is suspected, one should check a serum creatine phosphokinase.
- Additional evaluations
  - Acid/base status and urine pH
  - Renin and aldosterone levels may also aid in the evaluation of possible apparent or true aldosterone excess.
  - Measurement of serum magnesium should be considered, particularly in patients on chronic diuretic therapy, since hypomagnesemia can cause potassium loss.

Electrocardiography
ECG changes associated with hypokalemia include U waves, flat or inverted T waves and ST-segment depression, and PR prolongation. These changes do not correlate well with the degree of hypokalemia; however, with extremely low [K$^+$] levels, the PR and QRS intervals can lengthen and lead to ventricular fibrillation. Patients with severe hypokalemia should be monitored on telemetry.

TREATMENT

- The method and urgency of potassium repletion depend on the patient's clinical state. When patients have moderate to severe hypokalemia, are symptomatic, or have an acute myocardial infarction, treatment should be urgent.
- The approximate whole body **potassium deficit** as the plasma potassium level decreases from 4 to 3 mEq/L is in the range of 200–400 mEq, depending on the size of the patient. As the plasma level decreases to <3 mEq/L, the deficit can be >600 mEq but is unpredictable due to the potential release of potassium from cellular necrosis, which maintains and may even increase the [K$^+$]. These cellular shifts can mask a serious potassium deficit; levels should be checked frequently to ensure adequacy of replacement.
- **Potassium replacement** should be given orally whenever possible because of the potential cardiac risk of rapid IV K$^+$ administration, vein sclerosis, and cost. **Oral** doses of 40 mEq of potassium are generally well tolerated and can be given every 4 hours. Liquid potassium is generally unpalatable, and slow-release tablet forms should be avoided because of the risk of gastric ulceration. **Potassium chloride** is usually administered, as the chloride component helps to correct the often coinciding alkalosis and bicarbonaturia. **Potassium citrate** can be given **if hypokalemia associated with acidemia is present.**
- **IV potassium** can be administered in concentrations of up to 40 mEq/L via peripheral line or 40 mEq/100 mL via central venous line. High-concentration potassium chloride can cause severe phlebitis and tissue necrosis when extravasated. The rate of infusion should not exceed 20 mEq/h unless the clinical situation dictates otherwise (e.g., paralysis, malignant ventricular arrhythmias).
- Certain groups including those with heart failure or history of arrhythmias should be repleted more aggressively with a goal of >4 mmol/L. Care should be taken in potassium repletion in the setting of renal failure given the decreased capacity for excretion.

REFERENCES

1. Au BK, Dutton WD, Zaydfudim V, et al. Hyperkalemia following massive transfusion in trauma. *J Surg Res* 2009;157:284–9.
2. Kamel KS, Halperin ML. Intrarenal urea recycling leads to a higher rate of renal excretion of potassium: an hypothesis with clinical implications. *Curr Opin Nephrol Hypertens* 2011;20:547–54.
3. Gardiner GW. Kayexalate (sodium polystyrene sulphonate) in sorbitol associated with intestinal necrosis in uremic patients. *Can J Gastroenterol* 1997;11:573–7.
4. Kovesdy CP. Management of hyperkalemia: an update for the internist. *Am J Med* 2015;128:1281–7.

Approach to Hyponatremia and Hypernatremia

19

Asrar Khan and John J. Cras

Hyponatremia

GENERAL PRINCIPLES

- Hyponatremia is the most common abnormality of water and electrolyte homeostasis seen by clinicians. Prevalence rates of 30% or greater have been reported for hospitalized patients.[1] Although incidence rates >20% have been reported for inpatients, 5% is probably a more clinically accurate estimate.[2,3]
- Hyponatremia is independently associated with negative outcomes across a wide spectrum of acute and chronic conditions, and in the outpatient and inpatient settings.[4,5]
    - It has been associated with increased morbidity and mortality in patients with heart failure, pneumonia, cancer, cirrhosis, and stroke, to name only a few.[6–13]
    - It has been linked to gait instability and an increased risk of falls, osteoporosis, and femoral neck fractures, even in clinically asymptomatic patients.[14–17]
    - Preoperative hyponatremia increases perioperative complications and 30-day mortality rates in surgical patients.[18]
    - Severe hyponatremia (serum Na$^+$ <125 mmol/L) doubles the risk of in-hospital mortality in ICU patients.[19]
    - Length of stay, hospital costs, and 30-day readmission risk have all been shown to increase with hyponatremia.[20–22] The direct costs of treating hyponatremia have been estimated at $1.6–$3.6 billion.[23]
    - Thus, by virtually any measurement, hyponatremia places a significant burden on the U.S. health care system and should not be considered an innocuous condition.
- Hyponatremia is defined as a serum sodium (sNa$^+$) concentration <135 mmol/L. The measured serum Na$^+$ level does not reflect total body Na$^+$ as much as it represents the ratio of Na$^+$ to plasma volume. This is important to remember, as hyponatremia generally reflects problems of water homeostasis, rather than isolated sodium loss. There are, of course, exceptions to this rule. Note that, for purposes of this discussion, the terms plasma and serum are used interchangeably.

DIAGNOSIS

Clinical Presentation

History
- The initial evaluation of a patient with suspected or confirmed hyponatremia should include a detailed history.
- Patients with **acute onset of hyponatremia** (<48 hours) may initially complain of lethargy, weakness, nausea, and vomiting.
    - As the sodium levels fall below 125 mmol/L, cerebral edema worsens and neurologic symptoms predominate.

○ These may include obtundation, ataxia, hyporeflexia, seizures, coma, and ultimately respiratory arrest from brainstem herniation. If death is averted, permanent brain damage may still occur.
- **Chronic hyponatremia** (>48 hours) is generally better tolerated, but symptoms may include cognitive defects as well as nausea and vomiting, weakness, and headache. Recent or current use of glucocorticoids may cause adrenal suppression and should be considered. The syndrome of inappropriate antidiuretic hormone (SIADH) may manifest well before the onset of an otherwise unapparent malignancy.

Physical Examination
A major focus should be on assessing the patient's **volume status**. Orthostatic blood pressure and heart rate are neither highly sensitive nor specific markers of volume status, though many clinicians still rely on them. Skin turgor and the oropharyngeal mucosa may be useful surrogates for total body water (TBW). The presence or absence of edema should be carefully noted. A thorough neurologic evaluation should be performed as well.

Diagnostic Testing

See Figure 19-1 for evaluation of hyponatremia.
- The first step in the diagnostic workup of hyponatremia (Fig. 19-1) is determining effective osmolality (eOsm): eOsm = measured plasma osmoles − ([BUN/2.8] + [ethanol/4.6]), BUN, blood urea nitrogen.
- The normal eOsm range is 280–295 mOsm/kg H_2O. A low eOsm indicates hypo-osmolality, and, as sodium and its associated anions are the major effective plasma osmoles, hyponatremia and hypo-osmolality are often concurrent.[24]
- There are clinical conditions, however, where hyponatremia is present with high or normal tonicity (hypertonic hyponatremia, isotonic hyponatremia, and pseudohyponatremia). Each of the categories is further discussed below.

Hypotonic Hyponatremia (Decreased eOsm)
Hypotonic hyponatremia indicates excess of water relative to serum solute. It is important to remember that in the presence of a low osmolar state, urine should be maximally dilute.[25] Thus, measurement of urinary osmolality (uOsm) and urinary Na^+ (uNa^+) can help delineate the etiology.

- **Urine osmolality <100 mOsm/L** identifies patients with decreased effective antidiuretic hormone (ADH) activity such as primary polydipsia, beer potomania, and malnutrition. Such patients overwhelm their kidneys' capacity to excrete water, either because of excessive water intake or impaired water excretion.
- **Urine osmolality >100 mOsm/L** identifies patients with increased ADH activity and must be further defined depending on the patient's **volume status** and **urine sodium concentration** (see Fig. 19-1).
  ○ Hypervolemic
    ▪ uNa^+ **< 10 mEq/L:** These patients have **decreased effective circulating volume,** but extracellular fluid (ECF) and total body water (TBW) are significantly increased; total body Na^+ is also increased, but to a lesser degree than TBW, and Na^+ concentration is generally >125 mmol/L. Edema is usually apparent (e.g., congestive heart failure [CHF], cirrhosis, nephrotic syndrome).
    ▪ uNa^+ **> 20 mEq/L:** renal insufficiency
  ○ **Euvolemic:** Effective circulating volume is normal or slightly increased, but TBW and plasma volume are elevated. Thus, serum Na^+ concentration is decreased. No edema is present. **The uNa^+ is >20 mEq/L unless there is low Na^+ intake** (e.g., SIADH, hypothyroidism, adrenal insufficiency).

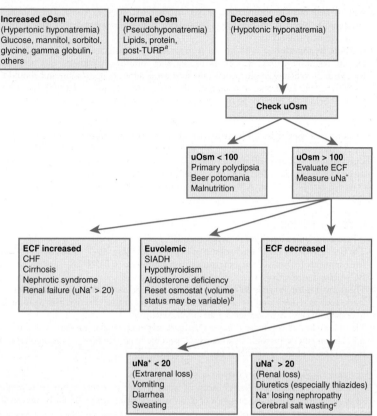

FIGURE 19-1 Evaluation of hyponatremia. ECF, extracellular fluid; eOsm, effective osmolality; uNa+, urinary sodium; uOsm, urinary osmolality; SIADH, syndrome of inappropriate antidiuretic hormone. [a]Actual plasma osmolality may be variable and occasionally cause symptomatic hyponatremia, especially in the setting of renal insufficiency. [b]Urine osmolality may be <100 mOsm/L after a water load. [c]May be indistinguishable from SIADH by laboratory data.

- See Table 19-1 for common causes of SIADH.
- The diagnosis of SIADH must involve exclusion of adrenal insufficiency and severe hypothyroidism. Furthermore, the diagnosis of SIADH cannot be reliably made in the setting of renal failure.
- **Reset osmostat** is a variant of SIADH but with a stable Na+. The key feature is the ability to appropriately dilute or concentrate the urine after water challenge or deprivation tests, respectively. It is common in pregnancy and can be seen in states of chronic decreased effective circulating volume such as CHF and, rarely, in severe malnutrition. Treatment is directed toward the underlying condition.
  - **Hypovolemic:** Effective circulating volume, TBW and ECF, and total body Na+ are all decreased, but Na+ depletion predominates. Edema is absent (e.g., gastrointestinal losses, osmotic diuresis, adrenal insufficiency, third-spacing conditions [e.g., ascites, burns, pancreatitis, peritonitis]).

TABLE 19-1 COMMON CAUSES OF THE SYNDROME OF INAPPROPRIATE ANTIDIURETIC HORMONE

CNS disorders	Hemorrhage, psychosis, infection, alcohol withdrawal
Malignancy (ectopic ADH)	Small cell lung cancer (most commonly implicated), CNS, leukemia, Hodgkin's, duodenal, pancreatic, etc.
Pulmonary	Infection, acute respiratory failure, mechanical ventilation
Miscellaneous	Pain, nausea (powerful stimulator of ADH), HIV (multifactorial), general postoperative state, cortisol deficiency, hypothyroidism
Pharmacologic agents (either mimic or enhance ADH)	Cyclophosphamide, vincristine, vinblastine, NSAIDs, "ecstasy" (also polydipsia)
	Tricyclics and related agents, serotonin reuptake inhibitors, chlorpropamide, nicotine, bromocriptine, oxytocin, desmopressin (deamino-8-D-arginine vasopressin)

ADH, antidiuretic hormone; CNS, central nervous system; HIV, human immunodeficiency virus; NSAIDs, nonsteroidal anti-inflammatory drugs.

- **uNa^+ > 20 mEq/L: renal Na^+ loss**. It is unusual for loop diuretics to produce significant hyponatremia owing to their effect on urine-concentrating ability. Thiazides more frequently cause hyponatremia. Sodium-wasting nephropathy can be seen with chronic kidney disease, polycystic kidney disease, obstructive uropathy, and nephritis induced by nonsteroidal anti-inflammatory drugs (NSAIDs).
- **uNa^+ < 20: extrarenal Na^+ loss** is seen with vomiting or diarrhea or conditions that lead to third spacing (such as pancreatitis or burns) and will be associated with a low uNa^+ and uCl^-. However, conditions that lead to alkalosis, and thus bicarbonaturia, may cause coelimination of significant Na^+ in the urine. Ketonuria can have the same effect on uNa^+. The urine chloride, however, should still be low in these situations.

Hypertonic Hyponatremia (Increased eOsm)
- Hypertonic hyponatremia is due to excess osmotically active substances, such as glucose or mannitol, drawing water into the **extracellular fluid (ECF)** and diluting serum Na^+ concentration. It is sometimes referred to as redistributive or translocational hyponatremia. This increases risk of cellular dehydration. See Figure 19-1 for specific etiologies.
- **Measured sodium must be corrected for hyperglycemia**. Historically, a correction factor of 1.6 mEq/L is added to the measured Na^+ for every 100 mg/dL rise in plasma glucose. However, more recent research suggests a correction factor of 2.4 mEq/L may be more accurate when dealing with **marked hyperglycemia** (>400 mg/dL).[26] Corrected Na^+ = measured Na^+ + (0.024)(measured glucose − 100).

Pseudohyponatremia or Isotonic Hyponatremia (Normal eOsm)
- Pseudohyponatremia occurs when older photometry or indirect potentiometry techniques are used to measure Na^+ concentration in whole plasma. If excess lipid, protein,

or white blood cells (WBCs) are present, the Na⁺ concentration is underestimated. However, serum sodium and osmolality are normal when they are measured by direct potentiometry. Pseudohyponatremia is a benign lab artifact requiring only recognition. It is seen with **hypertriglyceridemia**, with **paraproteinemia**, and sometimes with total parenteral nutrition.
- Isotonic hyponatremia may occur following laparoscopic surgery or transurethral resection of the prostate, due to the absorption of irrigants (glycine or sorbitol). The actual plasma osmolality can be variable and may occasionally cause symptomatic hyponatremia, especially in the setting of renal insufficiency.

TREATMENT

- The correction of hyponatremia, either acute or chronic in nature, which presents **with significant symptoms**, requires hypertonic saline.
  - Typically, 1 mL/kg/h of 3% saline will raise the serum Na⁺ by ~1 mmol/L/h.[27]
  - For patients with severe neurologic sequelae (seizures, coma), an initial infusion rate of 4–6 mL/kg/h may be used.
- A detailed approximation for the expected correction in serum Na⁺ by giving 1 L of infusate is as follows:

$$\frac{\text{Infusate Na}^+ \left(\text{mmol/L}\right) + \text{infusate K}\left(\text{mmol/L}\right) - \text{serum Na}^+ \left(\text{mmol/L}\right)}{\text{Estimated total body water}\left(\text{kg}\right) + 1}$$

  - Normal saline = 154 mmol Na⁺/L; 3% saline = 513 mmol Na⁺/L
  - Dividing the calculated volume by the desired time period gives the rate of infusion.
  - The addition of potassium (K⁺) to the solution is equivalent to adding sodium due to Na⁺/K⁺ exchange and needs to be included in calculations as well.
- Acute, severe central nervous system symptoms (e.g., coma, seizures) can often be reversed with a 5% increase in the serum Na⁺. Once symptoms are controlled, a **maximum serum Na⁺ increase in the first 24 hours of ~8–10 mmol/L** is recommended (including initial correction). At this point, hypertonic saline is usually no longer necessary. The subsequent correction rate should not exceed 18 mmol/L in any 48-hour period.[24]
  - Loop diuretics may be required either to prevent volume overload or to aid in the excretion of free water by lowering the urine osmolality (uOsm).
  - Calculations provide only a rough estimate to help initiate therapy and **do not replace frequent monitoring and adjustment.**
- Overly rapid correction may result in **central pontine myelinolysis** (also called osmotic demyelination syndrome). This is rare with acute hyponatremia (<48 hours in duration). Cognitive and movement disorders due to central pontine myelinolysis may not be apparent for days after correction of hyponatremia, and visible changes on magnetic resonance imaging may take weeks to appear. Risk factors include sodium concentration <120 mmol/L for >48 hours, recent liver transplantation, alcoholism, and severe malnutrition.[24,28]
- The treatment of accidental overcorrection with free water or ADH analogs to decrease the serum Na⁺ to the desired level of correction may be of benefit, especially if symptoms suggestive of osmotic demyelination appear.
- Chronic hyponatremia without acute neurologic events is best treated by fluid restriction or discontinuation of any pharmacologic culprits.
- For **SIADH**, free water restriction with high oral Na⁺ and protein intake are the mainstays of treatment.
  - The degree of **free water restriction** will depend on the uOsm present (as this will determine the amount of free water that can be excreted with the given osmotic load). The typical fluid restriction should be 500 mL/d less than the 24-hour urine output.[29]

- Fluid restriction alone is unlikely to be effective if the sum of urine Na^+ and urine K^+ exceeds the measured serum Na^+.[30]
- Use **hypertonic saline ± loop diuretics if symptoms are severe or uOsm is very high**. Administration of 0.9% (normal) saline in SIADH may worsen hyponatremia by allowing the kidney to extract the free water from the saline if uOsm is greater than the osmolarity of the infusate.
- **Oral urea** (30–60 g/d) may be the safest pharmacologic agent for the unusual case in which standard management is unsuccessful. However, it is not available in most US pharmacies and therefore rarely used here.[31]
- **Demeclocycline** and **lithium** have both been used to induce a nephrogenic diabetes insipidus. Lithium is unpredictable and has many side effects. Both are rarely used today.
- The V_2-receptor antagonists (conivaptan, tolvaptan, etc.) have been shown to be effective in raising serum sodium levels for patients with SIADH and CHF.[32-35] They should not be used in hypovolemic patients.
  - Due to an elevated risk of hepatic injury, tolvaptan should not be used in patients with chronic liver disease.[24,36]
  - Conivaptan should be used with extreme caution in cirrhotic patients, as it is also active at the V_{1a} receptor. Thus, there may be an increased risk of variceal bleeding and hepatorenal syndrome.[37]
  - Conivaptan is only available as an IV formulation and should be used for no more than 4 days.[24] Its use is limited to hospitalized patients.
  - Tolvaptan should be initiated in the hospital, but can used in the outpatient setting for up to 30 days.
- In hyponatremia from thiazides, complete resolution of the effect can sometimes take weeks after withdrawal. Patients who develop severe hyponatremia on a thiazide diuretic are at high risk of rapid recurrence and should not receive these agents again.[38]

Hypernatremia

GENERAL PRINCIPLES

- Hypernatremia is much less common than hyponatremia. It has been reported in 1–3% or more of general inpatients but may be present in over 25% of critically ill patients.[39,40]
- It is, however, a stronger signal of impending mortality than is hyponatremia. Left untreated, it can result in seizures, subarachnoid hemorrhage, coma, and death. Mortality rates range between 45 and 60% for all patients but may be as high as 80% for elderly patients.[41]
- As with hyponatremia, preoperative hypernatremia independently predicts 30-day mortality in surgical patients and increases the risk of perioperative myocardia infarction (MI), venous thromboembolism (VTE), and pneumonia.[42]
- It is rarely seen in alert patients with access to water, as even mild elevations in serum osmolality stimulate thirst and the repletion of free water. Thus, hypernatremia generally occurs in patients at the extremes of age and in those who are physically or cognitively debilitated.
- Risk factors for hypernatremia include the following:
  - Age > 65
  - Physical or cognitive impairment
  - Hospitalization
  - Nursing home residence
  - Osmotic diuresis (e.g., hyperglycemia, mannitol) or urinary concentrating defect (e.g., DI)
  - Intubation

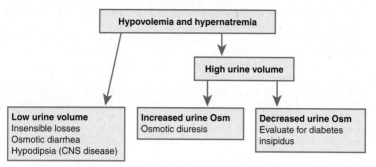

FIGURE 19-2 Differential diagnosis and evaluation of hypernatremia with volume depletion

Definition

Hypernatremia is defined as serum Na^+ > 145 mmol/L. Since sodium is the major extracellular osmole, hypernatremia is always a hyperosmolar state. Thus, it indicates a deficiency of water relative to total body solute.[43]

Pathophysiology

While hypernatremia may be caused by primary Na^+ gain, the vast majority of cases are due to the loss of free water, resulting in hypovolemia and dehydration.

- **Hypervolemic hypernatremia** is usually due to administration of hypertonic fluids but may also be caused by primary hyperaldosteronism.
- Hypernatremia of **varying volume status** may be caused by various mechanisms, such as:
  ○ Rapid shift of ECF to intracellular fluid due to rhabdomyolysis or prolonged seizures
  ○ Release of placental vasopressinase during pregnancy (rare)
- **Hypovolemic hypernatremia** etiologies are included in Figure 19-2.
  ○ **Osmotic diuresis** may be caused by diuretic drugs (loop diuretics > thiazides), hyperglycemia, high-protein diet, the diuretic phase of ATN, or postobstructive diuresis; in the latter two, accumulated urea leads to excretion of dilute urine.
  ○ **Central diabetes insipidus (DI)** is caused by disruption of the posterior pituitary by trauma, surgery, granulomatous diseases, meningitis, encephalitis, tumors, and pituitary apoplexy; it may rarely be hereditary.
  ○ **Nephrogenic DI** is often due to drugs (lithium, foscarnet, cidofovir), electrolytes (K^+ < 3.0, hypercalcemia), or kidney disease (obstructive uropathy, sickle cell disease, amyloidosis, Sjögren syndrome).

DIAGNOSIS

Clinical Presentation

History

- As with hyponatremia, the initial evaluation of a patient with suspected hypernatremia should include a detailed history, focusing on volume status and potential losses of free water.
- Symptoms include lethargy, irritability, weakness, and confusion. Seizures and coma may occur, but generally not until the serum Na^+ approaches 160 mmol/L.
- Try to determine the urine volume. Low urine volume is consistent with dehydration, but polyuria should raise suspicion for DI. Inquire about fluid intake as well.

Physical Examination

The physical exam should focus on assessing volume status. Look for signs of free water loss such as orthostasis, tachycardia, poor skin turgor, and dry mucous membranes. If DI is a consideration, a neurologic exam, including visual fields, is indicated.

Diagnostic Testing

History and physical exam will usually identify the cause of hypervolemic or euvolemic hypernatremia. Many patients with adequate thirst mechanisms may maintain volume status with DI. Hypovolemic hypernatremia may be evaluated as per Figure 19-2.

- With hypovolemia due to extrarenal free water loss, uOsm should be >600–800 mOsm/kg, and the uNa$^+$ should be <20 mmol/L; uOsm <300 mOsm/kg is consistent with renal free water loss.
- Release of a total of >1000 urine osmoles/day (uOsm × 24-hour urine output) is consistent with an osmotic diuresis.
- Patients with polyuria and hypernatremia may undergo a water-deprivation test to differentiate central from nephrogenic DI:
  ○ Water is withheld from the patient until three consecutive urine osmoles are stable (<30 mmol/kg increase).
  ○ The patient is given desmopressin (deamino-8-D-arginine vasopressin, DDAVP), 1 mcg SC with serum osmolality measured before injection and 45 minutes later.
  ○ **In central DI**, there is a >9% increase in uOsm with DDAVP.
  ○ With **nephrogenic DI**, there is little change.
  ○ Difficulty in diagnosis may arise in partial DI states.

TREATMENT

- As with hyponatremia, the rate of onset of hypernatremia is important in guiding the rate of correction.
- Acute hypernatremia develops in <48 hours and may be due to the administration of hypertonic fluids.
- After 48 hours of plasma hyperosmolality, brain cells generate organic osmolytes that restore and maintain normal brain volume.
- Overly rapid correction of serum osmolality and hypernatremia can result in significant cerebral edema with severe neurologic sequelae. Thus, in chronic hypernatremia (>48 hours), the free water must be repleted carefully over 48–72 hours. Correction of serum Na$^+$ at a **rate of <0.5 mmol/L/h** (<12 mmol per 24-hour period) has a low likelihood of causing complications.
- Calculating the **free water deficit** is important when addressing hypernatremia. The water deficit can be estimated with the following equation[44]:
  ○ Water deficit = current TBW × ([serum Na$^+$/140] − 1)
  ○ Note that TBW is roughly 60% of **body weight in kg** for nonelderly, euvolemic men. For women and older men, TBW is roughly 50% of lean body weight.[44] The percentages for TBW decrease in the elderly and volume-depleted patients.
- Once the water deficit has been calculated, it is imperative to determine the appropriate rate of correction.
  ○ In cases of acute hypernatremia (<48 hours), the water deficit should be corrected over 24 hours with electrolyte free water (e.g., 5% dextrose solution). Thus, the infusion rate can be estimated as: Infusion Rate (mL/h) = Water Deficit (mL)/24 h.
  ○ For patients with chronic hyponatremia, however, only enough water to lower the serum Na$^+$ 10–12 mmol/L is administered in the first 24 hours. The desired water replacement in the first day is then: (Water Deficit (mL) × 10–12 mmol/L)/(serum Na$^+$ − 140). The infusion rate is then calculated by dividing that value over 24 hours.

- The above calculations do not account for insensible and ongoing losses. An additional 30–40 mL/h should be added to the infusion rate to account for insensible losses. Ongoing urinary or gastrointestinal losses may require 25–50 mL/h further.
- A useful rule of thumb to remember is for every 3–4 mL of electrolyte–free water per kg body weight that is administered, the serum Na$^+$ concentration will fall by 1 mmol/L.[27]
  - Thus, when treating acute hypernatremia, it is reasonable to infuse water at 3–6 mL/kg/h initially. Once the serum Na$^+$ is down to 145 mmol/L, the infusion should be changed to 1 mL/kg/L, until normonatremia (serum Na$^+$ ~140 mmol/L) is reached.
  - Similarly, for patients with chronic hyponatremia, free water infusion can be started at 1.35 mL/kg/h.
- **These calculations DO NOT preclude the need for close monitoring and frequent measurement of the serum sodium levels.** If the sodium concentration is not changing at the desired rate, the clinician should adjust the free water infusion as appropriate.
- Normal saline (0.9%) should only be used in the hypernatremic patient with severe volume depletion requiring fluid resuscitation. Lesser degrees of clinical volume depletion can be treated with 0.22% ("quarter normal") or 0.45% ("half normal") saline solution (39 and 77 mmol/L Na$^+$, respectively). Once volume status has been restored, 5% dextrose solution alone should be used to correct hypernatremia.
- Central DI may be treated with subcutaneous desmopressin acetate (**DDAVP**) titrated to effect. There are several management options for nephrogenic DI. Thiazide diuretics ± NSAIDs cause volume depletion and increase renal Na$^+$ retention. Amiloride may block access of lithium to the Na$^+$ channel of the collecting tubule and is useful in lithium-induced nephrogenic DI. Consultation with colleagues experienced in treating patients with DI may prove invaluable.

REFERENCES

1. Upadhyay A, Jaber BL, Madias NE. Epidemiology of hyponatremia. *Semin Nephrol* 2009;29:227–38.
2. Hoorn EJ, Lindemans J, Zietse R. Development of severe hyponatremia in hospitalized patients: treatment-related risk factors and inadequate management. *Nephrol Dial Transplant* 2006;21:70–6.
3. Zilberberg MD, Exuzides A, Spalding J, et al. Epidemiology, clinical and economic outcomes of admission hyponatremia among hospitalized patients. *Curr Med Res Opin* 2008;24:1601–8.
4. Sajadieh A, Binici Z, Mouridsen MR, et al. Mild hyponatremia carries a poor prognosis in community subjects. *Am J Med* 2009;122:679–86.
5. Waikar SS, Mount DB, Curhan GC. Mortality after hospitalization with mild, moderate and severe hyponatremia. *Am J Med* 2009;122:857–65.
6. Balling L, Schou M, Videbaek L, et al. Prevalence and prognostic significance of hyponatraemia in outpatients with chronic heart failure. *Eur J Heart Fail* 2011;13:968–73.
7. Bettari L, Fiuzat M, Shaw LK, et al. Hyponatremia and long-term outcomes in chronic heart failure: an observational study from the Duke Databank for cardiovascular diseases. *J Card Fail* 2012;18:74–81.
8. Edmonds, ZV. Hyponatremia in pneumonia. *J Hosp Med* 2012;7:S11–3.
9. Doshi SM, Shah P, Lei X, et al. Hyponatremia in hospitalized cancer patients and its impact on clinical outcomes. *Am J Kidney Dis* 2012;59(2):222–8.
10. Ruf AE, Kremers WK, Chavez LL, et al. Addition of serum sodium into the MELD score predicts waiting list mortality better than MELD alone. *Liver Transpl* 2005;11(3):336–43.
11. Guevara M, Baccaro ME, Torre A, et al. Hyponatremia is a risk factor of hepatic encephalopathy in patients with cirrhosis: a prospective study with time-dependent analysis. *Am J Gastroenterol* 2009;104:1382–89.
12. Sigal SH. Hyponatremia in cirrhosis. *J Hosp Med* 2012;7:S14–7.
13. Rodrigues B, Staff I, Fortunato G, et al. Hyponatremia in the prognosis of acute ischemic stroke. *J Stroke Cerebrovasc Dis* 2014;23:850–4.
14. Renneboog B, Musch W, Vandemergel X, et al. Mild chronic hyponatremia is associated with falls, unsteadiness and attention deficits. *Am J Med* 2006;119(1):71.e1–8.

15. Verbalis JG, Barsony J, Sugimura Y, et al. Hyponatremia-induced osteoporosis. *J Bone Miner Res* 2010;25:554–63.
16. Jamal SA, Arampatzis S, Litwack-Harrison S, et al. Hyponatremia and fractures: findings from the MrOS study. *J Bone Miner Res* 2015;30:967–9.
17. Kengne FG, Andres C, Sattar L, et al. Mild hyponatremia and risk of fracture in the ambulatory elderly. *Q J Med* 2008;101:583–8.
18. Leung AA, McAlister FA, Rogers SO, et al. Preoperative hyponatremia and perioperative complications. *Arch Intern Med* 2012;171(19):1474–81.
19. Bennani SL, Abouqal R, Zeggwagh AA, et al. Incidence, causes and prognostic factors of hyponatremia in intensive care [French]. *Rev Med Interne* 2003;24:224–9.
20. Wald R, Jaber BL, Price LL, et al. Impact of hospital-associated hyponatremia on selected outcomes. *Arch Intern Med* 2010;170:294–302.
21. Amin A, Deitzelweig S, Christian R, et al. Evaluation of incremental healthcare resource burden and readmission rates associated with hospitalized hyponatremic patients in the US. *J Hosp Med* 2012;7:634–9.
22. Deitzelweig S, Amin A, Christian R, et al. Hyponatremia-associated healthcare burden among US patients hospitalized for cirrhosis. *Adv Ther* 2013;30:71–80.
23. Boscoe A, Paramore C, Verbalis JG. Cost of illness of hyponatremia in the United States. *Cost Eff Resour Alloc* 2006;4:10.
24. Verbalis JG, Goldsmith SR, Greenberg A, et al. Diagnosis, evaluation, and treatment of hyponatremia: expert panel recommendations. *Am J Med* 2013;126:S5–41.
25. Palmer BF. Diagnostic approach and management of inpatient hyponatremia. *J Hosp Med* 2010;5:S1–7.
26. Hillier TA, Abbott RD, Barrett EJ. Hyponatremia: evaluating the correction factor for hyperglycemia. *Am J Med* 1999;106:399–403.
27. Sterns RH, Silver SM. Salt and water: read the package insert. *QJM* 2003;96:549–52.
28. Singh TD, Fugate, JE, Rabinstein AA. Central pontine and extrapontine myelinolysis: a systematic review. *Eur J Neurol* 2014;21:1443–50.
29. Aylwin S, Burst V, Peri A, et al. 'Dos and Don'ts' in the management of hyponatremia. *Curr Med Res Opin* 2015;31:1755–61.
30. Furst H, Hallows KR, Post J, et al. The urine/plasma electrolyte ratio: a predictive guide to water restriction. *Am J Med Sci* 2000;319(4):240–4.
31. Sterns RH, Silver SM, Hix JK. Urea for hyponatremia? *Kidney Int* 2015;87:268–70.
32. Greenberg A, Verbalis JG. Vasopressin receptor antagonists. *Kidney Int* 2006;69:2124.
33. Udelson JE, Smith WB, Hendrix GH, et al. Acute hemodynamic effects of conivaptan, a dual V(1a) and V(2) vasopressin receptor antagonist, in patients with advanced heart failure. *Circulation* 2001;104:2417–23.
34. Schrier RW, Gross P, Gheorghiade M, et al. Tolvaptan, a selective oral vasopressin V_2-receptor antagonist for hyponatremia. *N Engl J Med* 2006;355:2099–112.
35. Konstam MA, Gheorghiade M, Burnett JC Jr, et al. Effects of oral tolvaptan in patients hospitalized for worsening heart failure: the EVEREST outcome trial. *JAMA* 2007;297:1319–31.
36. Torres VE, Chapman AB, Devuyst O, et al. Tolvaptan in patients with autosomal dominant polycystic kidney disease. *N Engl J Med* 2012;367:2407–18.
37. Krag A, Moller S, Henriksen JH, et al. Terlipressin improves renal function in patients with cirrhosis and ascites without hepatorenal syndrome. *Hepatology* 2007;46:1863–71.
38. Sonnenblick M, Friedlander Y, Rosin A. Diuretic-induced severe hyponatremia. Review and analysis of 129 reported patients. *Chest* 1993;103:601–6.
39. Palevsky PM, Bhagrath R, Greenberg A. Hypernatremia in hospitalized patients. *Ann Intern Med* 1996;124:197–200.
40. Poldermans KH, Schreuder WO, Strack van Schijndel RJ. Hypernatremia in the intensive care unit: an indicator of quality of care? *Crit Care Med* 1999;27:1105–8.
41. Snyder NA, Feigal DW, Arieff AI. Hypernatremia in elderly patients a heterogeneous, morbid, and iatrogenic entity. *Ann Intern Med* 1987;107:309–19.
42. Leung AA, McAlister FA, Finlayson SR, et al. Preoperative hypernatremia predicts increased perioperative morbidity and mortality. *Am J Med* 2013;126:877–86.
43. Verbalis JG. Disorders of body water homeostasis. *Best Pract Res Clin Endocrinol Metab* 2003;17:471–503.
44. Arora SK. Hypernatremic disorders in the intensive care unit. *J Intensive Care Med* 2013;28:37–45.

Approach to the Patient with Hematuria

20

Melissa DeFoe and Melvin Blanchard

GENERAL PRINCIPLES

- **Hematuria** is defined by the presence of abnormal number of red blood cells (RBCs) in the urine and may be microscopic or macroscopic.[1] A small number of RBCs may be found in the urine of normal individuals, usually ≤3 RBCs per high-power field in urinary sediment, although this level of hematuria does not exclude disease.
- **Microscopic hematuria** is defined by the American Urological Association (AUA) as ≥3 RBCs per high-power field on a single microscopic evaluation of urinary sediment.[1]
  - A positive dipstick does not define microscopic hematuria, nor should it prompt a workup without further microscopic evidence.[1]
  - The US Preventive Task Force has concluded that there is insufficient evidence to support screening urinalysis in the general population, so hematuria is generally found incidentally.[2]
- In macroscopic (gross) hematuria, the urine appears red, cola-colored, or brown. The dipstick is positive, and there is red sediment after light centrifugation.
- Hematuria may be due to an abnormality anywhere from the glomerulus to the distal tip of the urethra.
- Table 20-1 outlines etiologies of hematuria.[3–5]

DIAGNOSIS

Clinical Presentation

History
- Hematuria at the initiation of urinary stream is indicative of a urethral source.[6]
- If hematuria begins midway through, it suggests bladder origin.[6]
- The source may be in the upper urinary tract (kidney, ureter) or located diffusely in the bladder when hematuria occurs throughout urination.[6]
- In women, it is important to determine whether menstruation is contaminating the urinary specimen.
- A recent history of trauma, urinary catheterization, and exercise may indicate the cause of hematuria.
- An obstructing blood clot in the bladder may impair urination.
- A recent history of pharyngitis suggests a postinfectious glomerulonephritis, whereas a recent mucosal infection (upper respiratory infection, urinary tract infection [UTI], enteritis, etc.) may accompany IgA nephropathy. Recurrent sinusitis/otitis may suggest granulomatosis with polyangiitis.
- Bloody diarrhea may precede hemolytic uremic syndrome.
- Dysuria, urinary frequency/urgency, and flank pain may be clues to cystitis/pyelonephritis. Urethral discharge may or may not occur with urethritis.[6]
- Flank pain radiating to the groin may indicate nephrolithiasis or blood clot causing urethral obstruction.[6]
- Rash and arthralgias may point to lupus erythematosus.[6]

TABLE 20-1 DIFFERENTIAL DIAGNOSIS OF HEMATURIA

Glomerular		Nonglomerular	
Proliferative GN	**Nonproliferative GN**	**Neoplasms**	**Vascular**
IgA nephropathy	Minimal change disease	Renal cell carcinoma	Renal vein thrombosis
Postinfectious GN	Focal glomerulosclerosis	Transitional cell cancer	Renal infarction
Crescentic GN	Membranous nephropathy	Prostate carcinoma	Malignant hypertension
Membranoproliferative GN	Hemolytic uremic syndrome	Squamous cell cancer of the urethra	Arteriovenous malformation
Fibrillary GN	**Familial glomerular disease**	Wilms tumor	**Other**
Henoch-Schönlein purpura	Alport syndrome	Angiomyolipoma	Nephrolithiasis
Systemic lupus erythematosus	Familial benign hematuria	Multiple myeloma	Trauma
Anti-glomerular basement membrane nephritis	Fabry disease	**Infectious**	Vigorous exercise
Systemic vasculitides	Nail–patella syndrome	Acute cystitis	Cyclophosphamide
Chronic bacteremia		Prostatitis	Medullary sponge kidney
Mixed cryoglobulinemia		Urethritis	Loin pain hematuria syndrome
		Tuberculosis	
		Schistosomiasis	

GN, glomerulonephritis.

Adapted from Cohen R, Brown R. Microscopic hematuria. *N Engl J Med* 2003;348:2330–38; Vakili ST, Alam T, Sollinger H. Loin pain hematuria syndrome. *Am J Kidney Dis* 2014;64:460–72; Ziemba J, Guzzo TJ, Ramchandani P. Evaluation of the patient with asymptomatic microscopic hematuria. *Acad Radiol* 2015;22:1034–7, Refs.[4,5,9]

- Illegal drug use is a risk factor for human immunodeficiency virus (HIV), hepatitis, endocarditis, and (in those using IV heroin) focal segmental glomerular sclerosis (FSGS) versus membranoproliferative glomerulonephritis (MGPN).[7]
- Exposure to certain over-the-counter and prescription drugs can cause hematuria. These agents include analgesics (analgesic nephropathy), anticoagulants, and cyclophosphamide (cystitis).
- Risk factors for malignancy include age >50; cigarette smoking; occupational exposure to certain industries (leather, dye, rubber, or tire manufacturing); pelvic irradiation; high-dose cyclophosphamide; ingestion of aristolochic acid, which is found in some weight loss products; and recent gross hematuria.
- Dietary and medical history should be reviewed as ingestion of beets, blackberries, iron, and rifampin can alter urine color. Porphyria also can alter urine color.[6]

A family history should include inquiries about deafness and kidney disease (Alport syndrome), cerebral aneurysm and kidney disease (autosomal dominant polycystic kidney disease), sickle cell disease, and kidney stones. Patients of Asian heritage may be at higher risk for IgA nephropathy.[5,8]

Physical Examination

The physical examination may contribute to identifying the cause of hematuria.

- A markedly elevated blood pressure may indicate hypertensive emergency as the cause.
- The dermatologic exam may reveal rashes suggestive of vasculitis and autoimmune disease (systemic lupus erythematosus); palpable purpura on the buttocks suggests Henoch-Schönlein purpura; erythematous or painful lesions on the palmar surfaces of the hands, feet, or nail beds are stigmata of endocarditis.
- The joint exam may reveal signs of arthritis or synovitis suggesting an autoimmune etiology.
- A careful genitourinary exam is essential in the evaluation of hematuria.
  - In men, examine for prostatitis, prostate cancer, benign prostate hypertrophy, testicular masses, and signs of epididymitis.
  - In women, a pelvic exam is essential to assess for masses or malignancy.

Diagnostic Testing

- The AUA has developed guidelines for the evaluation of hematuria and is outlined in Figure 20-1.[3]
- There is debate about whether the 2012 AUA guidelines are more aggressive than necessary given the relatively high prevalence of microscopic hematuria (9–18%) compared with low prevalence of urothelial cancer in the general population (0.01–3%).[9,10]
- An alternative guideline based on risk model known as the Hematuria Risk Index has been suggested.[10] It characterizes patients based on risk of malignancy using a model based on an 11-point scale as follows:
  - 4 points each: history of gross hematuria, age > 50
  - 1 point each: history of smoking, male sex, and >25 RBC/high power field (HPF) on a recent urinalysis
  - Interpretation:
    - 0–4: low risk
    - 5–8: moderate risk
    - 9–11: high risk[10]
    - Microscopic hematuria is unreliable at predicting urinary tract malignancies, and it is suggested that patients < 50 with no history of gross hematuria may not benefit from further. Practitioners can use this scale to help guide decisions to refer patients to urology for further workup.[10]
- Hematuria in the setting of supratherapeutic anticoagulation or bleeding diathesis still requires a workup.[1]

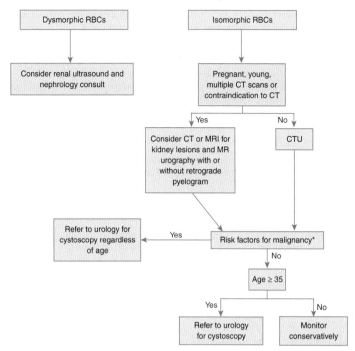

FIGURE 20-1 Evaluation of microscopic hematuria. *Risk factors for malignancy include recent gross hematuria, history of radiation, and smoking history. (Adapted from Niemi M, Cohen R. Evaluation of microscopic hematuria: a critical review and proposed algorithm. *Adv Chronic Kidney Dis* 2015;22:289–96.)

Laboratories
- Initial evaluation of hematuria should include evaluation after centrifugations (5 minutes at 3000 rpm) of a fresh urine specimen and examination of the sediment (macroscopic and microscopic). An unspun sample should be evaluated with the dipstick as well. The physician should not rely on the lab for this evaluation. The goal is to determine the source of the hematuria so that the patient can be quickly triaged.[11]
  - Macroscopic clues: RBCs collect in the supernatant after centrifugation. If the supernatant is red, myoglobin, hemoglobin, or pigments from medications may be the cause.[11]
  - Dipstick clues: Green color is positive for hemoglobin. Speckled patterns indicate intact RBCs, whereas uniform indicates free hemoglobin. Positive dipstick results for blood without RBCs on microscopy should prompt an evaluation for myoglobinuria.[6]
  - Microscopic analysis
    - If microscopy evaluation reveals dysmorphic RBCs (irregular cell membrane), red cell casts, and/or proteinuria, this suggests bleeding of glomerular origin.[11] Further testing should include the following serologies: antinuclear antibody (ANA), antineutrophil cytoplasmic antibody (ANCA), HIV, hepatitis panel, antiglomerular membrane, C3, C4, Venereal Disease Research Laboratory (VDRL) test, and antistreptolysin O titer.
    - If microscopy demonstrates isomorphic RBCs in the presence of pyuria, dysuria, or bacteriuria are likely related to a UTI. The presence of hematuria should be reevaluated after antibiotic therapy. In the absence of signs and symptoms of a UTI, the presence of isomorphic RBCs warrants evaluation for malignancy or renal calculi.[11]

- Other initial lab data should include basic chemistries, complete blood count, prothrombin time, partial thromboplastin time, and hepatic function panel.

Imaging
- As indicated in Figure 20-1, patients with dysmorphic RBCs or proteinuria should undergo a renal ultrasound with referral to nephrology.[5]
- Patients with reasonable suspicion of malignancy without contraindications to CT should undergo a CT urography. Patients with contraindications to CT can undergo MRI urography with or without retrograde pyelogram. If patient is of high risk for malignancy or aged 35 or greater, the AUA recommends referral to urology for cystoscopy.[1,5]

Diagnostic Procedures
The diagnosis of malignancy requires a tissue sample, usually obtained by biopsy performed by urology or other surgical specialists. Causes of glomerular bleeding are also often diagnosed by biopsy.

TREATMENT

- The treatment of hematuria is essentially entirely dependent on the cause. Thus, management of patients with hematuria lies mainly in establishing the origin of hematuria, determining malignancy versus benign origin, and rapid triage to the appropriate specialist.
- Any patient thought to have bleeding of glomerular origin (e.g., red cell casts, proteinuria, elevated creatinine) should be seen promptly by a nephrologist, particularly those patients who have evidence of renal dysfunction.
- Patients with renal calculi, masses, or positive cytology should be evaluated by a urologist.

MONITORING/FOLLOW-UP

In patients with persistent microscopic hematuria, yearly urinalysis should be conducted. If two consecutive annual urinalyses are negative for hematuria, no further screening urinalyses for detecting hematuria are required. In patients with persistent microscopic hematuria with an initial negative workup, clinicians should consider repeating workup every 3–5 years.[1]

REFERENCES

1. Davis R, Jones S, Barocas D, et al. AUA 2012 Guidelines. Diagnosis, Evaluation and Follow-up of Asymptomatic Microhematuria (AMH) in Adults. AUA GUIDELINE. May 2012. Available at: https://www.auanet.org/education/guidelines/asymptomatic-microhematuria.cfm (last accessed 2/7/16).
2. Moyer VA. Screening for bladder cancer: U.S. Preventive Services Task Force recommendation statement. *Ann Intern Med* 2011;155:246–51.
3. Cohen R, Brown R. Microscopic hematuria. *N Engl J Med* 2003;348:2330–8.
4. Vakili ST, Alam T, Sollinger H. Loin pain hematuria syndrome. *Am J Kidney Dis* 2014;64:460–72.
5. Ziemba J, Guzzo TJ, Ramchandani P. Evaluation of the patient with asymptomatic microscopic hematuria. *Acad Radiol* 2015;22:1034–7.
6. Tu WH, Shortliffe LD. Evaluation of asymptomatic, atraumatic hematuria in children and adults. *Nat Rev Urol* 2010;7:189–94.
7. Jaffe J, Kimmel P. Chronic nephropathies of cocaine and heroin abuse: a critical review. *Clin J Am Soc Nephrol* 2006;4:655–67.
8. Magistroni R, D'Agati VD, Appel GB, Kiryluk K. New developments in the genetics, pathogenesis, and therapy of IgA nephropathy. *Kidney Int* 2015;88:974–89.
9. Niemi, M, Cohen R. Evaluation of microscopic hematuria: a critical review and proposed algorithm. *Adv Chronic Kidney Dis* 2015;22:289–96.
10. Loo RK, Lieberman SF, Slezak JM, et al. Stratifying risk of urinary tract malignant tumors in patients with asymptomatic microscopic hematuria. *Mayo Clin Proc* 2013;88:129–32.
11. Mazhari R, Kimmel P. Hematuria: an algorithmic approach to finding the cause. *Cleve Clin J Med* 2002;69:870–84.

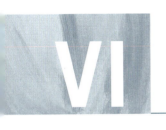

Infectious Disease

Infectious Diseases

Pneumonia

Indra Bole and Mark S. Thoelke

GENERAL PRINCIPLES

- Pneumonia is an inflammatory condition of the pulmonary parenchyma caused by an infection. The symptoms, treatment, and morbidity associated with the infection vary by the setting in which it is acquired.
- A classification system for pneumonia has been adopted by the Infectious Disease Society of America (IDSA) and the American Thoracic Society (ATS) as below[1]:
  - **Community-acquired pneumonia** (CAP): acquired as an outpatient, without any risk factors for HCAP, as below
  - **Hospital-acquired pneumonia** (HAP): acquired 48 hours or more after admission if not incubating at admission
  - **Health care–associated pneumonia** (HCAP): acquired in patients who were hospitalized in acute care hospitals for ≥2 days within 90 days of onset of infection, reside in a nursing home or long-term care facility, attended a hospital-based or hemodialysis clinic, or received recent wound care, chemotherapy, or intravenous IV antibiotics
  - **Ventilator-associated pneumonia** (VAP): pneumonia occurring in patients more than 48–72 hours after intubation
- Medical consultants will be asked to help manage pneumonia contracted from various locations, both in and out of the hospital.

Epidemiology

- Pneumonia is a significant contributor to morbidity and mortality worldwide. According to the 2010 US National Hospital Discharge Survey, pneumonia was the fifth most common major primary diagnosis at the time of discharge from inpatient care.
- The mortality associated with pneumonia increases drastically with age, from 2 annual deaths per 100,000 population for those aged 35–44 to 104 annual deaths per 100,000 population in those aged 75–84.[2]

Pathophysiology

- The etiology of pneumonia in a particular patient depends on a variety of factors, including host immune status and comorbidities including chronic respiratory disease and chronic liver disease and infection status of contacts.
- Viral pneumonias, such as influenza pneumonia, spread between hosts through multiple mechanisms including direct exposure of host mucosa with virus-inoculated bodily fluids of an infected contact, airborne inhalation of virus-inoculated droplets, and hand-to-mouth exposure of virus-inoculated secretions via direct contact or fomites.
- Bacterial pneumonias typically began as micro- or macroaspirations of nasopharyngeal or oropharyngeal bacteria. Rarely, bacteria can be transmitted through airborne droplets and lead to pneumonia after inhalation.
- After inoculation of alveoli with the causative agent of pneumonia, an inflammatory cascade is activated with subsequent chemotaxis and cytokine release. This process leads to symptoms typical of pneumonia including cough, fatigue, fever, dyspnea, and chest pain.

- Common pathogens of CAP include the following:
  - Bacteria
    - *Streptococcus pneumoniae* (most common)
    - *Haemophilus influenzae*
    - *Moraxella catarrhalis*
    - *Chlamydophila pneumoniae*
    - *Mycoplasma pneumoniae*
    - *Legionella* species and others
  - Viruses (influenza and others)
  - Fungi (e.g., *Histoplasma*)
- In cases of HCAP, HAP, and VAP, typical causative organisms are more likely to be bacteria with up to 70% of cases caused by gram-negative rods. Viral and fungal pathogens are unusual. HAP and VAP acquired early in the hospital course are less likely to involve multidrug-resistant (MDR) organisms, and the spectrum of organisms is closer to CAP.
  - Common bacterial pathogens include the following:
    - *Pseudomonas aeruginosa*
    - *Klebsiella pneumoniae*
    - *Escherichia coli*
    - *Acinetobacter* species
    - *Serratia* species
    - *Enterobacter* species
    - *Staphylococcus aureus*, including multidrug-resistant *S. aureus* (MRSA)

DIAGNOSIS

Clinical Presentation

History
- The initial presentation of patients with pneumonia can vary widely based on causative agent, comorbid conditions, and severity of infection.
- Symptoms typical of pneumonia include the following:
  - Cough
  - Dyspnea
  - Increased sputum production
  - Pleuritic chest pain
  - Fevers
  - Chills
  - Anorexia
  - Nausea and vomiting
  - Mental status changes, particularly in the elderly

Physical Examination
The physical examination for pneumonia should involve prompt evaluation of vital signs and stability of respiratory status. Findings typical of pneumonia can include rales, rhonchi, or evidence of consolidation with egophony and dullness to percussion.

Differential Diagnosis
There are several noninfectious etiologies that may mimic pneumonia.

- Aspiration pneumonitis
- Congestive heart failure (CHF)
- Pulmonary embolus
- Acute respiratory distress syndrome (ARDS)
- Malignancy

- Bronchiolitis obliterans organizing pneumonia (BOOP)
- Alveolar hemorrhage
- Vasculitis
- Drug reaction

Diagnostic Testing

- Initial diagnostic evaluation of suspected pneumonia in an acute care setting or hospital-based clinic should include chest radiograph and laboratory evaluation including the following:
  - Sputum Gram stain and culture and blood Gram stain and culture (positive in 10–20% of pneumonias) prior to antibiotic administration if feasible
  - *Legionella pneumophila* urine antigen and *S. pneumoniae* urine antigen tests if these infections as suspected and especially in the setting of critical illness
  - Complete blood cell count (CBC)
  - Lactic acid level if sepsis syndrome criteria are met
  - Procalcitonin level may be used to help differentiate between viral and bacterial etiologies of pneumonia and guide duration of antibiotic therapy.
- If a significant pleural effusion is present (>1 cm of fluid layers on a lateral decubitus), consider a diagnostic thoracentesis to rule out an empyema.
- In intubated patients, tracheal aspirate Gram stain and culture have been shown to correlate well with invasive quantitative cultures, with some loss of specificity.
- Nasopharyngeal respiratory viral pathogen multiplex polymerase chain reaction (PCR) and influenza virus PCR may help rapidly detect common respiratory viruses as causative or contributory agents in pneumonia.

TREATMENT

- Admission decision: The decision to admit a patient with CAP is complex. Multiple scoring systems have been established to aid risk stratification in this cohort of patients. The most frequently used prediction rules include the Pneumonia Severity Index (complex, but best supported by evidence), the CURB-65 score (easy to implement), and the severe CAP score (helpful in stratifying which patients may be best suited in an intensive care unit setting).
- The CURB-65 criteria have been used to predict 30-day mortality. A score of 2 points out of 5 warrants consideration for short-stay unit admission or close outpatient monitoring, and a score of 3 or more suggests need for inpatient hospitalization and consideration for ICU admission. CURB-65 criteria (0–1 points, outpatient; 2 points, medical floor admission; ≥ 3 points, ICU-level care).[3]
  - Confusion
  - Uremia (blood urea nitrogen [BUN] > 20 mg/dL)
  - Respiratory rate (>30 breaths/min)
  - Blood pressure (systolic < 90 mm Hg or diastolic <60 mm Hg)
  - Age ≥ 65 years
- If a patient is hospitalized, general supportive measures such as oxygen supplementation, pulmonary toilet, and prophylaxis for deep venous thrombosis should always be considered. Hospitalization also offers an opportunity to screen for pneumococcal infection and administer pneumococcal vaccine. Initial selection of antibiotic is discussed below. Pathogen-directed therapy is ideal if an organism is later obtained. Prompt initiation of antibiotics appears to improve outcomes.[4]
- Empiric recommendations for antibiotic therapy are guided by likely organisms and expected resistance patterns of these organisms. As above, it is important to tailor these recommendations based on location and temporal situation (know your antibiogram).

- **Community-acquired pneumonia**[5]
  - A β-lactam antibiotic plus a macrolide (e.g., ceftriaxone 1 g IV qday plus azithromycin 250 mg PO qday) **OR** a fluoroquinolone (e.g., moxifloxacin, 400 mg PO/IV qday)
  - In those patients ill enough to require ICU placement, fluoroquinolone therapy should be combined with a β-lactam agent.
  - A recent meta-analysis has shown that systemic corticosteroids in hospitalized patients with CAP may confer a modest mortality benefit and reduce hospital stay.[6]
- **Hospital- or ventilator-acquired pneumonia**, early onset: early HAP without risk factors for MDR may be treated as CAP above.
- **Hospital- or ventilator-acquired pneumonia**, late onset; health care–acquired pneumonia; or any risk for multidrug-resistant pathogens[1]
  - Antipseudomonal cephalosporin (e.g., cefepime) **OR** antipseudomonal carbapenem (e.g., meropenem) **OR** β-lactam/β-lactamase inhibitor (piperacillin–tazobactam); aztreonam can be substituted for penicillin allergic patients **PLUS**
  - Antipseudomonal fluoroquinolone **OR** aminoglycoside **PLUS**
  - Vancomycin or linezolid
- According to ATS/IDSA guidelines,[1] treatment of nosocomial pneumonias such as VAP, HCAP, and HAP should follow these general principles:
  - Avoid inadequate treatment given significant increase in mortality with undertreated health care infections.
  - Tailor antibiotic therapy based on region, hospital, location within hospital, and time period.
  - Avoid antibiotic overuse by tailoring therapy based on culture results and treating for minimum effective time period.
- Patients will usually respond to appropriate treatment within 3–4 days, even if they are bacteremic.[7] Nonresponders after this time should be evaluated for resistant organisms, empyema, or the alternate etiologies listed above. The IDSA and ATS recommend that CAP should be treated for a minimum of 5 days and until the patient is afebrile for 72 hours. Step-down to oral therapy and discharge from the hospital can occur when there is no more than one marker of clinical instability.[8] See Table 21-1 for markers of clinical stability.
- Duration of therapy for nosocomial pneumonias is uncertain, but shorter duration (8 vs. 15 days) has been shown to be as effective and to lead to less resistance.[9] *Pseudomonas* and *Staphylococcus* species warrant 14-day courses.[1] Negative growth in sputum or tracheal aspirate allows stopping treatment for *Staphylococcus*.

TABLE 21-1 MARKERS OF CLINICAL STABILITY

Temperature < 37.8°C
Pulse < 100 bpm
Respiratory rate < 24/min
O_2 saturation > 90%
Maintaining oral intake
Normal mental status

Adapted from Halm EA, Fine MJ, Kapoor WN, et al. Instability on hospital discharge and the risk of adverse outcomes in patients with pneumonia. *Arch Intern Med* 2002;162(11):1278–84.

- It is also advisable to repeat the chest x-ray in 6–12 weeks in older patients and chronic smokers to document resolution of pneumonia and exclude an associated malignancy leading to infection.

REFERENCES

1. ATS/IDSA Joint Statement. Guidelines for the management of adults with hospital-acquired, ventilator-associated, and healthcare-associated pneumonia. *Am J Respir Care Med* 2005;171: 388–416.
2. Heron M. Deaths: leading causes for 2012. *Natl Vital Stat Rep* 2015;64:1–93.
3. Lim WS, van der Eerden MM, Laing R, et al. Defining community acquired pneumonia severity on presentation to hospital: an international derivation and validation study. *Thorax* 2003;58:377–82.
4. Iregui M, Ward S, Sherman G, et al. Clinical importance of delays in the initiation of appropriate antibiotic treatment for ventilator-associated pneumonia. *Chest* 2002;122:262–8.
5. Mandell LA, Wunderink RG, Anzueto A, et al. Infectious Diseases Society of America/American Thoracic Society consensus guidelines on the management of community-acquired pneumonia in adults. *Clin Infect Dis* 2007;44(Suppl 2):S27–72.
6. Siemieniuk RA, Meade MO, Alonso-Coello P, et al. Corticosteroid Therapy for patients hospitalized with community-acquired pneumonia: a systematic review and meta-analysis. *Ann Intern Med* 2015;163:519–28.
7. Ramirez JA, Bordon J. Early switch from intravenous to oral antibiotics in hospitalized patients with bacteremic community-acquired *Streptococcus pneumoniae* pneumonia. *Arch Intern Med* 2001;161:848–50.
8. Halm EA, Fine MJ, Kapoor WN, et al. Instability on hospital discharge and the risk of adverse outcomes in patients with pneumonia. *Arch Intern Med* 2002;162(11):1278–84.
9. Chastre J, Wolff M, Fagon JY, et al. Comparison of 8 vs 15 days of antibiotic therapy for ventilator-associated pneumonia in adults: a randomized trial. *JAMA* 2003;290:2588–98.

Urinary Tract Infections

Caline S. Mattar and Stephen Y. Liang

GENERAL PRINCIPLES

- Urinary tract infections (UTIs) are the second most common cause for antibiotic prescription after upper respiratory infections.
- UTIs range from simple cystitis to pyelonephritis, bacteremia, and sepsis. Definitions include the following:
  - **Cystitis** is an infection of the bladder and the lower urinary tract.
    - **Uncomplicated cystitis** is an infection in women with a structurally normal urinary tract system.
    - **Complicated cystitis** is an infection in men, in pregnant women, or in the setting of obstruction, immunosuppression, renal failure, indwelling urinary catheter or nephrostomy tube or other recent instrumentation/urological procedure, renal transplant, urinary retention, and other metabolic abnormalities or infections with unusual pathogens.
  - **Pyelonephritis** is an infection involving the kidney. Similar definitions exist for **uncomplicated** and **complicated pyelonephritis**. Namely, patients with a structurally abnormal genitourinary tract have complicated pyelonephritis.
- Uncomplicated cystitis is especially frequent in women and generally responds readily to antibiotics.
- UTIs also account for 40% of all hospital-acquired infections, typically in the setting of an indwelling urinary catheter, and contribute significant morbidity and mortality.
- Decreased urine flow (e.g., outflow obstruction, prostatic disease, strictures, calculus, neurogenic bladder, inadequate fluid intake)[1]
- Increased urinary tract colonization (e.g., sexual activity, estrogen depletion, or use of spermicides or systemic antibiotics)[1]
- Bacterial ascent (e.g., urinary catheterization or instrumentation)[1]

DIAGNOSIS

Clinical Presentation

History

- It is important to distinguish simple cystitis from a complicated UTI and pyelonephritis. It may be difficult to differentiate cystitis from pyelonephritis in many patients because signs and symptoms may be nonspecific.
- It is important to discern historical information that would differentiate uncomplicated versus complicated infection as UTIs are classified based on patient characteristics.
- Typical symptoms such as dysuria, urinary frequency, and urinary urgency are common in all types of UTI.
- Fever, back pain, nausea, vomiting, and malaise suggest pyelonephritis, but these symptoms are neither sensitive nor specific.

Physical Examination
- Patients with cystitis may have suprapubic tenderness.
- Fever and tenderness at the costovertebral angle indicate pyelonephritis.
- Men should have a prostate exam to rule out prostatitis and genital exams to rule out orchitis or epididymitis.

Diagnostic Testing
Laboratories
- Diagnosis is made with appropriately collected urinalysis and urine culture. A clean-catch midstream urine specimen is preferred to minimize contamination, particularly in women. In catheterized patients, urine should be collected from the drainage catheter (many systems have a needleless port for this purpose) and not the drainage bag.
- Pyuria: >10 leukocytes per high-power field on microscopy. Specificity for UTI increases to 99% when pyuria is associated with a bacterial colony count of >10^5 colony-forming units (CFU)/mL from an accompanying urine culture; however, sensitivity remains low at 51%.[1]
- Nitrite test: effective at detecting gram-negative infections in first-morning voids; however, during later voids, the bacteria do not have adequate time to reduce nitrate to nitrite.

Imaging
Imaging of the urinary tract should be considered for all men, women with treatment failure, and in those with persistent pyuria or hematuria.[1]

TREATMENT

- **Cystitis**
  - **Uncomplicated cystitis** is generally monomicrobial and most commonly caused by *Escherichia coli* (*E. coli*) followed by *Staphylococcus saprophyticus* and *Enterococcus* species. Empiric therapy includes trimethoprim–sulfamethoxazole (TMP–SMX), nitrofurantoin, fluoroquinolones (e.g., ciprofloxacin given its high urinary concentration), and fosfomycin.[2] Local antibiotic susceptibility patterns should be considered when selecting empiric therapy. Standard duration of therapy is 3–7 days.[2]
  - In **complicated cystitis**, in addition to those bacteria, a wider spectrum of organisms including *Pseudomonas*, *Serratia*, *Providencia*, and fungi may be encountered. Longer durations of therapy may be necessary in patients with delayed response to treatment or complicated cystitis. Generally, a 14-day course of antibiotics is recommended for a complicated UTI.
- **Pyelonephritis**
  - *E. coli* and *Enterococcus* are the most common organisms implicated in uncomplicated, community-acquired pyelonephritis. In addition to these organisms, patients with complicated UTI, with recurrent infection, or who are hospitalized may have a greater risk of infection due to antibiotic-resistant organisms (e.g., *Proteus*, *Klebsiella*, *Enterobacter*, and *Pseudomonas*).
  - Imaging is recommended if symptoms persist after 48–72 hours of appropriate antibiotic therapy. Renal ultrasonography and CT scan are useful modalities for evaluating the urinary tract.
  - Uncomplicated pyelonephritis in patients able to tolerate oral intake can be treated with fluoroquinolones specifically ciprofloxacin or TMP–SMX. If a gram-positive organism is suspected, amoxicillin–clavulanate is an acceptable alternative.[2]
  - If the patient is ill with leukocytosis, high fever, signs of sepsis, or nausea and vomiting, intravenous antibiotics such as a fluoroquinolone with or without an aminoglycoside or third- or fourth-generation cephalosporin with or without an aminoglycoside should be used.

- In patients with complicated pyelonephritis where an antibiotic-resistant organism is suspected, initial treatment should consist of a beta-lactam/beta-lactamase inhibitor, a carbapenem, or an aminoglycoside.
- Duration of therapy for pyelonephritis is 7–14 days with more recent data demonstrating that 7 days of therapy is adequate.[3]

SPECIAL CONSIDERATIONS

Renal and Perinephric Abscesses

- Can be a complication of UTI or result from hematogenous spread.
- Risk factors include diabetes, pregnancy, and anatomic abnormalities.[4]
- Symptoms include fever, chills, abdominal pain, and less commonly dysuria. Costovertebral angle tenderness may be present on physical examination.[5]
- Contrast CT is the best imaging modality for evaluation of renal abscess. Ultrasonography can also be used.[4,5]
- Empiric therapy should be directed toward the suspected causative agents. If the abscess is thought to be due to pyelonephritis, therapy should be directed against gram-negative organisms. If hematogenous spread is suspected, antibiotics should cover the organism infecting the bloodstream.
- Drainage is required for all perinephric abscesses. For renal abscesses, size > 5 cm warrants drainage.[4]

Catheter-Associated UTI

- Catheter-associated UTI (CAUTI) is defined as growth of $\geq 10^3$ CFU/mL of bacteria with signs and symptoms suggestive of UTI, such as suprapubic discomfort or costovertebral angle tenderness, or unexplained systemic symptoms (e.g., altered mental status, hypotension, fever, or leukocytosis),[6] in the setting of an indwelling urinary catheter (e.g., urethral, suprapubic, or intermittent straight catheterization).
- Duration of urinary catheterization is the most important risk factor for developing a CAUTI. Discontinuation of the urinary catheter as early as possible is an effective CAUTI prevention measure.
- *E. coli* is the most common pathogen, followed by *Enterococcus* species, *Candida*, *Pseudomonas*, and *Klebsiella*.[6]
- Empiric therapy should consist of a third-generation cephalosporin (e.g., ceftriaxone) or a fluoroquinolone. In critically ill patients or if an antibiotic-resistant organism is suspected, coverage should be expanded to include *Pseudomonas* as well as gram-positive bacteria.
- Duration of therapy is generally 7 days for patients who exhibit prompt resolution of symptoms. It may be expanded to 10–14 days for patients with a delayed response to therapy.

Asymptomatic Bacteriuria

- Defined as the isolation of $>10^5$ CFU/mL of the same organism in the urine in a single clean-catch specimen for men or in two clean-catch specimens for women in the absence of symptoms (fever, chills, leukocytosis, flank pain, dysuria, frequency).
- Treat if the patient is pregnant or if the patient will undergo a urological intervention where mucosal bleeding is expected.[7]
- Treatment is not indicated in the elderly, spinal cord injury patients, patients with a urinary catheter, or those with diabetes mellitus.[7]

Asymptomatic Bacteriuria and UTI in Pregnancy

- Screen all pregnant women between 12 and 16 weeks of gestation for asymptomatic bacteriuria by urine culture.

- Treat if bacteriuria is present; asymptomatic bacteriuria in pregnancy has been associated with an increased risk of pyelonephritis and adverse outcomes (e.g., preterm delivery, low birth weight).
  - Antibiotic therapy should be tailored toward the susceptibility pattern of the recovered organism. The suggested duration of therapy is 3–7 days.[7]
  - A follow-up urine culture should be obtained a week after therapy to document clearance of bacteriuria.
- UTI symptoms such as dysuria, frequency, and urgency should prompt empiric antibiotic therapy as well as urinalysis and urine culture.[7]
- Pregnant women with pyelonephritis can be systemically ill and are at an increased risk for obstetrical complications as well as sepsis and septic shock. Pyelonephritis is typically treated with parenteral antibiotics during pregnancy. Duration of treatment should be 7–14 days.
- Safe antibiotics to treat UTI during pregnancy include penicillins, cephalosporins, aztreonam, carbapenems (except imipenem–cilastatin), nitrofurantoin, and fosfomycin. TMP–SMX should be avoided during early pregnancy as it is a folic acid antagonist.[1]

Recurrent UTI

- Recurrent UTI is defined as having three or more infections per year.[8]
  - Risk factors include spermicide use, new sexual partner, urinary incontinence, and increased postvoid residual urine.
  - Prevention strategies include postcoital voiding, increased fluid intake, and avoidance of contraceptive spermicides.
- Suppressive or postcoital antibiotic prophylaxis may be considered as a last resort for UTI prevention, but may promote antibiotic resistance.[8]

REFERENCES

1. Chambers ST. Cystitis and urethral syndromes. In: Cohen J, Opal SM, Powderly WG, eds. *Cohen & Powderly: Infectious Diseases*. 3rd ed. United Kingdom: Elsevier Ltd., 2010:589–97.
2. Warren JW, Abrutyn E, Hebel JR, et al. Guidelines for antimicrobial treatment of uncomplicated acute bacterial cystitis and acute pyelonephritis in women. Infectious Diseases Society of America (IDSA). *Clin Infect Dis* 1999;29:745–58.
3. Eliakim-Raz N, Yahav D, Paul M, Leibovici L. Duration of antibiotic treatment for acute pyelonephritis and septic urinary tract infection—7 days or less versus longer treatment: systematic review and meta-analysis of randomized controlled trials. *J Antimicrob Chemother* 2013;68:2183–91.
4. Drekonja DM, Johnson JR. Pyelonephritis and Abscesses of the Kidney. In: Cohen J, Opal SM, Powderly WG, eds. *Cohen & Powderly: Infectious Diseases*. 3rd ed. United Kingdom: Elsevier Ltd., 2010:605–13.
5. Lee BE, Seol HY, Kim TK, et al. Recent clinical overview of renal and perirenal abscesses in 56 consecutive cases. *Korean J Intern Med* 2008;23:140–8.
6. Hooton TM, Bradley SF, Cardenas DD, et al. Diagnosis, prevention, and treatment of catheter-associated urinary tract infection in adults: 2009 International Clinical Practice Guidelines from the Infectious Diseases Society of America. *Clin Infect Dis* 2010;50:625–63.
7. Nicolle LE, Bradley S, Colgan R, et al. Infectious Diseases Society of America Guidelines for the diagnosis and treatment of asymptomatic bacteriuria in adults. *Clin Infect Dis* 2005;40:643–54.
8. Albert X, Huertas I, Pereiró I. Antibiotics for preventing recurrent urinary tract infection in non-pregnant women. *Cochrane Database Syst Rev* 2004;(3):CD001209.

Cellulitis

Brett W. Jagger and Myra L. Rubio

GENERAL PRINCIPLES

- Cellulitis is defined as an infection of the skin and underlying subcutaneous tissue.
- Prior skin breakdown in the involved area from trauma, surgery, animal or insect bites, underlying eczema, or edema may predispose the skin to develop cellulitis.
- However, in some instances, no identifiable portal of entry of bacteria from skin breakdown or trauma may be identified.
- As with any infectious process, the patient's history and physical exam are essential in determining whether a patient will improve clinically with outpatient versus inpatient antibiotic treatment.
- Thus, a focus on background comorbidities as well as risk factors including immunocompromised states remains an important foundation in assessing the overall clinical risk of the patient with cellulitis.
- The most common organisms causing cellulitis in the general population are typically gram-positive cocci arising from the skin flora.
  - *Staphylococcus aureus*, including methicillin-resistant *Staphylococcus aureus* (MRSA) isolates
  - *Streptococcus* species (β-hemolytic, groups A, B, C, and G)
- If the cellulitis occurs after an animal bite, as from a cat or dog, organisms may also include anaerobic bacteria such as *Pasteurella multocida*, *Bacteroides*, or *Fusobacterium*.
- Necrotizing infections may be caused by *Streptococcus pyogenes*, *Vibrio vulnificus*, or *Aeromonas hydrophila*.
- Gas gangrene infections may be caused by *Clostridium perfringens* or other *Clostridium* species.
- In immunocompromised patients, unusual bacterial, fungal, or viral causes should also be considered.

DIAGNOSIS

Clinical Presentation

History
- Cellulitis may affect any area of the skin. However, the most commonly affected areas include the extremities, head and neck, and abdomen.
- Risk factors for developing an extremity cellulitis, such as venous or arterial insufficiency, peripheral neuropathy, eczema, or lymphedema, should be explored.
- Immunocompromising states, such as diabetes mellitus, human immunodeficiency virus (HIV) infection, chronic steroid or immunosuppressant medication usage, history of recent radiation or chemotherapy treatment, should also be investigated.
- A history of any recent trauma to the affected skin should be elicited, including the mechanism of injury, for example, animal bite, and the possibility of an indwelling foreign body.
- The presence of systemic symptoms, such as fevers, rigors, and malaise, is relevant for determining the severity of the infection and assessing the risk of necrotizing fasciitis, gas gangrene, toxic shock syndrome, or deep tissue involvement.

Physical Examination
- Cellulitis usually manifests as warm, tender, and erythematous skin.
- In contrast to erysipelas, the erythema in cellulitis is not raised or sharply demarcated.
- The involved area of cellulitis should be delineated with a marking pen on presentation so that subsequent physical examinations can determine whether the cellulitis is improving.
- Regional draining lymph nodes should be palpated.
- Examine the patient for the presence of an abscess, subcutaneous foreign body, and skin necrosis.
- Pain and tenderness out of proportion to other signs of infection, as well as the presence of subcutaneous crepitation, are concerning for necrotizing fasciitis.
- If the cellulitis involves the lower extremity, examine the toes for tinea pedis, diabetic foot ulcerations, edema, or other potentially reversible risk factors. Monofilament examination can be helpful in revealing an underlying sensory neuropathy, which can predispose to infections.

Diagnostic Testing
Laboratories
- For patients whose cellulitis warrants inpatient admission, a routine complete blood count (CBC) should be obtained and may show a leukocytosis with a left shift.
- Blood and cutaneous aspirate cultures need not be obtained routinely but should be considered if the patient is immunocompromised, shows systemic signs of infection, or has an exposure history that would suggest an unusual pathogen (e.g., water immersion or animal bite).[1]
- Abscess or other purulent drainage, if present, should be evaluated by Gram stain and bacterial culture.
- A creatine kinase may be elevated in patients showing systemic toxicity, especially those that may have a deeper infection such as pyomyositis or necrotizing fasciitis.

Imaging
- Plain films should be considered of an involved extremity if the clinical picture is concerning for osteomyelitis or retained foreign body. Plain films may demonstrate gas within the soft tissues, which is concerning for a necrotizing infection.
- Computed tomography (CT) or magnetic resonance imaging (MRI) of the involved extremity can be of use in diagnosing necrotizing fasciitis and ruling out underlying osteomyelitis.
- A venous Doppler ultrasound may be useful to rule out the presence of a deep venous thrombosis and associated thrombophlebitis when the cellulitis involves an extremity.

TREATMENT

- Any concern for necrotizing fasciitis or gas gangrene should prompt an emergent surgical consultation, which should not be withheld pending imaging or laboratory studies.
- Orthopedic or plastic surgery expertise may be indicated when the cellulitis involves the hand or fingers to ensure that there is no compartment syndrome, septic arthritis, or tenosynovitis, which could require surgical incision and drainage. Infectious diseases consultation should be pursued for complicated cellulitis or whenever management questions arise.
- Important considerations in the antimicrobial treatment of cellulitis include the presence or absence of purulence, which is an indication for empiric MRSA coverage, and the severity of infection, which determines the treatment setting of inpatient versus outpatient.[1]

- Purulent infections include furuncles, carbuncles, and abscesses. **Any abscesses or purulent fluid collections should be incised and drained**, and foreign bodies should be removed if possible.
  - Mild infections may respond incision and drainage alone.[1]
  - Moderate infections should be incised and drained as above, and the fluid sent for Gram stain and culture. Empiric antibiotics should be started and target community-acquired MRSA (CA-MRSA), including trimethoprim–sulfamethoxazole (TMP–SMX) and doxycycline.[1]
  - Severe infections should be incised and drained and fluid sent for Gram stain and culture and IV antibiotics started targeting MRSA, including vancomycin, daptomycin, linezolid, telavancin, or ceftaroline.[1]
- **Mild, nonpurulent cellulitis in an immunocompetent patient** can be treated with oral antibiotics with outpatient follow-up. Empiric coverage against MRSA is unnecessary in patients with uncomplicated, nonpurulent cellulitis.[2] Choices in this setting include the following:
  - Cephalexin 500 mg PO q6h
  - Dicloxacillin 500 mg PO q6h
  - Clindamycin 450–600 mg PO q8h
- **Empiric CA-MRSA coverage** is recommended whenever cellulitis is associated with purulent drainage.[3] Outpatient treatment options include the following:
  - Clindamycin 450–600 mg PO q8h
  - TMP–SMX 1–2 double strength (DS) tabs PO q12h
  - Doxycycline 100 mg PO q12h
- Risk factors for treatment failure include morbid obesity and recent prior antibiotic treatment. In patients with morbid obesity, lower doses of clindamycin and TMP–SMX were also associated with higher risk of clinical failure. Therefore, in the absence of a contraindication, higher doses (e.g., clindamycin 600 mg PO q8h or TMP–SMX 2 DS tabs PO q12h) of these medications are preferred in this patient population.[4]
- Inpatient management is indicated for patients with the systemic inflammatory response syndrome (SIRS), hemodynamic instability, deep or necrotizing infection, significant immune compromise, or prior outpatient treatment failure.[1] Initial therapies for nonpurulent cellulitis in a hemodynamically stable, nontoxic-appearing hospitalized patient include the following:
  - Oxacillin 1–2 g IV q6h
  - Cefazolin 1–2 g IV q8h
  - Clindamycin 600 mg IV q8h
- For patients with **severe cellulitis**, as defined by the presence of SIRS, organ dysfunction, bullae, skin sloughing, or an immunocompromised state, empiric treatment with IV vancomycin is recommended. The initial dose is typically 15–20 mg/kg q12h, although an initial one-time loading dose of 25 mg/kg may be considered in seriously ill patients. Vancomycin dosing is dependent on renal function, and trough levels should be monitored closely. In patients with purulent cellulitis, alternatives to vancomycin include the following:
  - Daptomycin 4–6 mg/kg IV q24h
  - Linezolid 600 mg IV q12h
  - Ceftaroline 600 mg IV q8h
- Empiric coverage for severe, nonpurulent cellulitis, including necrotizing fasciitis, is typically vancomycin and piperacillin–tazobactam[1] or vancomycin and meropenem. However, it should be noted that treatment of necrotizing fasciitis is primarily surgical and a surgical consultation should be obtained emergently.[1]
- In all types of cellulitis, isolation of a causative organism may prompt directed therapy on the basis of susceptibility testing.[1]

- An appropriate antibiotic for a localized cellulitis arising from a cat or dog bite is amoxicillin–clavulanate to cover for *P. multocida*. Rabies postexposure prophylaxis may be necessary in the patient who presents with a cellulitis after a dog, cat, bat, or other animal bite; infectious diseases consultation may be appropriate in this circumstance. Similarly, tetanus immunization status should be reviewed, and immunization given if indicated, when the cellulitis is attributable to a penetrating injury.
- Treatment duration for mild, uncomplicated cellulitis is 5 days.[1]
  - A variety of factors may prompt an extension of antibiotic treatment, including slow or incomplete clinical response during this time period, vascular insufficiency or edema in the affected area, severe or recurrent disease, or associated bacteremia.
  - Patients found to be bacteremic with *S. aureus* should receive an infectious disease consultation and an extended course of IV antibiotics.[5]
- Serial clinical assessments should be performed after treatment has been initiated. Typically, there will be an improvement in erythema, warmth, and tenderness within 24 hours, though the rate of improvement can vary widely between patients. Serial examinations are important to aid in distinguishing cellulitis from rapidly progressive, subcutaneous infections such as necrotizing fasciitis. If the patient exhibits hemodynamic instability or the cellulitis appears rapidly progressive, a surgical consult should be obtained immediately.

REFERENCES

1. Stevens DL, Bisno AL, Chambers HF, et al. Practice guidelines for the diagnosis and management of skin and soft tissue infections: 2014 update by the Infectious Diseases Society of America. *Clin Infect Dis* 2014;59:147.
2. Pallin DJ, Binder WD, Allen MB, et al. Clinical trial: comparative effectiveness of cephalexin plus trimethoprim-sulfamethoxazole versus cephalexin alone for treatment of uncomplicated cellulitis: a randomized controlled trial. *Clin Infect Dis* 2013;56:1754.
3. Liu C, Bayer A, Cosgrove SE, et al. Clinical practice guidelines by the Infectious Diseases Society of America for the treatment of methicillin-resistant *Staphylococcus aureus* infections in adults and children. *Clin Infect Dis* 2011;52:e18.
4. Halilovic J, Heintz BH, Brown J. Risk factors for clinical failure in patients hospitalized with cellulitis and cutaneous abscess. *J Infect* 2012;65:128.
5. Robinson JO, Pozzi-Langhi S, Phillips M, et al. Formal infectious diseases consultation is associated with decreased mortality in *Staphylococcus aureus* bacteraemia. *Eur J Clin Microbiol Infect Dis* 2012;31:2421–8.

Osteomyelitis

24

Kevin Hsueh

GENERAL PRINCIPLES

- Osteomyelitis, infection of the bone or bone marrow, results from direct infection of bone from a contiguous infectious source, or hematogenous seeding from a distant primary source.
- Its clinical manifestations are manifold, sometimes presenting as a vigorous acute illness or smoldering as a subacute or chronic ailment.
- In children, osteomyelitis generally presents acutely, the result of bacteremic seeding of highly vascular forming bone.[1]
- In adults, osteomyelitis is more often subacute or chronic, frequently due to a contiguous infection, although metastatic blood-borne infections, particularly to the vertebral column, are still quite common.[2]
- Risk factors for osteomyelitis generally come in three categories:
  - Conditions that result in damaged or abnormal bone
  - Conditions of large or chronic pathogen exposure
  - Immunosuppressive conditions
- Diabetics are particularly prone to bone infections as they carry all types of risk. Diabetic ulcers expose ischemic bone to large amounts of bacteria in the context of innate immunity impaired by hyperglycemia. Osteomyelitis secondary to diabetic foot ulcers is the leading cause of nontraumatic amputation.[3]
- Prevention of osteomyelitis in at-risk patients is critical, as osteomyelitis is one of the most difficult types of infection to treat, requiring weeklong courses of systemic antibiotics.
- Bone infections are intrinsically difficult to clear; infected bone results in sequestra and abscesses, which act as foci for persistent infection.[4]
- The longer osteomyelitis persists, the more devitalized bone results and the more frequent treatment failure and recurrence become.
- Antibiotic therapy should be chosen carefully and directed toward culture-proven pathogens.[5,6]
- Surgical debridement is as much a part of chronic osteomyelitis treatment as antibiotic therapy; removal of necrotic debris and infected material has clearly been shown to improve likelihood of treatment success.[7]
- Treatment for acute osteomyelitis is generally relatively successful; however, long-term recurrence rates in chronic osteomyelitis are estimated to be between 20% and 30%, and recurrences have been noted decades after treatment.[8,9]
- The organisms of osteomyelitis vary widely depending upon clinical context. It is most often caused by pyogenic bacteria, but many other pathogens such as mycobacteria and fungi may also infect bone.
- *Staphylococcus aureus* is the most common causal organism, found in over 50% of culture-positive osteomyelitis of all types.[2,10]
- Streptococci and coagulase-negative staphylococci are the next most common infective agents.
- *Kingella kingae* is frequently found in very young children.

- Tuberculous osteomyelitis is also frequent in populations at risk for *Mycobacterium tuberculosis*.
- The involvement of other pathogens in osteomyelitis is highly associated with the route of bone exposure, degree of patient vulnerability, and other patient risk factors.
- **Conditions of abnormal bone are associated with the following pathogens:**
  - Trauma (e.g., fractures, punctures, Charcot joints): *S. aureus*
  - Sickle cell disease: *Salmonella* species or *Streptococcus pneumoniae*
  - Surgical manipulation/prosthetic implantation: coagulase-negative staphylococci, enterobacteriaceae, or *Propionibacterium* species
- **Conditions of pathogen exposure are associated with the following pathogens:**
  - Chronic ulcer disease (diabetic, decubitus, vascular): Streptococci, Enterobacteriaceae, *Pseudomonas* species, nonfermenting gram-negative bacteria, anaerobes
  - Bite wounds: Streptococci, *Pasteurella* species, *Eikenella corrodens*
  - IV drug use: *S. aureus*, *Pseudomonas aeruginosa*
- **Immunosuppressive conditions are associated with the following pathogens:**
  - Hematologic malignancy: *Aspergillus* species, *Candida* species, *Mycobacterium* species, other fungal pathogens
  - HIV/AIDS: *Bartonella henselae*, *Bartonella quintana*

PRESENTATION

Clinical Presentation

History
- Localized pain is common to both acute and chronic osteomyelitis.
- Acute osteomyelitis typically arises over <2 weeks and is accompanied by systemic symptoms such as fever, chills, and malaise.
- Chronic osteomyelitis is often indolent, arising over the course of months, with few constitutional symptoms but often a history of a predisposing trauma or soft tissue lesion.
- Vertebral osteomyelitis is a particularly vexing condition to diagnose, typically presenting as new or worsening back pain refractory to conventional therapy that may or may not be associated with fever or new neurologic deficits.[5,11]

Physical Examination
- Swelling, tenderness, and erythema are much more pronounced in acute rather than chronic osteomyelitis, where localized findings are usually blunted, though occasionally draining sinus tracts can be seen.
- Patients with chronic osteomyelitis often do not appear ill. For contiguous infections, a soft tissue ulcer that can be probed to the bone should be treated as osteomyelitis unless proven otherwise.[12]
- Size of the ulcer may also be predictive, with ulcers >2 cm^2 found to correlate with diagnosis of osteomyelitis.[13]
- A thorough neurologic exam should be performed in those with vertebral osteomyelitis to rule out impingement of nerve roots or spinal cord.

Diagnostic Testing

Laboratories
- WBC is frequently normal in chronic osteomyelitis.
- Superficial cultures of contiguous ulcers are rarely concordant with the invasive bone pathogen(s). They are not recommended, as they can be misleading.[14,15]
- Blood cultures should be drawn prior to antibiotics. They have a low diagnostic yield, but can be critical in identifying an organism for pathogen-directed therapy.

- In chronic osteomyelitis, a **bone biopsy for culture** and sensitivities is extremely important to ensure proper pathogen-directed therapy. Ideally, they are **performed before** antibiotic therapy unless there is evidence of true cellulitis or sepsis (in which case empiric coverage should be started). Bone biopsy can also be diagnostic, if it shows pathologic signs of osteomyelitis.
- Elevations in **erythrocyte sedimentation rate (ESR)** and **C-reactive protein (CRP)** tests are nonspecific, though an ESR >70 mm/h is relatively sensitive in detecting osteomyelitis. Both ESR and CRP can be used as part of treatment monitoring.[16]

Imaging
- **Plain films** are not particularly sensitive for osteomyelitis diagnosis, as changes can take 3–6 weeks to become visible, but if characteristic findings are noted (destructive changes, radiolucencies, cortical defects, involucrum), they are moderately specific.
- **Computed tomography (CT)** is better able to identify extent and severity of disease than plain film, especially the degree of soft tissue involvement; however, it is not clear how sensitive or specific it is for the diagnosis of osteomyelitis.
- **Magnetic resonance imaging (MRI)** is considered the gold standard test for osteomyelitis, with high sensitivity as well as specificity. Like CT, MRI can clearly define additional soft tissue involvement; however, expense and contraindications do not always allow for its use.
- **Triple-phase bone scans** (technetium-99) and **tagged white blood cell scans** (indium-111) are both relatively sensitive, and negative tests can be useful in the rule-out of osteomyelitis. Positive tests are less useful, as sensitivity is poor.
- **18-fluorodeoxyglucose positron emission tomography (PET)** imaging may be extremely sensitive and specific for osteomyelitis; however, experience and availability are limited at this time.

TREATMENT

Medications
- At least 4–6 weeks of antibiotic therapy is recommended for both acute and chronic osteomyelitis, starting from the date of last debridement (if performed).
- Extension of therapy is based on clinical response; some treatment courses last up to 12 weeks.
- Traditionally, therapy is parenteral; however, for **highly bioavailable oral antibiotics**, conversion to oral antibiotic therapy after 2–4 weeks of IV therapy is safe and equally efficacious.[9,17]
- **Antibiotic selection should be guided by results of bone cultures.** Blood cultures may also be used, if the organism isolated is typical for osteomyelitis.
- Parenteral regimens for common pathogens (should be tailored to specific resistances)
  ○ Methicillin-sensitive *S. aureus* (MSSA)
    - **Nafcillin** or **oxacillin** (2 g IV q4–6h or continuous infusion) **OR**
    - **Cefazolin** (2 g IV q8h) **OR**
    - **Ceftriaxone** (2 g IV q24h)
    - **Rifampin** (600 mg PO qday) sometimes added for biofilm penetration especially with retained prosthetic material
  ○ Methicillin-resistant *S. aureus* (MRSA) or coagulase-negative staphylococci
    - **Vancomycin** (15 mg/kg IV q12h) with trough monitored for goal of 15–20 mg/dL
    - **Rifampin** (600 mg PO qday) sometimes added for biofilm penetration especially with retained prosthetic material
  ○ Streptococci
    - **Penicillin G** (2–4 million units IV q4–6h or continuous infusion) **OR**

- **Cefazolin** (2 g IV q8h) **OR**
- **Ceftriaxone** (2 g IV q24h)
  - P. aeruginosa
    - **Cefepime** (2 g IV q12h).
    - **Ciprofloxacin** (400 mg IV q8–12h) or **levofloxacin** (750 mg IV q24h) if isolate sensitive
  - Anaerobic bacteria
    - **Metronidazole** (500 mg IV q6h) **OR**
    - **Clindamycin** (600 mg IV q6h)
    - β-Lactam/β-lactamase inhibitor combinations (such as **piperacillin–tazobactam** or **ampicillin–sulbactam**) or carbapenems (such as **meropenem** or **ertapenem**) cover anaerobes and eliminate the need for separate antianaerobic agents.
- **High-bioavailability oral agents** for common pathogens (pathogen must be sensitive to be used)
  - Staphylococci
    - **Trimethoprim–sulfamethoxazole** (2 DS tabs PO q8–12h) **OR**
    - **Doxycycline** or **minocycline** (100 mg PO daily) **OR**
    - **C**lindamycin (300–450 mg PO q6h)
  - Gram-negative bacilli: **Ciprofloxacin** (750 mg PO q12h) **or levofloxacin** (750 mg PO q24h)

Surgical Management

- **Surgical debridement of bone and surrounding tissue greatly increases the chances of treatment success for chronic osteomyelitis** and should be performed if at all possible at the start of antimicrobial therapy.
- Contiguous osteomyelitis requires treatment of associated infection or wounds. Diabetic or pressure ulcers need to be aggressively debrided and offloaded, and ulcers from ischemia should be considered for revascularization. Infected prosthetic materials must also be removed if possible.
- Surgical amputation may be necessary if treatment fails to cure or suppress infections.

REFERENCES

1. Ferroni A, Al Khoury H, Dana C, et al. Prospective survey of acute osteoarticular infections in a French paediatric orthopedic surgery unit. *Clin Microbiol Infect* 2013;19:822–8.
2. Grammatico-Guillon L, Baron S, Gettner S, et al. Bone and joint infections in hospitalized patients in France, 2008: clinical and economic outcomes. *J Hosp Infect* 2012;82(1):40–8.
3. Lipsky BA, Berendt AR, Cornia PB, et al. 2012 Infectious Diseases Society of America clinical practice guideline for the diagnosis and treatment of diabetic foot infections. *Clin Infect Dis* 2012;54:e132–73.
4. Lew DP, Waldvogel FA. Osteomyelitis. *Lancet* 2004;364:369–79.
5. Berbari EF, Kanj SS, Kowalski TJ, et al. 2015 Infectious Diseases Society of America (IDSA) clinical practice guidelines for the diagnosis and treatment of native vertebral osteomyelitis in adults. *Clin Infect Dis* 2015;6:1:e26–46.
6. Osmon DR, Berbari EF, Berendt AR, et al. Diagnosis and management of prosthetic joint infection: clinical practice guidelines by the Infectious Diseases Society of America. *Clin Infect Dis* 2013;56:e1–25.
7. Simpson AH, Deakin M, Latham JM. Chronic osteomyelitis—the effect of the extent of surgical resection on infection-free survival. *J Bone Joint Surg Br* 2001;83:403–7.
8. Lazzarini L, Lipsky BA, Mader JT. Antibiotic treatment of osteomyelitis: what have we learned from 30 years of clinical trials? *Int J Infect Dis* 2005;9:127–38.
9. Conterno LO, da Silva Filho CR. Antibiotics for treating chronic osteomyelitis in adults (review). *Cochrane Database Syst Rev* 2009;(3):CD004439.

10. Tice AD, Hoaglund PA, Shoultz DA. Risk factors and treatment outcomes in osteomyelitis. *J Antimicrob Chemother* 2003;51:1261–8.
11. Gasbarrini AL, Bertoldi E, Mazzetti M, et al. Clinical features, diagnostic and therapeutic approaches to haematogenous vertebral osteomyelitis. *Eur Rev Med Pharmacol Sci* 2005;9:53–66.
12. Dinh MT, Abad CL, Safdar N. Diagnostic accuracy of the physical examination and imaging tests for osteomyelitis underlying diabetic foot ulcers: meta-analysis. *Clin Infect Dis* 2008;47:519–27.
13. Butalia S, Palda VA, Sargeant RJ, et al. Does this patient with diabetes have osteomyelitis of the lower extremity? *JAMA* 2008;299:806–13.
14. Senneville E, Melliez H, Beltrand E, et al. Culture of percutaneous bone biopsy specimens for diagnosis of diabetic foot osteomyelitis: concordance with ulcer swab cultures. *Clin Infect Dis* 2006;42:57–62.
15. Zuluaga AF, Galvis W, Jaimes F, Vesga O. Lack of microbiological concordance between bone and non-bone specimens in chronic osteomyelitis: an observational study. *BMC Infect Dis* 2002;2:8.
16. Carragee EJ, Kim D, van der Vlugt T, Vittum D. The clinical use of erythrocyte sedimentation rate in pyogenic vertebral osteomyelitis. *Spine* 1997;22:2089–93.
17. Zaoutis T, Localio AR, Leckerman K, et al. Prolonged intravenous therapy versus early transition to oral antimicrobial therapy for acute osteomyelitis in children. *Pediatrics* 2009;123:636–42.

Approach to the Patient with Fever

Anupam S. Pande and Stephen Y. Liang

GENERAL PRINCIPLES

- Fever is a common symptom in the hospital setting.
- Incidence of fever during hospitalization ranges from 2% to 17%. Infection is implicated as the cause of fever in 37–74% of reported cases.[1]
- Common infectious causes of fever acquired in the hospital include urinary tract infections, pneumonia, bloodstream infections, and sinusitis.
- Common noninfectious causes of fever include malignancy, ischemic events, and procedures such as blood transfusion.
- In 2008, the Society of Critical Care Medicine and the Infectious Diseases Society of America agreed that the definition of fever was somewhat arbitrary depending on the host; however, fever has been previously defined as a core body temperature of >38.0°C (100.4°F), whereas other sources define it as two consecutive core body temperatures of >38.3°C (101.0°F).[2]
- In neutropenic patients, fever has been defined as a single oral temperature of ≥38.3°C (101.0°F) in the absence of an obvious environmental cause or a temperature elevation of ≥38.0°C (100.4°F) for 1 hour.[2]
- Temperature is most accurately measured from an intravascular or bladder catheter; however, oral, rectal, or external auditory canal measurements are also relatively accurate. Axillary temperature measurements and chemical dot thermometry of the forehead are unreliable owing to poor reproducibility.
- Two specific populations are important to highlight for the consultant, including fever of unknown origin (FUO) and postoperative fever.
- **FUO**
  - FUO was originally defined in 1961 as a temperature of ≥38.3°C on several occasions for >3 weeks with no identified etiology after 1 week of inpatient evaluation.[3]
  - In order to reflect recent medical and technological progress, FUO has now been defined as persistent fever ≥38.3°C for 3 weeks and failure to establish a diagnosis with three outpatient visits or 3 days of inpatient investigation.[4]
  - The causes of FUO are typically classified into the following groups: infectious, inflammatory (collagen–vascular), malignancy, miscellaneous, and undetermined. Table 25-1 lists the most common causes of FUO but is not meant to be all inclusive, as more than 200 different causes have been identified.
  - Historically, infection has been implicated in 28% of cases, inflammatory disease in 21%, and malignancy in 17%; in 19% of cases, a cause remains undetermined.[5] Disseminated tuberculosis and intra-abdominal abscess are the most commonly cited infectious causes. The incidence of cytomegalovirus (CMV) has been increasing, possibly secondary to improved polymerase chain reaction (PCR)-based detection methods. Temporal arteritis is the most common inflammatory cause of FUO in the elderly. Malignancy may be declining as a cause for FUO, owing to improved screening procedures and diagnostic imaging resulting in earlier diagnosis.

TABLE 25-1 COMMON CAUSES OF FEVER OF UNKNOWN ORIGIN

Diagnosis	Clinical Syndrome	Diagnostic Tests
Infections		
Tuberculosis disseminated or extrapulmonary	Patients from endemic areas, prisoners, those with HIV Chronic pericardial or pleural exudative effusion or ascites with lymphocyte predominance and negative bacterial cultures Chronic meningitis with elevated protein, decreased glucose, and lymphocytic CSF pleocytosis and negative bacterial culture	Chest radiograph (often negative) PPD/IGRA Biopsies and mycobacterial cultures of appropriate site PCR detection may help with certain specimens
Intra-abdominal abscess	Abdominal pain with localizing signs	CT abdomen/pelvis with contrast
CMV	Infectious mononucleosis-like illness (sore throat, viral prodrome, lymphadenopathy, splenomegaly)	Blood CMV PCR or serum CMV IgM
Infectious endocarditis	New murmurs, signs of valvular dysfunction, peripheral stigmata of endocarditis—Janeway lesions, Osler nodes, Roth spots, glomerulonephritis	Several sets of blood cultures. Echocardiography (TEE if TTE unrevealing) *Coxiella burnetii* serology if blood cultures negative
ENT/dental infections	Mastoiditis, sinusitis, otitis, dental abscesses	CT sinuses, temporal bone, maxillofacial Dental panoramic radiograph
Prostatitis	Urinary symptoms with negative urine culture; digital rectal exam painful in acute infection	Urine culture after prostatic massage
Osteomyelitis	Usually in vertebral or pelvic bones from hematogenous seeding; may also be related to traumatic or surgical wounds	Imaging of affected area Biopsy for culture and pathology
Prosthetic joint infections	Usually presents with signs that can be localized to prosthesis	Imaging of affected joint Arthrocentesis for synovial fluid analysis and culture
Tick-borne illnesses	Fever (often accompanied by rash), history of antecedent tick exposure, often leukopenia, thrombocytopenia, and transaminitis	Relevant serology/PCR for tick-borne pathogens endemic to area (e.g., RMSF serology, *Ehrlichia* PCR, Lyme serology)

Diagnosis	Clinical Syndrome	Diagnostic Tests
Inflammatory conditions		
Temporal arteritis	Jaw claudication, headaches, visual field defects (particularly in the elderly)	ESR Temporal artery biopsy
Adult-onset Still disease	Once or twice daily high fever, disappearing rash, and arthritis/arthralgia	Diagnosis of exclusion
Systemic lupus erythematosus	Malar rash, photosensitivity, arthritis, pleuropericardial effusions, seizures, nephritic/nephrotic syndrome	ANA and its subsets Biopsy of affected tissues
Rheumatoid arthritis	Arthritis of small joints, morning stiffness	RA factor, anti-CCP
Inflammatory bowel disease	Bloody diarrhea, malabsorption, abdominal strictures, fistulae, abscesses	Biopsy of colonic tissue
Malignancies		
Lymphoma; leukemia	Night sweats, chills, weight loss, anorexia (B symptoms)	Bone marrow/lymph node biopsy. Flow cytometry
Solid tumors, often with metastases	Symptoms depend on site of primary malignancy (e.g., hepatocellular carcinoma, renal cell carcinoma, colon cancer) and sites of metastases	CT chest/abdomen/pelvis
Miscellaneous		
Drug fever	Commonly due to captopril, erythromycin, hydralazine, hydrochlorothiazide, and penicillins; however, virtually any drug can cause fever	Diagnosis made by cessation of drug
	Well-appearing patient with temporal association of fever and drug administration	
Hematomas, deep venous thrombosis	Symptoms related to site Thrombophlebitis and pontine hemorrhage are common causes	Venous ultrasound or CT suspected focus of hematoma

ANA, antinuclear antibodies; CT, computerized tomography; CCP, cyclic citrullinated peptide; CMV, cytomegalovirus; CSF, cerebrospinal fluid; ESR, erythrocyte sedimentation rate; HIV, human immunodeficiency virus; IGRA, interferon-gamma release assay; PCR, polymerase chain reaction; PPD, purified protein derivative; RA, rheumatoid arthritis; RMSF, Rocky Mountain spotted fever; TEE, transesophageal echocardiography; TTE, transthoracic echocardiography.

TABLE 25-2 DIFFERENTIAL DIAGNOSIS OF POSTOPERATIVE FEVER

Onset Time, Postoperative	Common Etiologies
<24 h	Cytokine release from direct trauma to surgical site, rarely necrotizing wound infection (*Streptococcus* or *Clostridium*) or intestinal leak after abdominal surgery, thyroid storm, addisonian crisis, drug fever, transfusion reaction, malignant hyperthermia
24–48 h	Instrumentation-related infection, including urinary tract infection associated with Foley catheter and central line–associated bloodstream infection
Postoperative days 3–5	Surgical site infection, sinusitis (if nasogastric tube in situ), hospital-acquired pneumonia (especially if mechanically ventilated), systemic candidiasis (if patient is on total parenteral nutrition), *C. difficile*–associated diarrhea, deep venous thrombosis or pulmonary embolism, acalculous cholecystitis, pancreatitis, alcohol withdrawal, acute gout
Postoperative days 6 and beyond	Deep wound infection and abscess, hospital-acquired pneumonia with multidrug-resistant organisms, urinary tract infection with multidrug-resistant organisms

- **Postoperative fever**
  - A limited differential diagnosis for postoperative fever is provided in Table 25-2.
  - It is important to note that timing after surgery is a key factor in the evaluation of postoperative fever.
  - Fever occurs with high incidence in the first 24–48 hours after surgery. Infection is implicated in <10% of cases. Fever may be mediated by release of inflammatory cytokines due to tissue injury at the surgical site.[6] In general, fever during this period in the absence of other symptoms (e.g., mental status changes, tachycardia, hyperventilation, hypotension) is common and usually resolves without intervention.
  - Fever present 48–72 hours after surgery may be indicative of infection and requires further evaluation.
  - The type, extent, and duration of surgery as well as any perioperative complications all impact risk of postoperative infection and should be identified on review of the operative note and in discussion. The surgical site should be surveyed daily for the development of erythema, fluctuance, purulent drainage, and wound dehiscence.
  - **Atelectasis should no longer be considered a typical cause of fever**, as studies have failed to show a relationship between the presence of atelectasis and fever.[7] Pulmonary toilet and incentive spirometry, however, should still be utilized during this time to reduce the risk of later postoperative pneumonia.
- **Pathophysiology of fever**
  - Temperature regulation is determined within the hypothalamus.
  - Elevated levels of prostaglandin E_2 (PGE_2) in the hypothalamus lead to an increase in the body set point temperature.

- Endogenous (e.g., interleukin-1, interleukin-6, and tumor necrosis factor alpha) and exogenous pyrogens (e.g., microbial products like lipopolysaccharide) stimulate PGE_2 synthesis by the arachidonic acid pathway.
- Antipyretics such as aspirin, acetaminophen, and nonsteroidal anti-inflammatory drugs (NSAIDs) are thought to act centrally on the arachidonic acid pathway to reduce PGE_2 synthesis.

DIAGNOSIS

Clinical Presentation

History
- Determine if fever was subjective or measured. Obtain details of all constitutional as well as localizing symptoms.
- Characterize chronology of progression (magnitude, frequency, duration) of fever and correlate with other symptoms.
- Determine if the patient is at risk of being immunocompromised (e.g., malignancy, chemotherapy, HIV, chronic use of immunosuppressants or corticosteroids).
- A careful history should include a complete past medical and surgical history, current medication list (including over-the-counter medications), and social history identifying travel, occupational, sexual, environmental (including animal and insect exposure), dietary, and recreational exposures as well as sick contacts.
- The review of systems should be repeated every day, as accompanying symptoms for various diseases may not be present at the time of the initial fever.

Physical Examination
- A thorough physical examination is essential. Listed below are common physical examination findings that may help narrow diagnostic considerations (Table 25-3).
- For hospitalized patients, close monitoring of all indwelling catheters (e.g., urinary, intravascular) is required.
- For postoperative patients, the surgical site must be frequently assessed for signs of infection.
- For all patients, a physical examination should be repeated daily to identify new and potentially relevant findings not be present at the time of the initial fever.
- All patients with evidence of systemic infection should be classified along the continuum of sepsis spanning from systemic inflammatory response syndrome (SIRS) to multiorgan dysfunction syndrome (MODS) in order to determine the appropriate level of care. Please see Table 25-4.

Diagnostic Testing
- Laboratory evaluation varies based upon the suspected sources of fever. Basic laboratory evaluation for fever should include complete blood count, routine serum chemistry and liver function tests, urinalysis, and blood cultures (preferably while the patient is not receiving antibiotics).
- Lumbar puncture should be considered in the presence of fever with altered mental status and/or meningeal signs.
- Chest radiography should be performed if pneumonia is suspected.
- An HIV test is necessary in all patients with risk factors for exposure.
- Stool testing for *Clostridium difficile* toxin should be pursued in the setting of fever, diarrhea, and recent antibiotic exposure.
- Skin testing with purified protein derivative (PPD) for tuberculosis or interferon-gamma release assay (IGRA) can be considered if initial evaluation is unremarkable or in patients with exposure to tuberculosis.

TABLE 25-3 IMPORTANT PHYSICAL EXAMINATION FINDINGS IN PATIENTS PRESENTING WITH FEVER

Location	Physical Exam Findings and Diagnostic Associations
Eyes	Conjunctival suffusion, uveitis, endophthalmitis, retinitis, Roth spots
Ears	Mastoid tenderness, otitis externa/media
Face/head	Temporal artery enlargement and tenderness, sinus tenderness, parotid swelling
Nose	Turbinate hypertrophy, purulent discharge
Throat	Thrush, pharyngeal erythema, tonsillar hypertrophy/abscess, periodontitis, dental abscess
Neck	Meningismus, thyromegaly, tenderness along internal jugular (septic thrombophlebitis)
Heart	Murmurs, rubs, distant sounds
Lungs	Crackles, rhonchi, dullness to percussion
Abdomen	Focal tenderness, peritoneal signs, hepatomegaly, splenomegaly, ascites
Genitourinary: male	Urethral discharge, testalgia, prostatic tenderness, epididymal enlargement, Fournier gangrene
Genitourinary: female	Cervical/vaginal discharge, adnexal mass/tenderness, retained tampon
Rectum	Perirectal fluctuance, ulcers, fistulae
Back	Spinal tenderness, pressure sores, costovertebral angle tenderness
Extremities	Signs of thrombosis/thrombophlebitis, stigmata of endocarditis (e.g., Osler nodes, Janeway lesions, splinter hemorrhages), clubbing, track marks (intravenous drug use)
Neurologic	Altered mental status, focal deficits
Skin	Rash, crepitus, sinus tracts
Musculoskeletal	Joint effusions, septic arthritis, tenosynovitis
Lymph	Lymphadenopathy, drainage/abscess

- Initial laboratory evaluation for inflammatory causes includes antinuclear antibodies, rheumatoid factor, and erythrocyte sedimentation rate.
- Computerized tomography (CT) imaging is warranted if abscess or malignancy is suspected. Fluid collections should be drained and cultured if feasible.
- Cultures of open wounds are of limited utility in determining antibiotic treatment.
- Radionuclide imaging with technetium-99m–labeled antigranulocyte antibodies or indium-labeled leukocytes can potentially highlight foci of inflammation, aiding in diagnosis.
- The evaluation of a patient with an FUO should, at minimum, include the following[9]:
  - Comprehensive history and physical examination
  - Complete blood count with differential
  - Routine blood chemistries including lactate dehydrogenase and liver function tests
  - Urinalysis and microscopic examination

TABLE 25-4 THE CONTINUUM OF HOST INFLAMMATORY RESPONSE

SIRS	≥2 of the following: Temperature >38.3°C or <36°C Heart rate >90 beats/min Respiratory rate >20 breaths/min WBC >12,000 cells/cc or <4000 cells/cc or >10% bands
Sepsis	SIRS with documented infection
Severe sepsis	Sepsis with evidence of organ dysfunction or tissue hypoperfusion in the form of any of the following: Systolic blood pressure <90 mm Hg or diastolic blood pressure <70 mm Hg Urine output <0.5 mL/kg for >2 h despite adequate fluid resuscitation Lactate above upper limits of laboratory normal Creatinine >2 mg/dL Acute lung injury with PaO_2/FiO_2 without pneumonia, or <200 with pneumonia Platelet count <100,000 cells/cc International normalized ratio >1.5 Bilirubin >2 mg/dL Evidence of disseminated intravascular coagulation
Septic shock	Severe sepsis with hypotension that is unresponsive to fluid resuscitation
Refractory septic shock	Septic shock unresponsive to vasopressors
MODS	Altered organ function of two or more organ systems

Adapted from Dellinger R, Levy M, Rhodes A, et al. Surviving sepsis campaign: international guidelines for management of severe sepsis and septic shock, 2012. *Intensive Care Med* 2013;39:165–228, Ref. [8].

- Inflammatory markers, antinuclear antibodies and rheumatoid factor, angiotensin-converting enzyme level
- Human immunodeficiency virus antibody, CMV IgM antibodies, or virus detection in blood; heterophile antibody test in children and young adults
- Chest radiograph
- PPD or IGRA
- CT scan of the abdomen (or radionuclide scan)
- Three sets of blood cultures (off antibiotics)

TREATMENT

- Management is determined by the suspected cause of fever.
- If the patient is febrile but is otherwise stable, it is reasonable to treat with antipyretics alone.

- In this situation, avoid empiric antibiotics until a clear source of infection is ascertained.
- Remember, there are multiple potential noninfectious causes of fever and SIRS (e.g., trauma, burns, pain, postoperative state, and pancreatitis).
- Also, as previously noted, almost one-fifth of FUOs have no determined cause after workup.
- If there is clinical evidence of sepsis, empiric broad-spectrum antibiotics should be initiated after blood and urine cultures have been collected. Mortality from sepsis decreases if effective antibiotic therapy is initiated early. The choice of antibiotics is dictated by the likeliest source of infection and local antibiotic resistance patterns.
- For suspected hospital-acquired pneumonia (developing after 48 hours of hospitalization or in the setting of recent prior hospitalization), empiric antibiotic coverage should include *Pseudomonas* species and methicillin-resistant *Staphylococcus aureus* (MRSA).[10]
- For intra-abdominal infections, antibiotic coverage should also address potential anaerobic infection.
- Suspected *C. difficile*–associated diarrhea may be empirically treated with metronidazole while *C. difficile* stool toxins are being collected.
- Quickly de-escalate and tailor antibiotic therapy to specific cover pathogens as culture data permits.

REFERENCES

1. Kaul DR, Flanders SA, Beck JM, Saint S. Brief report: incidence, etiology, risk factors, and outcome of hospital-acquired fever: a systematic, evidence-based review. *J Gen Intern Med* 2006;21:1184–7.
2. O'Grady NP, Barie PS, Bartlett JG, et al. Guidelines for evaluation of new fever in critically ill adult patients: 2008 update from the American College of Critical Care Medicine and the Infectious Diseases Society of America. *Crit Care Med* 2008;36:1330–49.
3. Petersdorf RG, Beeson PB. Fever of unexplained origin: report on 100 cases. *Medicine (Baltimore)* 1961;40:1–30.
4. Jitendranath L, Slim J. Work-up of fever of unknown origin in adult patients. *Hosp Physician* 2005;41:9.
5. Mourad O, Palda V, Detsky AS. A comprehensive evidence-based approach to fever of unknown origin. *Arch Intern Med* 2003;163:545–51.
6. Athanassious C, Samad A, Avery A, et al. Evaluation of fever in the immediate postoperative period in patients who underwent total joint arthroplasty. *J Arthroplasty* 2011;26:1404–8.
7. Engoren M. Lack of association between atelectasis and fever. *Chest* 1995;107:81–4.
8. Dellinger R, Levy M, Rhodes A, et al. Surviving sepsis campaign: international guidelines for management of severe sepsis and septic shock, 2012. *Intensive Care Med* 2013;39:165–228.
9. Williams J, Bellamy R. CME: clinical practice and its basis. Fever of unknown origin. *Clin Med* 2008;8:526–30.
10. American Thoracic Society; Infectious Diseases Society of America. Guidelines for the management of adults with hospital-acquired, ventilator-associated, and healthcare-associated pneumonia. *Am J Respir Crit Care Med* 2005;171:388–416.

Bacteremia

26

Shadi Parsaei

GENERAL PRINCIPLES

- Nearly 600,000 individuals in North America are diagnosed with a bloodstream infection (BSI) annually.[1]
- Associated with significant morbidity and mortality, it is the seventh leading cause of death in the United States.[2]
- While bacteremia and BSI are sometimes used interchangeably, it is important to understand that they are not synonymous in meaning.
  - **Bacteremia** refers to the presence of cultivatable organism in the blood.[3] **Transient bacteremia** can be a frequent event and often inconsequential in the immunocompetent host; occurring in the setting of brushing one's teeth or with minor abrasions, it is often eliminated by the host immune system.[4]
  - **BSI** is bacteremia associated with signs and symptoms of infection or a positive blood culture with an organism associated with disease (i.e., *Staphylococcus aureus*).[5]
    - In order for a BSI to be present, one or more blood cultures must be positive; however, a single positive blood culture does not necessarily imply the presence of BSI.[5]
    - This can be seen in the setting of **pseudobacteremia** or **contamination**, when blood cultures are positive with an organism (i.e., skin commensals such as *S. epidermidis*, *Bacillus* species, *Corynebacterium* species not *C. jeikeium*, or *P. acnes*) not originating from the bloodstream, despite efforts for careful culture acquisition and processing techniques.[5]
    - **Primary** BSI is an intravascular source of infection that includes infections due to indwelling prosthetic devices such as intravenous catheters (please refer to Chapter 27).
    - **Secondary** BSI stems from an infection originating at a distant site (i.e., pneumonia, urinary tract infection/pyelonephritis, or intra-abdominal abscess).
    - BSI can also be classified as **community onset** (identified in the outpatient setting or within the first 48 hours of hospital admission) or **hospital acquired/nosocomial** (identified > 48 hours of hospital admission); however, this binary classification is falling out of favor, as pathogens previously associated as nosocomial (i.e., methicillin-resistant *Staphylococcus aureus* [MRSA] and extended spectrum β-lactamases [ESBL] organisms) are increasingly identified as community-onset infections given shifts in the health care delivery models.[5,6]

Epidemiology

- A meta-analysis of population-based studies demonstrate the most common causes of BSI overall to be *Escherichia coli* (35 per 100,000 population), *S. aureus* (25 per 100,000 population), and *S. pneumoniae* (10 per 100,000 population).[7] Some studies have identified coagulase-negative staphylococci (CoNS) or *Klebsiella* species to be the most commonly encountered organisms behind *E. coli* and *S. aureus*. The incidence of infecting organisms varied among regions in part due to study methodology (some excluded skin

commensals or contaminants such as CoNS), regional differences in patient demographics, and patient risk factors.[7]
- Over the past two decades, **gram-positive organisms** have become an increasingly frequent cause of community-onset infections and nosocomial BSI secondary to the increased use of intravascular catheters[8] and exposure to health care–associated settings.[5] The proportion of nosocomial BSI due to MRSA has increased from 27% to 54%.[9]
  - CoNS is often a contaminant, but this organism does account for up to 30% of nosocomial BSI.[10]
  - Enterococci comprise 10% of all BSI, with the greatest majority originating from genitourinary and gastrointestinal (GI) sources.
  - An endovascular source was seen in 25% of community-onset BSI.[11]
  - Infections due to enterococci are predominantly due to *E. faecalis* with a smaller proportion due to *E. faecium*.[11]
- In terms of gram-negative organism:
  - The most common community-acquired **gram-negative bacilli (GNB)** are *E. coli*, *Klebsiella pneumoniae*, *Proteus mirabilis*, *Haemophilus influenzae*, and *Bacteroides*.
  - **Nosocomial GNB** commonly include *E. coli*, *K. pneumoniae*, *Enterobacter aerogenes*, *Serratia marcescens*, and *Pseudomonas aeruginosa*.[12] Mortality rates of nosocomial GNB BSI appear to increase with the severity of illness, ranging from 14% for non-ICU patients[8] up to 60% of ICU patients.[13]
- **Fungemia** is most commonly caused by *Candida* species.[4]

Risk Factors

- Colonization of the skin and nasopharynx by gram-positive organisms are common, and breaching of natural mechanical barriers can predispose to infection.
  - The presence of an intravascular catheter is the largest risk factor for gram-positive bacteremia.[14]
  - Neutropenia, abnormal heart valves, and presence of prosthetic devices and foreign material also increase this risk.
  - Higher rates of colonization and thus infection with *S. aureus* occur in the settings of insulin-dependent diabetics, chronic hemodialysis, dermatologic conditions, IV drug abuse, human immunodeficiency virus (HIV) infection, and the postoperative state.
  - Risk factors for enterococcal BSI include prior GI colonization, serious underlying disease, prolonged hospital stay, neutropenia, transplantation, HIV, IV drug abuse, urinary or vascular catheters, and recent stay in an intensive care unit (ICU).
- Risk factors identified for GNB bacteremia include neutropenia (most significant), corticosteroid use, advanced age, prolonged hospitalization, prior antimicrobial use, and severe underlying comorbid conditions and skin lesions (decubitus ulcers, burns). GNB bacteremia is also associated with surgical procedures, urinary tract and respiratory tract manipulation.
- Risk factors associated with candidemia are the following: hyperalimentation, presence of central venous catheters, prolonged use of antibiotics, malignancy, colonization, surgery (especially involving the GI tract), and prolonged ICU stay.[4,15]

DIAGNOSIS

Clinical Presentation

History
- All patients with known or suspected BSI should be admitted to the hospital for further evaluation. A thorough history and physical examination is tantamount.
- Past medical history should include any recent infections, particularly those caused by resistant pathogens.

- The history should evaluate for recent health care system exposure, ascertain the likely source of infection, and assess for potential complications from hematogenous seeding (i.e., endocarditis, osteoarticular infections, epidural abscess, and endophthalmitis) especially in cases in which *S. aureus* or *Candida* species are involved.

Physical Examination
- Fever is the most common presenting sign; however, this may be absent in elderly or immunocompromised populations.
- Shock can be present in GNB and *S. aureus* BSI.
- A new murmur or evidence of an embolic phenomenon (splinter hemorrhages, Janeway lesions, Osler nodes) on the physical exam can be clinical clues for subacute infective endocarditis.
- In patients with central lines, carefully examine for signs of erythema, tenderness, or drainage from the site of catheter insertion as these may indicate infection. Make note of any implantable devices or presence of prosthetic material and assess for their involvement.
- Evaluate the joints for evidence of swelling, erythema, or pain with range of motion.
- Examine the skin for evidence of cellulitis or wound infections.

Diagnostic Testing
- Blood cultures remain the gold standard in diagnosis of BSI. At least two sets of blood cultures from **separate** venipuncture sites should be obtained optimally **prior to the start of antimicrobial therapy**.
  - If a catheter is present, a peripheral and central culture should be obtained.
  - Once a BSI has been identified, repeat blood cultures must be obtained in order to document resolution.
  - Despite careful culture acquisition and sterile technique, contamination of blood cultures (pseudobacteremia) with skin commensals can occur. In studies that examine rates of contamination due to CoNS, a single positive blood culture may represent contamination in 75–95% of cases.[5,16,17] If multiple cultures are positive, susceptibility patterns can be compared to determine whether the organisms recovered represent the same or different strains. The likelihood of BSI increases if a second blood culture results the same organism with the same susceptibility pattern as the initial blood cultures.
- There has been keen interest in non–culture-based molecular testing such as polymerase chain reaction (PCR) and matrix-assisted laser desorption/ionization-time of flight (MALDI-TOF) in order to improve time-to-organism identification. In addition to rapid diagnostic capability, these tests have demonstrated high sensitivity and high specificity. It is important to highlight that these methods can be subject to false-positive results; this technology is likely to complement, rather than replace blood cultures.[18] Further studies are needed to evaluate the impact of non–culture-based molecular diagnostics on the management of BSI in clinical practice.
- If clinically indicated, laboratory testing or diagnostic imaging such as UA, CXR, CT may be indicated to assess for pneumonia, urinary tract, intra-abdominal/pelvic, hepatobiliary tract, or musculoskeletal infections in cases of secondary BSI.
- Further testing with transesophageal echocardiography (TEE) or ultrasound is often needed to rule out endocarditis or septic thrombophlebitis in the setting of *S. aureus* or *Candida* species BSI or if fever or blood cultures remain persistently positive despite appropriate antibiotic treatment. Abdominal ultrasound or a computed tomography (CT) scan may aid in the detection of occult splenic, hepatic, or renal abscesses. If *Candida* species or persistent *S. aureus* BSI is noted, ophthalmologic consultation should be obtained to assess for endophthalmitis.

TREATMENT

- Determining the probable source of infection will help direct the empiric antibiotic regimen and may provide clues on the possible organism(s) involved. The source will also help guide the duration of antibiotic therapy. In this section, we examine certain considerations in choosing antibiotic therapy based on patient population, source of infection, and specific organisms.
- **Empiric antibiotics** should be individualized based on the suspected clinical diagnosis, patient risk factors and comorbidities, severity of infection, and the prevalence of antimicrobial resistance.[19]
  - The treatment is later narrowed to **definitive** therapy once the causative organism is identified.
  - Please refer to Table 26-1 for empiric treatment of specific patient populations and sources of BSI.
- If **coagulase-negative** *Staphylococcus* is present in a stable asymptomatic patient with a single positive culture, repeat cultures and consider **observation** rather than empiric therapy. If true BSI is identified (usually in the context of a line-associated infection), then narrow to definitive therapy based on susceptibilities (change to β-lactam if the isolate is β-lactamase negative). Please refer to Chapter 27 for further details.
- *S. aureus* BSI should be treated promptly and not considered a contaminant. The presence of *S. aureus* bacteriuria should always prompt an evaluation for *S. aureus* BSI. Duration of treatment is dependent on whether the bacteremia is **uncomplicated** versus **complicated**.

TABLE 26-1 EMPIRIC TREATMENT OF SPECIFIC PATIENT POPULATIONS AND SOURCES OF BLOOD STREAM INFECTIONS (BSIs)

Patient Population	Suspected Organisms	Empiric Regimens
Critically ill/ICU	• Gram positives • Gram negatives • If risk factors present, consider *Candida* species	• Vancomycin + 4th-gen. cephalosporin • Vancomycin + β-lactam + β-lactamase inhibitor • Vancomycin + carbapenem if MDRO of concern
Neutropenic	• Gram negatives, including *Pseudomonas* • If vascular catheter present, consider *Staphylococcus* species	• Please refer to Chapter 38
Health care associated	• Gram positives • Gram negatives	• Vancomycin + 4th-gen. cephalosporin • Vancomycin + β-lactam + β-lactamase inhibitor

Suspected Sources	Suspected Organisms	Empiric Regimens
Skin and soft tissue	• Gram positives such as *Staphylococcus* and *Streptococcus*	• 1st-gen. cephalosporin • Semisynthetic penicillins • Lincomycin (i.e., clindamycin) • If MRSA prevalent, consider vancomycin
Vascular catheter	• Gram positives such as *Staphylococcus*	• Please refer to Chapter 27
Genitourinary	• Gram negatives • Occasionally *Enterococcus* if risk factors present	• Fluoroquinolone • 3rd-gen. cephalosporin
Intra-abdominal (community acquired)	• Gram negatives • Anaerobes • Occasionally *Enterococcus* (hepatobiliary infections) • If risk factors present	• 3rd-gen. cephalosporin + metronidazole • β-Lactam + β-lactamase inhibitor • Fluoroquinolone + metronidazole

MDRO, multidrug-resistant organism; MRSA, methicillin-resistant *Staphylococcus aureus*.

- Uncomplicated *S. aureus* BSI is defined as positive blood cultures with: (1) exclusion of endocarditis (TEE), (2) no implanted prosthesis, (3) sterile blood cultures performed 2–4 days after the initial set, (4) defervescence within 72 hours of initiating appropriate antibiotic therapy, and (5) no evidence of metastatic infection.[20] If ALL of the above criteria are fulfilled, the treatment duration is a *minimum* of 2 weeks of therapy.
- Complicated *S. aureus* BSI is defined as community-acquired infection[21] or any patient who does not meet all of the criteria for uncomplicated infection.[20] Treatment duration will range from 4 to 6 weeks (depending on whether endovascular infection such as endocarditis or evidence of metastatic infection is present).
- As a rule, *S. aureus* BSI should not be treated with oral antibiotics. In the majority of cases, vancomycin should be started empirically. After sensitivities return, if MSSA is identified, replace vancomycin with a semisynthetic penicillin (nafcillin, oxacillin) or cephalosporin (cefazolin or ceftriaxone). β-Lactams have better bactericidal activity than vancomycin and demonstrate improved outcomes in cases of MSSA BSI.[22] In certain settings, use of alternative antibiotics such as daptomycin, linezolid, or ceftaroline may be indicated. The treatment of endocarditis is discussed in Chapter 28.
- An infectious diseases consultation for *S. aureus* BSI is strongly encouraged as studies have demonstrated improved patient morbidity and mortality.[23]
- **Enterococcal** BSI if susceptible should be treated with penicillin/ampicillin, otherwise, vancomycin is an option. Treatment of **vancomycin-resistant enterococcus** requires careful susceptibility testing, but daptomycin, linezolid, and dalfopristin–quinupristin have demonstrated some success.
  - Daptomycin should not be used in cases of pulmonary involvement (inactivated by pulmonary surfactant) or in cases of CNS involvement (poor penetration of blood–brain barrier).

- The most common toxicity of linezolid is thrombocytopenia (usually seen after 2 weeks); beyond 4 weeks of therapy, it has been associated with the rare occurrence of peripheral and optic neuropathies.
- Dalfopristin–quinupristin is associated with significant myalgias.
- In **Candida** BSI, the choice of empiric therapy should take into account the severity, source, and prevalence of nonalbicans *Candida* species. Most *C. albicans* are susceptible to fluconazole.
  - Echinocandin therapy is preferred for *C. krusei* and *C. glabrata*.
  - *C. parapsilosis* is less susceptible to this class of antifungals, and use of fluconazole is preferred.[4]
  - Empiric fluconazole may be suitable in less critically ill patients without risk factors for resistant candidiasis (e.g., azole use in the preceding 30 days).
  - Echinocandins should not be used for BSI that may have a CNS or urinary tract source of infection given lack of sufficient drug penetration. Amphotericin B is usually recommended as empiric therapy for suspected or confirmed fungal endocarditis, please refer to chapter 28 for further details.
- **Persistent BSI** after 48 hours of antibiotics requires catheter removal, a search for infectious complications, and **surgical consultation** may be required for assistance in source control in the setting of septic thrombophlebitis and persistently positive blood cultures, deep tissue metastatic infections requiring debridement, endocarditis with need for valve replacement, septic arthritis, or epidural abscesses, or intra-abdominal abscess drainage.
- **Duration of therapy** is dependent on the source of infection. For GNB BSI, antibiotics should continue for at least 14 days, but the patient may require a longer duration based on the source, such as if an abscess or an endovascular infection is present.

REFERENCES

1. Watson CM, Al-Hasan MN. Bloodstream infections and central line-associated bloodstream infections. *Surg Clin North Am* 2014;94:1233–44.
2. Goto M, Al-Hasan MN. Overall burden of bloodstream infection and nosocomial bloodstream infection in North America and Europe. *Clin Microbiol Infect* 2013;19:501–9.
3. Munford RS, Suffredini AF. Sepsis, Severe Sepsis, and Septic Shock. In: Mandell GL, Bennett JE, Dolin R, eds. *Mandell, Douglas, and Bennett's Principles and Practice of Infectious Diseases*. 7th ed. Philadelphia, PA: Elsevier, 2010:987–8.
4. Wieland BW, Presti R. Bacteremia and Infections of the Cardiovascular Systems. In: Kirmani N, Woeltje K, Babcock H, eds. *Infectious Diseases Subspecialty Consult*. 2nd ed. Philadelphia, PA: Lippincott Williams & Wilkins, 2013:39–75.
5. Laupland KB, Church DL. Population-based epidemiology and microbiology of community-onset bloodstream infections. *Clin Microbiol Rev* 2014;27:647–64.
6. Friedman ND, Kaye KS, Stout JE, et al. Health care–associated bloodstream infections in adults: a reason to change the accepted definition of community-acquired infections. *Ann Intern Med* 2002;137:791–7.
7. Laupland KB. Incidence of bloodstream infection: a review of population-based studies. *Clin Microbiol Infect* 2013;19:492–500.
8. Marschall J, Agniel D, Fraser VJ, et al. Gram-negative bacteraemia in non-ICU patients: factors associated with inadequate antibiotic therapy and impact on outcomes. *J Antimicrob Chemother* 2008;61:1376–83.
9. Klevens RM, Edwards JR, Gaynes RP, et al. The impact of antimicrobial-resistant, health care–associated infections on mortality in the United States. *Clin Infect Dis* 2008;47:927–30.
10. Thylefors JD, Harbarth S, Pittet D. Increasing bacteremia due to coagulase-negative staphylococci: fiction or reality? *Infect Control Hosp Epidemiol* 1998;19:581–9.
11. Pinholt M, Ostergaard C, Arpi M, et al. Incidence, clinical characteristics and 30-day mortality of enterococcal bacteraemia in Denmark 2006–2009: a population-based cohort study. *Clin Microbiol Infect* 2014;20:145–51.

12. Diekema DJ, Beekmann SE, Chapin KC, et al. Epidemiology and outcome of nosocomial and community-onset bloodstream infection. *J Clin Microbiol* 2003;41:3655–60.
13. Gardiner DF, Scholand SJ, Babinchak T. Mortality and gram-negative rod bacteraemia in the intensive care unit. *J Hosp Infect* 2006;62:453–7.
14. Yasmin M, El Hage H, Obeid R, et al. Epidemiology of bloodstream infections caused by methicillin-resistant Staphylococcus aureus at a tertiary care hospital in New York. *Am J Infect Control* 2016;44:41–6.
15. Pongrácz J, Juhász E, Iván M, Kristóf K. Significance of yeasts in bloodstream infection: epidemiology and predisposing factors of Candidaemia in adult patients at a university hospital (2010–2014). *Acta Microbiol Immunol Hung* 2015;62:317–29.
16. Beekmann SE, Diekema DJ, Doern GV. Determining the clinical significance of coagulase-negative staphylococci isolated from blood cultures. *Infect Control Hosp Epidemiol* 2005;26:559–66.
17. Hall KK, Lyman JA. Updated review of blood culture contamination. *Clin Microbiol Rev* 2006;19:788–802.
18. Opota O, Jaton K, Greub G. Microbial diagnosis of bloodstream infection: towards molecular diagnosis directly from blood. *Clin Microbiol Infect* 2015;21:323–31.
19. Huttunen R, Syrjänen J, Vuento R, Aittoniemi J. Current concepts in the diagnosis of blood stream infections. Are novel molecular methods useful in clinical practice? *Int J Infect Dis* 2013;17:e934–8.
20. Liu C, Bayer A, Cosgrove SE, et al. Clinical practice guidelines by the Infectious Diseases Society of America for the treatment of methicillin-resistant Staphylococcus aureus infections in adults and children: executive summary. *Clin Infect Dis* 2011;52:285–92.
21. Fowler VG Jr, Olsen MK, Corey GR, et al. Clinical identifiers of complicated Staphylococcus aureus bacteremia. *Arch Intern Med* 2003;163:2066–72.
22. Kim SH, Kim KH, Kim HB, et al. Outcome of vancomycin treatment in patients with methicillin-susceptible Staphylococcus aureus bacteremia. *Antimicrob Agents Chemother* 2008;52:192–7.
23. Honda H, Krauss MJ, Jones JC, et al. The value of infectious diseases consultation in Staphylococcus aureus bacteremia. *Am J Med* 2010;123:631–7.

Intravascular Catheter Infections

27

Lemuel R. Non and Gerome V. Escota

GENERAL PRINCIPLES

- Intravascular devices/central lines are frequently necessary in treating critically ill patients and those requiring regular venous access.
- However, these devices carry some risk given their association with infection.
- Both local infectious complications and bloodstream infections can occur in relation to the intravascular catheter.

Definition

- **Catheter-related bloodstream infection** (CRBSI) is defined as bacteremia/fungemia in a patient with an intravascular catheter, with at least one positive blood culture obtained percutaneously, accompanied by clinical manifestations of infection (e.g., fever, chills, hypotension), and no other apparent source of infection besides the catheter.[1] Definitive diagnosis requires that the same organism grow from at least one peripherally obtained blood culture and from a catheter tip culture or that at least two blood cultures, obtained from a peripheral vein and from a catheter hub, meet criteria for **positive quantitative blood culture** and **differential time to positivity (DTP).**
  - A positive quantitative blood culture is defined as at least threefold greater colony count of microbes in blood obtained through the catheter hub than in blood obtained from a peripheral vein.
  - For DTP, a positive result requires that the culture from the catheter hub grow at least 2 hours before the blood culture obtained from a peripheral vein.
  - Alternatively, diagnosis can be made on two blood cultures obtained from different catheter hubs when the colony count on one blood sample obtained through one catheter hub is threefold greater than another blood sample obtained from a different catheter lumen.[1]
- The delineation between short-term and long-term catheters is not exact. Most, however, define short-term catheters as staying for <6 weeks, while long-term catheters usually stay for more than 6 weeks to months.[2]
- Local infections that can result from intravascular catheters include[1] the following:
  - **Phlebitis**: signs of infection (erythema, warmth, and tenderness) involving the tract of a catheterized vein
  - **Exit site infection**: signs of infection, including purulent drainage, within 2 cm of the catheter exit site
  - **Tunnel infection**: signs of infection more than 2 cm from the catheter exit site, involving the subcutaneous portion of a tunneled catheter
  - **Pocket infection**: signs of infection, usually including presence of infected fluid, in the subcutaneous pocket of a totally implanted intravascular device

Epidemiology

- CRBSIs are common and costly, leading to a high level of morbidity. In the United States, the annual incidence of CRBSI is estimated to be between 4.3 and 7.0 cases per

10,000 persons,[3] while the median rate of CRBSI in various types of ICUs ranged from 1.8 to 5.2 per 1000 catheter.[4]
- The estimated attributable mortality rate for CRBSI is reported to be 1.8%.
- CRBSI is also associated with significant increases in duration of mechanical ventilations, duration of ICU and hospital stays, and total hospital cost.[5] Risks of infection vary according to the type of catheter, location and duration of catheter use, catheter care, and materials.[6]

Etiology

- Migration of skin organisms at the insertion site into the cutaneous catheter tract with colonization of the catheter tip is the most common mechanism of infection. Other putative mechanisms include contamination of the catheter hub, hematogenous seeding from other sites of infection, and, rarely, infusate contamination.[7,8]
- In order for infection to be established in the catheter, microorganisms must first gain access to the extraluminal or intraluminal surface of the catheter and form a biofilm that allows persistence of the infection and hematogenous dissemination.[7]
- Determinants of catheter-related infection include the material from which the catheter is made and also the intrinsic virulence of the infecting organism. Thrombosis may also predispose to catheter infection.[9]
- The most common organisms are gram-positive aerobes (coagulase-negative staphylococci, *Staphylococcus aureus*, and *Enterococcus*), gram-negative bacilli (*Escherichia coli*, *Klebsiella* species, *Pseudomonas aeruginosa*, *Enterobacter* species, *Serratia* species, *Acinetobacter baumannii*), and *Candida* species.[10]

DIAGNOSIS

Clinical Presentation

Fever is the most sensitive sign. Inflammation and purulence of the catheter site are more specific but less sensitive. Look for evidence of infection other than the catheter for secondary bacteremia and for evidence of metastatic infection, such as osteomyelitis or endocarditis.[1]

Diagnostic Testing

- Paired blood cultures should be obtained under sterile conditions: at least one from a peripheral vein and one from the catheter before initiating antibiotics. If blood cannot be obtained from a peripheral vein, ≥2 blood samples should be drawn from different catheter lumens.[1]
- When a catheter is removed because of suspected CRBSI (i.e., based on signs and symptoms), culture of the catheter should be performed. For central venous catheters, the catheter tip should be sent for culture, whereas for pulmonary artery catheter, the introducer tip should be cultured. If a venous access subcutaneous port is removed for suspected CRBSI, send both the port and tip for cultures. Two catheter culturing techniques are commonly used: semiquantitative (roll plate) and quantitative (vortex, sonification). Growth of >15 colony-forming units (cfu) by semiquantitative culture or >10^2 cfu by quantitative culture is indicative of catheter colonization.[1]
- When there is catheter exit site exudate, swab the purulent material and send for Gram stain and culture.[1]
- Echocardiography should be considered in the following instances: patients with *S. aureus* bacteremia in which duration of therapy <4–6 weeks is being considered and those with findings suggestive of endocarditis, such as persistent fevers or positive blood cultures >72 hours after removal of catheter and initiation of antibiotic therapy, presence of new murmur, septic emboli, or the presence of prosthetic valve, cardiovascular implantable electronic devices, or other endovascular hardware. Transesophageal

echocardiography is the preferred study for ruling out endocarditis, and ideally should be performed 5–7 days after the onset of bacteremia.[1,11]

TREATMENT

- In general, removal of the central venous catheter (CVC) is recommended in patients with severe sepsis, thrombophlebitis, infective endocarditis, or prolonged bacteremia of >72 hours despite appropriate antibiotic therapy.
  - Removal of long-term CVCs should also be done in those with CRBSI due to *S. aureus*, *P. aeruginosa*, fungi, or mycobacteria.
  - Additionally, for short-term CVCs, removal should be done in CRBSI due to *S. aureus*, gram-negative bacilli, *Enterococcus*, fungi, or mycobacteria.
  - Removal is also indicated in CRBSI from difficult to eradicate organisms, such as *Bacillus* species, *Micrococcus* species, and *Propionibacteria*.[1]
- Empiric coverage is usually with vancomycin at 15 mg/kg IV q12h (adjust based on renal function). Additional therapy for gram-negative bacteria, targeting potentially multidrug-resistant strains, with fourth-generation cephalosporin, carbapenem, or β-lactam/β-lactamase inhibitor, with or without aminoglycoside (choice is based on antibiotic susceptibility data), should be considered in patients who are severely ill and immunocompromised and those with femoral catheters. Empiric antifungal therapy, usually with an echinocandin, can be considered in septic patients who have risk factors for *Candida* infection (e.g., total parenteral nutrition, hematologic malignancy, receipt of transplantation, presence of femoral catheter). De-escalate to narrower therapy when the organism and its susceptibilities are known.[1]
- For CRBSI involving short-term catheters, the recommended duration of antibiotic therapy for uncomplicated CRBSI (no other intravascular device and no evidence of endocarditis, suppurative thrombophlebitis, or osteomyelitis) after removal of catheter in patients without active malignancy or immunosuppression is as follows:
  - Coagulase-negative staphylococci: 5–7 days
  - Enterococcus: 7–14 days
  - Gram-negative bacilli: 7–14 days
  - *S. aureus*: ≥ 14 days
  - *Candida* species: 14 days[1]
- For uncomplicated CRBSI involving long-term catheters, recommended duration of treatment is as follows (for all CRBSI, day 1 starts on the day of first negative blood culture[1]):
  - Coagulase-negative staphylococci: 10–14 days
  - *S. aureus*: 4–6 weeks
  - Enterococcus: 7–14 days
  - Gram-negative bacilli: 10–14 days
  - *Candida* species: 14 days
- For complicated CRBSI, such as those associated with septic thrombophlebitis, endocarditis, and osteomyelitis, the infected catheter should be removed, and duration of treatment is at least 4–6 weeks for thrombophlebitis, 6 weeks for endocarditis, and 6–8 weeks for osteomyelitis.[1]
- Of note, a dilated ophthalmologic examination should be performed on all patients with candidemia.[12]
- Patients with local infections, particularly tunnel infection or port abscess, and no concomitant bacteremia/fungemia, require removal of the catheter and 7–10 days of antibiotics. Catheter salvage may be attempted in patients with uncomplicated CRBSI, but additional blood cultures should be obtained. Antibiotic lock therapy should be used with systemic antibiotics for catheter salvage; however, if this cannot be used, then the antibiotics should be given through the infected catheter. If blood cultures remain persistent >72 hours despite appropriate therapy, then the catheter should be removed.[1,13]

SPECIAL CONSIDERATIONS

- The availability of specialized teams of experienced staff has decreased the complications and costs associated with CRBSIs.
- The site of catheter insertion plays a role, with the subclavian site being superior to the internal jugular, which in turn is superior to femoral in terms of having low infection rates.[6] However, other factors such as potential for mechanical complications or the skill of the catheter operator must also be considered.
- The type of catheter also plays a role, with Teflon or polyurethane catheters having lower rates of infection than polyvinyl chloride, Silastic, or polyethylene. The use of catheters coated with antiseptics or antimicrobials, such as chlorhexidine/silver sulfadiazine or minocycline/rifampin, has also been shown to reduce rates of infection.
- Skin antisepsis with 2% chlorhexidine is superior to other skin antisepsis, such as povidone–iodine.
- Hand hygiene and maximal sterile barrier precautions (e.g., cap, mask, sterile gown, sterile gloves, sterile large drape) have been shown to decrease rates of CRBSI and should be used with insertion of CVCs.[9]
- Systemic antimicrobial prophylaxis has not been shown to improve outcomes. There is no evidence that changing catheters on a schedule as opposed to when needed reduces infection rates. Also, catheters exchanged over a guidewire do not decrease infection risk and should not be performed to replace nontunneled catheters suspected of infection.[9]

REFERENCES

1. Mermel LA, Allon M, Bouza E, et al. Clinical practice guidelines for the diagnosis and management of intravascular catheter-related infection: 2009 update by the Infectious Diseases Society of America. *Clin Infect Dis* 2009;49:1–45.
2. Galloway S. Long-term central venous access. *Br J Anaesth* 2004;92:722–34.
3. Daniels KR, Frei CR. The United States' progress toward eliminating catheter-related bloodstream infections: incidence, mortality, and hospital length of stay from 1996 to 2008. *Am J Infect Control* 2013;41:118–21.
4. National Nosocomial Infections Surveillance System. National Nosocomial Infections Surveillance (NNIS) System Report, data summary from January 1992 through June 2004, issued October 2004. *Am J Infect Control* 2004;32:470–85.
5. Blot SI, Depuydt P, Annemans L, et al. Clinical and economic outcomes in critically ill patients with nosocomial catheter-related bloodstream infections. *Clin Infect Dis* 2005;41:1591–8.
6. Goetz AM, Wagener MM, Miller JM, Muder RR. Risk of infection due to central venous catheters: effect of site of placement and catheter type. *Infect Control Hosp Epidemiol* 1998;19:842–45.
7. Safdar N, Maki DG. The pathogenesis of catheter-related bloodstream infection with noncuffed short-term central venous catheters. *Intensive Care Med* 2004;30:62–7.
8. Moro ML, Viganò EF, Cozzi Lepri A. Risk factors for central venous catheter-related infections in surgical and intensive care units. The Central Venous Catheter-Related Infections Study Group. *Infect Control Hosp Epidemiol* 1994;15:253–64.
9. O'Grady NP, Alexander M, Burns L, Dellinger P. Guidelines for the prevention of intravascular infections. *Clin Infect Dis* 2011;52:e1–e32.
10. Wisplinghoff H, Bischoff T, Tallent SM, et al. Nosocomial bloodstream infections in US hospitals: analysis of 24,179 cases from a prospective nationwide surveillance study. *Clin Infect Dis* 2004;39:309–17.
11. Baddour LM, Wilson WR, Bayer AS, et al. Infective endocarditis in adults: diagnosis, antimicrobial therapy, and management of complications: a scientific statement for healthcare professionals from the American Heart Association. *Circulation* 2015;132:1435–86.
12. Pappas PG, Kauffman CA, Andes D, et al. Clinical practice guidelines for the management of candidiasis: 2009 update by the Infectious Diseases Society of America. *Clin Infect Dis* 2009;48:503–35.
13. Justo JA, Bookstaver PB. Antibiotic lock therapy: review of technique and logistical challenges. *Infect Drug Resist* 2014;7:343–63.

Endocarditis

28

Courtney D. Chrisler

GENERAL PRINCIPLES

- The clinical spectrum of infective endocarditis (IE) has changed over the decades for numerous reasons, such as decreased incidence of rheumatic fever, extended life expectancy (and, therefore, increased degenerative valve disease), expanded use of prosthetic heart valves and other intravascular devices, intravenous drug use (IDU), and the emergence of antibiotic resistance.[1]
- Risk factors include IDU, chronic valvular disease (degenerative disease now more common than rheumatic heart disease), prior valve replacement, congenital heart disease (e.g., congenital aortic stenosis and ventriculoseptal defect), hypertrophic obstructive cardiomyopathy, prior endocarditis, intravascular devices, poor dental hygiene (although most feel the association with dental procedures per se is overemphasized), hemodialysis, increasing age, and human immunodeficiency virus (HIV).[2,3]
- **Most cases are not directly attributable to invasive procedures.**
- Despite antibiotic treatment, IE continues to have a high morbidity and mortality.
- The incidence of native valve IE ranges from 1.7 to 6.2 per 100,000 patient-years; for prosthetic valve IE, the figure is roughly 1 per 100,000 patient-years or 1% at 12 months and 2–3% at 60 months. With IDU, the incidence is markedly higher, at about 150–2000 per 100,000.[3]
- A myriad of different bacteria are capable of causing IE, but the large majority of cases are caused by viridans group streptococci and staphylococci. Overall, *Staphylococcus aureus* is the most common organism.[4,5] Coagulase-negative staphylococci and enterococci are the next most common.
- The clinical scenario can be used to some extent in narrowing the possibilities:
  - **Acute IE** rapidly progresses over 1–2 days, and the infecting organism is highly pathogenic (e.g., *S. aureus*). It is less likely to present with embolic and immunologic phenomena.
  - **Subacute IE** symptoms evolve over weeks to months, and the infecting organism is less virulent (e.g., viridans group streptococci). Embolic and immunologic phenomena are more likely to be seen in left-sided subacute IE.
  - **Native valve endocarditis** in adults 15–60 years old, excluding IDU and nosocomial infection, most commonly occurs in the setting of mitral valve prolapse with an associated regurgitation and murmur. Congenital heart disease accounts for up to a quarter of cases. *S. aureus* and viridans group streptococci and are the most common organisms.
  - **IDU** is associated with a high risk for IE; about 75% of cases occur on the right side (tricuspid). The cause for this right-sided predilection is not entirely clear. *S. aureus* causes 60–70% of cases; streptococci account for most of the remainder; less frequently, gram-negative organisms (e.g., *Pseudomonas aeruginosa*) and fungi are causative.
  - **Early prosthetic valve IE** occurring within 2 months of surgery is most commonly caused by coagulase-negative staphylococci.

- **Late prosthetic valve IE** is most commonly caused by viridans group streptococci. It is believed to be related to incidental bacteremias and not associated with the original surgery.
- **Nosocomial endocarditis** is probably more frequent than previously suspected. The most common offending organisms are *S. aureus*, enterococci, gram-negative bacilli, and *Candida* species.
- Other important organisms include *Streptococcus bovis* (associated with colon cancer), other nonviridans/nonenterococcal streptococci, and diphtheroids.
- "Culture-negative" endocarditis may be caused by "HACEK" organisms (*Haemophilus parainfluenzae, H. paraphrophilus, H. aphrophilus, Actinobacillus actinomycetemcomitans, Cardiobacterium hominis, Eikenella corrodens, Kingella kingae*), Mycoplasma species, *Bartonella* species, *Brucella* species, and *Coxiella burnetii*.[5] **In many cases of "culture-negative" IE, blood cultures are obtained after antibiotics were started.**

DIAGNOSIS

Clinical Presentation

History

- **Fever occurs in 90%** of patients (along with a new murmur the most common presentation). While obvious, it is important to note that up to 10% of patients will, in fact, be afebrile.
- Rash, chills, diaphoresis, malaise, anorexia, and weight loss may occur.
- The elderly and immunocompromised may have more atypical presentations.
- Any history of preexisting or prior cardiac abnormalities should be carefully elucidated.
- Symptoms of congestive heart failure (CHF) may develop and may be quite important with regard to possible surgery.
- Pulmonary symptoms are important in association with IDU because septic emboli may occur from right-sided endocarditis. Peripheral embolic phenomena generally do not occur in right-sided IE.

Physical Examination

An especially thorough physical examination is indicated whenever there is any concern for IE.[6]

- Cardiac exam should focus on **new or changing murmur(s) and signs of CHF**.
- In addition to conjunctival petechiae, a funduscopic exam should be done to look for retinal hemorrhages, **Roth spots**, and evidence of endophthalmitis. Roth spots are retinal lesions with a pale center surrounded by a red halo.
- **Petechiae** are the most common rash seen in IE. In addition to occurring on the conjunctivae of the lids, they may also be seen on the palate and above the clavicles at the base of the neck. Purpuric lesions may occur as well.
- **Osler nodes** are ephemeral, painful, and very tender erythematous/bluish-purple nodules, usually on the pads of the fingers and toes, which may have pale central areas without necrosis. They may also occur on the palms, soles, and elsewhere. Each lesion may last from hours to days. Osler nodes are thought to be immunologic in origin, a sterile vasculitis.
- **Janeway lesions** are also thought to be immunologic in origin. They are painless, flat, pink/red irregular spots that blanch with pressure and are found on the palms and soles of some patients.
- **Splinter hemorrhages** (subungual hemorrhages) can be detected on the fingernails with the background of a penlight. They are red (then brown or black), oriented along the long axis of the distal third of the nail, and generally 1–3 mm long.

- **Splenomegaly** is relatively common.
- **Neurologic findings** are not unusual and include confusional states, focal neurologic findings from emboli, hemorrhages from mycotic aneurysms, and cerebritis symptoms.
- Look for physical evidence of IDU.

Diagnostic Testing

Evaluation should be guided by the **modified Duke criteria** (Tables 28-1 and 28-2),[1] but these should not exclude best clinical judgment.

Laboratories
- **Blood cultures**, if at all possible, are of the utmost importance, **before** antibiotics are given. A minimum of three sets should be obtained over no <1 hour from separate sites. In subacute cases, this time frame can be safely expanded to a few days. Save the cultures for 2–3 weeks to isolate fastidious organisms.
- **Urinalysis** may reveal a microscopic hematuria and proteinuria. Immune complex glomerulonephritis is associated with red blood cell (RBC) casts, gross proteinuria, and decreased total complement levels. Renal infarction from embolic disease may manifest as gross hematuria.
- The **complete blood count** may reveal anemia and leukocytosis.

TABLE 28-1 MODIFIED DUKE CRITERIA OF INFECTIVE ENDOCARDITIS

Definite Infective Endocarditis

Pathologic criteria

Microorganisms demonstrated by culture or histologic examination of a vegetation, a vegetation that has embolized, or an intracardiac abscess specimen or

pathologic lesions; vegetation or intracardiac abscess confirmed by histologic examination showing active endocarditis

Clinical criteria

2 major criteria, or

1 major criterion and 3 minor criteria, or

5 minor criteria

Possible infective endocarditis

1 major criterion and 1 minor criterion, or

3 minor criteria

Infective endocarditis rejected

Firm alternative diagnosis explaining evidence of IE, or

Resolution of IE syndrome with antibiotic therapy for ≤4 d, or

No pathologic evidence of IE at surgery or autopsy, with antibiotic therapy for ≤4 d, or

Does not meet criteria for possible IE as above

Modified from Li JS, Sexton DJ, Mick N, et al. Proposed modifications to the Duke criteria for the diagnosis of infective endocarditis. *Clin Infect Dis* 2000;30:633–8.

TABLE 28-2 MODIFIED DUKE CRITERIA TERMS

Major Criteria

Blood culture positive for infective endocarditis (IE)

Typical microorganisms consistent with IE from two separate blood cultures: viridans streptococci, *S. bovis*, HACEK group, *S. aureus*; or community-acquired enterococci in the absence of a primary focus; or

Microorganisms consistent with IE from persistently positive blood cultures defined as follows: at least 2 positive cultures of blood samples drawn <12 h apart; or all of 3 or a majority of ≤4 separate cultures of blood (with first and last sample drawn at least 1 h apart)

Single positive blood culture for *Coxiella burnetii* or anti–phase 1 IgG antibody titer ≥1:800

Evidence of endocardial involvement

Echocardiogram positive for IE (TEE recommended for patients with prosthetic valves, rated at least "possible IE" by clinical criteria, or complicated IE [paravalvular abscess]; TTE as first test in other patients) defined as follows: oscillating intracardiac mass on valve or supporting structures, in the path of regurgitant jets, or on implanted material in the absence of an alternative anatomic explanation; or abscess; or new partial dehiscence of prosthetic valve; new valvular regurgitation (worsening or changing or preexisting murmur not sufficient)

Minor Criteria

Predisposing heart disease or IV drug user

Fever >38°C

Vascular phenomena, major arterial emboli, septic pulmonary infarcts, mycotic aneurysm, intracranial hemorrhage, conjunctival hemorrhages, and Janeway lesions

Immunologic: Osler nodes, Roth spots, rheumatoid factor, glomerulonephritis

Immunologic phenomena: glomerulonephritis, Osler nodes, Roth spots, and rheumatoid factor

Microbiologic evidence: positive blood culture but not meeting a major criterion as noted above (excludes single positive cultures for coagulase-negative staphylococci and organisms that do not cause endocarditis) or serologic evidence of active infection with organism consistent with IE

TEE, transesophageal echocardiography; TTE, transthoracic echocardiography.

Modified from Li JS, Sexton DJ, Mick N, et al. Proposed modifications to the Duke criteria for the diagnosis of infective endocarditis. *Clin Infect Dis* 2000;30:633–8.

- Elevations in nonspecific markers of inflammation (**erythrocyte sedimentation rate, C-reactive protein, and rheumatoid factor**) are common.

Electrocardiography

An **electrocardiogram** should be obtained to look for evidence of embolic disease to coronary arteries and to assess for conduction delays suggestive of abscess formation.

Imaging

- A **chest radiograph** should be obtained in all patients.
- Echocardiography should be performed on all patients with suspected IE.
  - A **transthoracic echocardiogram (TTE)** is a rational choice when the images are likely to be of good quality or initial clinical suspicion is fairly low.
  - If the echo images are likely to be poor (e.g., with chronic obstructive pulmonary disease, severe obesity, prior thoracic surgery) or the clinical suspicion of IE and/or its complications is high (e.g., prosthetic valve, staph bacteremia, new atrioventricular [AV] block), then **transesophageal echocardiography (TEE)** is the best first test. However, in some clinical situations, it may not be possible to obtain a TEE relatively urgently (<12 hours after initial evaluation), in which case a TTE should be obtained.
  - If an initial TTE discloses high-risk findings (e.g., large and/or mobile vegetations, valvular insufficiency, indications of perivalvular extension, or secondary ventricular dysfunction), then a TEE should subsequently be done to better delineate these abnormalities.
  - Repeat echocardiography may be warranted if the first study is negative but clinical suspicion remains or when the initial echocardiogram is positive and the patient subsequently deteriorates despite treatment (e.g., progression of CHF, change in murmur, new AV block, or other arrhythmia). Intraoperative echocardiography may be helpful in cases that go to surgery. All patients should have a repeat echo in the posttreatment phase to define the new baseline.

TREATMENT

- In general, high doses of antibiotics are required for prolonged periods in order to effect a cure. Therapy should be directed by culture and sensitivity results whenever possible. In the majority of cases, an infectious diseases consultation is desirable.
- At least two sets of blood cultures should be obtained every 24–48 hours during the initial stages of antibiotic therapy until negative.
- Total recommended duration of therapy begins on the first day the cultures are sterile.
- When the recommended regimen calls for the use synergistic antibiotics, these should be given as close together as possible.
- Baseline audiometry should be obtained for patients who will receive 7 or more days of aminoglycoside.
- Patients should defervesce and clinically improve within about 3–10 days of appropriate therapy. If they are still spiking fevers, then assess them for potential complications, such as abscess, and reassess the sensitivity of the pathogen.
- **Empiric therapy** may be required for acute IE, while the etiologic organism and antibiotic susceptibilities are being determined. Of course, the clinical scenario may provide clues as to the likely organism (see above).
  - For **acute IE**, a reasonable empiric regimen is vancomycin 30 mg/kg/day divided twice per day plus gentamicin 3 mg/kg/day divided two or three times per day. **Therapy should then be modified on the basis of culture and susceptibility data**.
  - In many cases of subacute IE, antibiotics may be withheld until the organism is identified.
- The 2015 American Heart Association guidelines[1] (endorsed by the Infectious Diseases Society of America) recommend the following regimens for the most common forms of IE:
  - **NATIVE valve viridans group streptococci and *S. bovis* IE and penicillin minimum inhibitory concentration (MIC) ≤0.12 mcg/mL**
    - Penicillin G 12–18 million U/day IV (continuously or divided equally four to six times per day) for 4 weeks **OR**

- Ceftriaxone 2 g/day IV/IM (in one dose) for 4 weeks
- Two weeks of either may be sufficient if given in combination with gentamicin 3 mg/kg/day IV (in one dose).
- Vancomycin may be used in those intolerant of both penicillin and ceftriaxone.
- **NATIVE valve viridans group streptococci and *S. bovis* IE and penicillin MIC >0.12 to ≤0.5 mcg/mL**
  - Penicillin G 24 million U/day IV (continuously or divided equally four to six times per day) for 4 weeks **OR**
  - Ceftriaxone 2 g/day IV/IM (in one dose) for 4 weeks **PLUS**
  - Gentamicin 3 mg/kg/day IV (in one dose) for 2 weeks
  - Vancomycin may be used in those intolerant of both penicillin and ceftriaxone.
- **PROSTHETIC valve viridans group streptococci and *S. bovis* IE and penicillin MIC ≤0.12 mcg/mL**
  - Penicillin G 24 million U/day IV (continuously or divided equally four to six times per day) for 6 weeks **OR**
  - Ceftriaxone 2 g/day IV/IM (in 1 dose) for 6 weeks **WITH OR WITHOUT**
  - Gentamicin 3 mg/kg/day IV (in one dose) for the first 2 weeks
  - Vancomycin may be used in those intolerant of both penicillin and ceftriaxone.
- **PROSTHETIC valve viridans group streptococci and *S. bovis* IE and penicillin MIC >0.12 mcg/mL**
  - Penicillin G 24 million U/day IV (continuously or divided equally four to six times per day) for 6 weeks **OR**
  - Ceftriaxone 2 g/day IV/IM (in one dose) for 6 weeks **PLUS**
  - Gentamicin 3 mg/kg/day IV (in one dose) for 6 weeks
  - Vancomycin may be used in those intolerant of both penicillin and ceftriaxone.
- **NATIVE valve *S. aureus* IE**
  - **Oxacillin-sensitive *S. aureus* (OSSA)**
    - Nafcillin or oxacillin 12 g/day (divided equally four to six times per day) for 6 weeks **PLUS OPTIONAL**
    - Gentamicin 3 mg/kg/day IV (divided equally two to three times per day) for 3–5 days
    - Skin testing should be done in those with a questionable history of penicillin allergy. A first-generation cephalosporin may be substituted in patients with non-anaphylactoid reactions.
    - Vancomycin can be used for those with anaphylactoid reactions.
  - **Oxacillin-resistant *S. aureus* (ORSA)**: Vancomycin 30 mg/kg/day (divided equally twice per day) for 6 weeks. Adjust doses for a peak level of 30–45 mcg/mL and a trough level of 10–15 mcg/mL.
- **PROSTHETIC valve *S. aureus* IE**
  - **Oxacillin-sensitive *S. aureus* (OSSA)**
    - Nafcillin or oxacillin 12 g/24 hours (divided equally six times per day) for at least 6 weeks **PLUS**
    - Rifampin 900 mg/day IV/PO (divided equally three times per day) for at least 6 weeks **PLUS**
    - Gentamicin 3 mg/kg/day IV (divided equally two to three times per day) for the first 2 weeks
  - **Oxacillin-resistant *S. aureus* (ORSA)**
    - Vancomycin 30 mg/kg/day (divided equally twice per day) for at least 6 weeks **PLUS**
    - Rifampin 900 mg/day IV/PO (divided equally three times per day) for at least 6 weeks **PLUS**

- Gentamicin 3 mg/kg/day (divided equally two to three times per day) for the first 2 weeks
- Adjust vancomycin doses for a peak level of 30–45 mcg/mL and a trough level of 10–15 mcg/mL
- **Coagulase-negative staphylococcal IE**
  - The majority of coagulase-negative staph are resistant to penicillin; therapy should proceed under this assumption unless sensitivity can be definitely demonstrated.
  - Treatment is essentially as described above for oxacillin-resistant *S. aureus*.
- **Surgery** is ultimately required in approximately one-third of patients. It is more commonly needed in prosthetic valve IE than in native valve IE. Decisions regarding surgery are quite complex and must be informed by expert clinical judgment. The major indications for surgery include refractory CHF, fungal IE, infection with antibiotic-resistant organisms, persistent bacteremia despite 1 week of antibiotics, left-sided IE with gram-negative bacteria, one or more embolic events in the first 2 weeks, and echocardiographic evidence of valve obstruction, dehiscence, perforation, rupture, or fistula or a large perivalvular abscess. Other potential indications for surgery include anterior mitral valve leaflet vegetation >10 mm, persistent vegetation after systemic embolization, and increasing vegetation size despite antibiotics. Surgical removal of implanted cardiac devices is also indicated for patients with IE.[7]

SPECIAL CONSIDERATIONS

- **In 2007, the American Heart Association (AHA) released its most recent guideline[8] regarding IE prophylaxis; it contains major changes compared to prior guidelines**.
- There is a notable lack of data supporting the use of antibiotic prophylaxis in the setting of dental, gastrointestinal (GI), and genitourinary (GU) procedures, and evidence of causation is circumstantial. In fact, there has been no prospective, placebo-controlled, multicenter, randomized, double-blind study of the efficacy of IE antibiotic prophylaxis.
- Based on a synthesis of available data, it is likely that **most cases of IE are not directly caused by dental or other procedures** and that even if antibiotic prophylaxis were completely effective, a very large number prophylactic doses would be needed to prevent a very small number of cases or IE.
- **The cumulative risk for IE is much greater with ordinary daily activities** (chewing, brushing, and flossing). On the other hand, the risks associated with single-dose antibiotic prophylaxis are quite low, but they do exist (e.g., increased antibiotic resistance and rare cases of anaphylaxis). The AHA suggests that there be greater emphasis on oral health in individuals with high-risk cardiac conditions.
- The guidelines conclude that **antibiotic prophylaxis is reasonable in very few clinical situations**. Prophylaxis is now recommended (despite the lack of conclusive evidence) **only** for patients with cardiac conditions associated with the highest risk of adverse outcome who are undergoing certain dental procedures (Table 28-3).[8] This **does not** include patients with mitral valve prolapse.
- **Only** dental procedures that involve manipulation of the gingival tissue or the periapical region (i.e., near the roots) of teeth or perforation of the oral mucosa warrant prophylaxis. Tooth extractions and cleanings are included. In these instances, prophylactic antibiotics should be directed against viridans streptococci. Despite known resistance patterns, the recommended regimens for **dental procedures** are as follows:
  - **Amoxicillin 2 g PO 30–60 minutes before the procedure.**
  - **If unable to take PO,** ampicillin 2 g IM/IV **or** cefazolin 1 g IM/IV **or** ceftriaxone 1 g IM/IV 30–60 minutes before the procedure.
  - **If allergic to penicillins,** cephalexin 2 g PO (do not use if there is a history of anaphylactoid reactions) **or** clindamycin 600 mg PO **or** azithromycin/clarithromycin

TABLE 28-3 CARDIAC CONDITIONS WITH THE HIGHEST RISK OF ADVERSE OUTCOME FROM INFECTIVE ENDOCARDITIS

Prosthetic valve or prosthetic material used for valve repair

Previous infective endocarditis

Congenital heart disease (CHD)

Unrepaired cyanotic CHD, including palliative shunts and conduits

Completely repaired CHD with prosthetic material or device, whether placed by surgery or by catheter intervention, during the first 6 months after the procedure

Repaired CHD with residual defects at the site or adjacent to the site of a prosthetic patch or prosthetic device (which would inhibit endothelialization)

Cardiac transplantation recipients who develop cardiac valvulopathy

Modified from Wilson W, Taubert KA, Gewitz M, et al. Prevention of infective endocarditis: guidelines from the American Heart Association. *Circulation* 2007;116:1736–54.

---

500 mg PO 30–60 minutes before the procedure. Another first- or second-generation cephalosporin may be used in doses equivalent to cephalexin.

- For patients who are **penicillin allergic and cannot take PO**, cefazolin/ceftriaxone 1 g IM/IV (do not use if there is a history of anaphylactoid reactions) **or** clindamycin 600 mg IM/IV 30–60 minutes before the procedure.
- IE prophylaxis may also be reasonable for high-risk patients (Table 28-3) having **procedures on the respiratory tract involving incision or biopsy of the respiratory mucosa**. The same regimens recommended above for dental procedures should be used.
- **For procedures on infected skin, skin structures, or musculoskeletal tissue**, it is reasonable that treatment for the infection itself should be active against staphylococci and β-hemolytic streptococci (e.g., an antistaphylococcal penicillin or cephalosporin). For patients unable to tolerate penicillins or who are suspected or known to have an ORSA infection, vancomycin or clindamycin may be used.
- **Antibiotics solely for the purpose of IE prophylaxis are no longer recommended for GI (including endoscopy) or GU procedures on any patient.**

REFERENCES

1. Baddour LM, Wilson WR, Bayer AS, et al. Infective endocarditis: diagnosis, antimicrobial therapy, and management of complications: a scientific statement for healthcare professionals from the American Heart Association: endorsed by the Infectious Diseases Society of America. *Circulation* 2015;132(15):1435–86.
2. Lockhart PB, Brennan MT, Thornhill M, et al. Poor oral hygiene as a risk factor for infective endocarditis-related bacteremia. *J Am Dent Assoc* 2009;140(10):1238–44.
3. Hill EE, Herijgers P, Claus P, et al. Infective endocarditis: changing epidemiology and predictors of 6-month mortality: a prospective cohort study. *Eur Heart J* 2007;28(2):196–203.
4. Fowler VG, Miro JM, Hoen B, et al. *Staphylococcus aureus* endocarditis: a consequence of medical progress. *JAMA* 2005;293:3012–21.
5. Pierce D, Calkins BC, Thornton K. Infectious endocarditis: diagnosis and treatment. *Am Fam Physician* 2012;85(10):981–6.
6. Murdoch DR, Corey GR, Hoen B. Clinical presentation, etiology, and outcome of infective endocarditis in the 21st century: the International Collaboration on Endocarditis Prospective Cohort Study. *Arch Intern Med* 2009;169(5):463–73.

7. Baddour LM, Epstein AE, Erickson CE, et al. Update on cardiovascular implantable electronic device infections and their management: a scientific statement from the American Heart Association. *Circulation* 2010;121:458–77.
8. Wilson W, Taubert KA, Gewitz M, et al. Prevention of infective endocarditis: guidelines from the American Heart Association: a guideline from the American Heart Association Rheumatic Fever, Endocarditis, and Kawasaki Disease Committee, Council on Cardiovascular Disease in the Young, and the Council on Clinical Cardiology, Council on Cardiovascular Surgery and Anesthesia, and the Quality of Care and Outcomes Research Interdisciplinary Working Group. *Circulation* 2007;116:1736–54.

Meningitis

Steven H. Borson and Hilary E. L. Reno

GENERAL PRINCIPLES

- Meningitis is an inflammation of the meninges caused by bacteria, viruses, fungi, parasites, or noninfectious etiologies.
- Bacterial meningitis still has a high mortality rate (up to 12%).
- Early diagnosis and therapy are critical for improving outcomes.

Epidemiology
- Meningitis has an annual incidence of ~1.38 per 100,000 people.[1]
- Risk factors include extremes of age, immunocompromised states, traumatic or surgical breakdown of the blood–brain barrier, and infectious exposure.

Etiology
See Table 29-1 for a differential diagnosis of aseptic meningitis and Table 29-2 for the most common causes of bacterial meningitis.

- **Bacterial meningitis**
  - *Streptococcus pneumoniae* is the most common cause of bacterial meningitis in the United States.
  - *Neisseria meningitidis* most often occurs in children, young adults, and those with terminal complement deficiencies. Outbreaks may occur.
  - *Listeria monocytogenes* develops in neonates, older adults (>50 years old), and those who are immunocompromised.
  - Health care–associated meningitis usually occurs in the setting of head trauma, recent neurosurgery, or placement of a ventricular drain; it is usually caused by *Staphylococcus* species, aerobic gram-negative bacilli, or *Propionibacterium acnes*.
- **Aseptic meningitis/other infectious etiologies**: Aseptic meningitis is defined by clinical and laboratory evidence for meningeal inflammation, but negative routine bacterial cultures.
  - Etiologies include viruses, such as enterovirus (most common), HIV, herpes simplex virus (HSV), mumps virus, arthropod-borne viruses, West-Nile virus, St. Louis encephalitis virus, varicella-zoster virus (VZV), Epstein-Barr virus (EBV), cytomegalovirus (CMV), and human herpesvirus 6 (HHV6).[2]
  - Additional infectious etiologies of meningitis include the following:
    - Spirochetes, such as syphilis
    - Tick-borne diseases such as Lyme disease, Rocky Mountain spotted fever (RMSF), or ehrlichiosis
    - Fungal meningitis, which can be caused by cryptococcus and coccidiomycosis

TABLE 29-1 ETIOLOGIC DIFFERENTIAL DIAGNOSIS OF ASEPTIC MENINGITIS

Partially Treated Bacterial Meningitis (Most Common)
Carcinomatous meningitis
Kawasaki disease
Wegener granulomatosis
Spirochetes
Vaccines (MMR, polio)
Sarcoidosis
Lupus and Sjögren syndrome
Brucella
Mollaret meningitis (benign recurrent aseptic meningitis)
Behçet disease
Toxins

Drugs
Azathioprine
Penicillin
IV immune globulin
TMP–SMX
Isoniazid
Carbamazepine
NSAIDs and COX-2 inhibitors
Muromonab-CD3

COX-2, cyclooxygenase-2; MMR, measles, mumps, rubella; NSAIDs, nonsteroidal anti-inflammatory drugs; TMP–SMX, trimethoprim–sulfamethoxazole.

TABLE 29-2 LIKELY BACTERIAL PATHOGENS AND EMPIRIC THERAPY BASED ON CLINICAL CHARACTERISTICS

Age or Risk Factor	Bacterial Pathogens	Empiric IV Therapy
3 mo to 18 y	*S. pneumoniae* *N. meningitidis* *Haemophilus influenzae*	Ceftriaxone, 2 g q12h, + vancomycin, 15 mg/kg IV q8h to q12h
18–50 y	*N. meningitides* *S. pneumoniae* *Haemophilus influenzae*	Ceftriaxone, 2 g q12h, + vancomycin, 15 mg/kg IV q8h to q12h
>50 y	*S. pneumoniae* *L. monocytogenes* Gram-negative bacilli	Ceftriaxone, 2 g q12h, + ampicillin, 2 g q4h, + vancomycin, 15 mg/kg IV q8h to q12h
Immunocompromised	Varied but includes *Listeria*, *Pseudomonas* With AIDS, *Cryptococcus* is very likely	Ceftriaxone, 2 g IV q12h or ceftazidime, 2 g q8h, + ampicillin, 2 g q4h, + vancomycin, 15 mg/kg IV q8h to q12h
Recent neurosurgery, CSF shunts, penetrating head trauma	*Staphylococcus aureus* diphtheroids Gram-negative bacilli (including *Pseudomonas*)	Cefepime or ceftazidime, 2 g q8h, + vancomycin, 15 mg/kg IV q8h to q12h

AIDS, acquired immunodeficiency syndrome; CSF, cerebrospinal fluid.
From Sinner SW, Tunkel AR. Antimicrobial agents in the treatment of bacterial meningitis. *Infect Dis Clin North Am* 2004;18:581.

DIAGNOSIS

Clinical Presentation

History
- Patients usually present with a combination of fever, headache, meningismus, and signs of cerebellar dysfunction (confusion, delirium, seizure, or decreased level of consciousness).[3]
- In cases of bacterial meningitis, these symptoms present within hours to days, while symptoms of fungal or tuberculous meningitis present within days to weeks of infection.
- The headache that is often described is very common and is characterized as severe and generalized.
- Older adults may present more insidiously with lethargy, without fever, or meningismus.
- It is important to pay attention to any history suggestive of a possible etiology.
  - A history of **immunosuppression** (HIV status, splenectomy, end-stage renal disease [ESRD], cirrhosis, or alcoholism)
  - **Time of year/outdoor exposures** (summer to fall is more likely to include enteroviruses, arboviruses, or West Nile virus)
  - **A cancer history** (consider carcinomatous meningitis), where neurologic symptoms predominate; leg weakness or numbness, ataxia, or cranial nerve symptoms may be the only clue
  - **Recent upper respiratory infection** (more likely viral etiology)

Physical Examination
- Physical examination should include investigation for findings associated with meningitis; meningismus and photophobia are common.
- **Kernig** sign can be performed as follows: flex thigh on the abdomen with knee also in flexed position and then extend the knee. It is positive if it elicits pain or resistance.
- **Brudzinski** sign can be performed as follows: flexion of the neck leads to flexion of the hips and/or knees.
- Neurological examination should be complete.
  - Cranial nerve palsies can be seen in 10–15% of bacterial infections (cranial nerves III, IV, VI, and VII are most commonly affected).
  - Papilledema or absent retinal venous pulsations, obtundation, bilateral cranial nerve III palsies, and Cushing response (bradycardia, hypertension, erratic respirations) suggest greatly increased intracranial pressure.
  - Cerebellar ataxia is seen in VZV encephalitis.
  - Asymmetric flaccid paralysis suggests West Nile viral infection.
- A skin examination will evaluate for rashes associated with certain etiologies of meningitis.
- Petechial rash suggests meningococcus, but this can also be seen in pneumococcal disease and others.
- Maculopapular rashes are common with viral infections.

Diagnostic Testing
- A complete blood count (CBC) will usually show leukocytosis; complete metabolic profile, prothrombin time/partial thromboplastin time, and urinalysis should be performed. Obtain blood, urine, and sputum cultures; also consider HIV testing and throat and stool cultures for a viral source.
- Performing a lumbar puncture (LP) to examine the cerebral spinal fluid (CSF) is crucial for establishing the diagnosis, identifying the causative organism, and performing in vitro susceptibility testing.[4]
  - The most serious complication of LP is cerebral herniation, prompting many to obtain a noncontrast head CT to evaluate risk for elevated intracranial pressure.
  - It is recommended by the Infectious Disease Society of America (IDSA) that for those patients who present with concern for meningitis, **a noncontrast head CT should be**

TABLE 29-3 COMMON CEREBROSPINAL FLUID PATTERNS IN NORMAL AND DISEASE STATES

Condition	Color	Pressure (mm H$_2$O)	Cells/mL	Protein (mg/dL)
Normal	Clear	10–180	0–5 mononuclear	15–45
Viral meningitis	Clear or opalescent	Normal	>5–2000, >50% lymphocytes, may be PMNs early in course	20–200
Bacterial meningitis	Opalescent	Increased (may be normal)	Increased with PMNs	50–1500
Tuberculous meningitis	Clear or opalescent	Usually increased	50–500 lymphocytes	45–500
Fungal meningitis	Clear or opalescent	Normal or increased	5–800 lymphocytes	Normal or increased
Carcinomatous meningitis	Clear or opalescent	Normal or increased	5–1000 mononuclear	Up to 500
Subarachnoid hemorrhage	Bloody or xanthochromic	Normal or increased	Many RBCs, with WBC: RBC same as blood	Up to 2000

PMNs, polymorphonuclear neutrophils; RBCs, red blood cells; WBC, white blood cell.

    reserved for those who have an immunocompromised state, history of CNS disease, new-onset seizure, papilledema, altered consciousness, or focal neurological deficit.[5]
- One should always be aware of clinical signs of impending herniation regardless of CT scan findings (pupillary changes, posturing, or very recent seizure) and avoid LP.
- If LP is delayed for head CT, blood cultures and antimicrobial therapy should be administered empirically before the imaging study.[5]
- Table 29-3 elucidates common patterns of CSF studies in normal and disease states; Gram stain is always recommended.[6]
- Two thirds of patients with viral meningitis have polymorphonuclear leukocyte (PMN) predominance in the CSF when examined early in the course of the illness. This generally evolves to a lymphocytic predominance.
- HSV may be associated with hemorrhagic CSF.
- If a traumatic LP is suspected and the peripheral WBC count is not abnormally low or high, a method for estimating the adjusted WBC count is to subtract 1 WBC for every 500–1500 red blood cells measured in the CSF.
- Other CSF tests to consider include the following:
  - Acid-fast (for *Mycobacterium tuberculosis*) and India Ink (for *Cryptococcus neoformans*), and venereal disease research laboratory (VDRL) test and fluorescent treponema antibody absorption (FTA-ABS) test for syphilis.

- Fungal serologic testing: cryptococcal antigen, *Histoplasma* antigen, *Blastomyces* and coccidioides complement-fixation antibody
- Polymerase chain reaction (PCR) for HSV, CMV, VZV, EBV, HHV6, JC virus
- Latex agglutination testing for *S. pneumoniae*, *N. meningitidis*, *H. influenzae*, *Escherichia coli*, and group B streptococcus has good sensitivity, but its use does not modify the administration of antibiotic therapy. The IDSA practice guidelines for meningitis do not recommend routine use of latex agglutination testing in the diagnosis of meningitis,[7] but it may be most useful in patients who received antibiotics prior to LP and have a negative Gram stain and culture.
- Cytology and flow cytometry

TREATMENT

- Empiric treatment consists of supportive measures and antimicrobial therapy.
- Whenever acute bacterial meningitis is suspected, high-dose parenteral antimicrobial therapy should be started as soon as possible. Tailor therapy is based on Table 29-2.[8]
- Until the etiology of the meningitis is known, an empiric regimen should be based on patient risk factors and Gram stain of the CSF.
- Duration of therapy is 10–14 days; most physicians treat for 14 days.
- Gram-negative and *L. monocytogenes* infections may require 21–28 days of therapy.
- Adjunctive dexamethasone
  - Animal models have shown decreased subarachnoid space inflammation with administration of adjunctive dexamethasone.
  - The administration of dexamethasone reduces the risk of poor neurologic outcome (hearing loss and sequelae but does not affect mortality) in patients with meningitis from *S. pneumoniae*.[9]
  - Recommended dosing of dexamethasone is 0.15 mg/kg q6 for 2–4 days with the first dose administered 10–20 minutes before or concomitant with the first dose of antimicrobial therapy.
  - Only continue steroids if CSF Gram stain reveals gram-positive diplococci and/or positive culture for *S. pneumoniae*.
  - Dexamethasone may reduce CSF vancomycin penetration, and therefore, addition of rifampin to empirical vancomycin and cephalosporin may be reasonable pending culture results.[7]
- Tailored treatment
  - Gram stain will be the first test to return and will influence therapy (Table 29-4).[10]
  - Therapy can then be tailored to cultures and susceptibility results. For presumed and/or confirmed HSV meningitis, IV acyclovir at 10 mg/kg q8h for a total of 10–14 days of treatment is appropriate.
  - If tuberculous meningitis is suspected, treatment involves a four-drug therapy with a tailored regimen that is continued for 6–12 months.

Other Nonpharmacologic Therapies

- **Indication for repeat LP:** No clinical response after 48 hours of appropriate empiric antimicrobials should warrant a repeat LP.[7]
- **Isolation**
  - All patients with meningitis should be initially placed in respiratory isolation for at least 24 hours of effective therapy pending testing results given the concern for *N. meningitidis* infectivity.
  - Patients with measles, mumps, or influenza should be placed in respiratory isolation throughout the duration of illness.

TABLE 29-4 EMPIRIC THERAPY BASED ON CEREBROSPINAL FLUID GRAM STAIN RESULTS

Gram-positive cocci	Ceftriaxone, 2 g q12h, or ceftazidime, 2 g IV q8h, + vancomycin, 15 mg/kg q8h to q12h
Gram-negative cocci	Ceftriaxone, 2 g IV q12h, or ceftazidime, 2 g IV q8h
Gram-positive bacilli	Ampicillin, 2 g q4h, + consideration of gentamicin, 1 mg/kg q8h
Gram-negative bacilli	Ceftriaxone, 2 g q12h, or ceftazidime, 2 g q8h, + in children, gentamicin, 1 mg/kg q8h

From Brouwer MC, Tunkel AR, van de Beek D. Epidemiology, diagnosis, and antimicrobial treatment of acute bacterial meningitis. *Clin Microbiol Rev* 2010;23:467–92.

REFERENCES

1. Thigpen MC, Whitney CG, Messonnier NE, et al. Bacterial meningitis in the United States, 1998–2007. *N Engl J Med* 2011;364:2016.
2. Connolly KJ, Hammer SM. The acute aseptic meningitis syndrome. *Infect Dis Clin North Am* 1990;4:599.
3. Attia J, Hatala R, Cook DJ, Wong JG. The rational clinical examination. Does this adult patient have acute meningitis? *JAMA* 1999;282:175.
4. Kaplan SL. Clinical presentations, diagnosis, and prognostic factors of bacterial meningitis. *Infect Dis Clin North Am* 1999;13:579.
5. Hasbun R, Abrahams J, Jekel J, Quagliarello VJ. Computed tomography of the head before lumbar puncture in adults with suspected meningitis. *N Engl J Med* 2001;345:1727.
6. Spanos A, Harrell FE Jr, Durack DT. Differential diagnosis of acute meningitis. An analysis of the predictive value of initial observations. *JAMA* 1989;262:2700.
7. Tunkel AR, Hartman BJ, Kaplan SL, et al. Practice guidelines for the management of bacterial meningitis. *Clin Infect Dis* 2004;39(9):1267–84.
8. Sinner SW, Tunkel AR. Antimicrobial agents in the treatment of bacterial meningitis. *Infect Dis Clin North Am* 2004;18:581.
9. Brouwer MC, McIntyre P, Prasad K, van de Beek D. Corticosteroids for acute bacterial meningitis. *Cochrane Database Syst Rev* 2015;(9):CD004405.
10. Brouwer MC, Tunkel AR, van de Beek D. Epidemiology, diagnosis, and antimicrobial treatment of acute bacterial meningitis. *Clin Microbiol Rev* 2010;23:467–92.

VII Neurology

Approach to Altered Mental Status

Vaiibhav Patel and Thomas M. De Fer

GENERAL PRINCIPLES

- **Altered mental status is an imprecise term** that could be used to describe essentially any deviation from a normal alert state. While delirium is definitely a state of altered mental status, **not all altered mental status is delirium** (e.g., coma, dementia, postictal state, etc.). In the context of internal medicine, altered mental status is often taken to imply delirium but certainly not always. The term **encephalopathy** also encompasses delirium and connotes global brain dysfunction that is often reversible, generally due to metabolic and/or toxic causes, and not caused by a focal brain lesion.
- **Delirium is common**, affecting up to 29% of elderly hospitalized patients.[1] Postoperatively, the incidence may approach 60% in the elderly.[2] In patients who require an intensive care unit, the incidence of delirium reaches 70%.[3]
- These patients are at risk for complications including increased length of stay, malnutrition, decubitus ulcers, and death.[2,4] They are also at an increased risk of new nursing home placement and functional decline, even up to 3 months after discharge.[5] With these complications, delirium results in an enormous burden on health care resources, with estimated costs up to 150 billion dollars per year.[6]
- The *Diagnostic and Statistical Manual of Mental Disorders*, fifth edition (DSM-5) characterizes delirium as follows[7]:
  - There is a disturbance in **attention** (reduced ability to direct, focus, sustain, and shift attention) and awareness.
  - The disturbance develops over a **short period of time** (hours to days), represents a change from baseline, and tends to fluctuate during the course of the day.
  - There is an additional **disturbance in cognition** (memory deficit, disorientation, language, visuospatial ability, or perception).
  - The disturbances are not better explained by another preexisting, evolving, or established neurocognitive disorder and do not occur in the context of a severely reduced level of arousal such as coma.
  - The history, physical, and laboratories suggest that the disturbance is caused by a medical condition, substance intoxication or withdrawal, or medication side effect or from multiple etiologies
- The **Confusion Assessment Method** (CAM) diagnostic algorithm is sensitive (94–100%) and specific (90–95%) for the diagnosis of delirium and requires the presence of the following:[8]
  - Acute onset with a fluctuating course **AND**
  - Inattention **PLUS**
  - Disorganized thinking **OR**
  - Altered level of consciousness/alertness
- Table 30-1 presents a comparison of the characteristics of delirium and dementia.[9,10]
- Patients with preexisting dementia, advanced age (>65 years old), neurological disease, chronic kidney or hepatic disease, history of falls and immobility are at greater risk for delirium.[9,11,12]

TABLE 30-1 CHARACTERISTICS OF DELIRIUM AND DEMENTIA

Delirium	Dementia
Acute confusional state	Chronic confusional state
Abrupt onset, fluctuating, short duration	Insidious, slowly progressive, very chronic
Inattention	Normally attentive until later stages
Impaired recent and immediate memory	Prominent, progressive memory disturbance
Global cognitive and/or perceptual disturbances not accounted for by dementia	Other cognitive dysfunction such as aphasia, apraxia, and agnosia
Altered level of consciousness ("clouded")	Normal consciousness until very late stages
Fluctuating alertness (hypo- or hyperactive)	Normal alertness until very late stages
Disorientation	Orientation maintained until middle to late stages
Disorganized, distorted, and fragmented thinking	Impaired executive functioning (e.g., planning, organizing, abstraction) and judgment
Psychomotor agitation/retardation	
Hallucinations (particularly visual)	May have apraxia
Sleep–wake disturbance	Misperceptions usually absent

- The well-described syndrome of **sundowning** is not delirium per se but is a clinical diagnosis thought to be related to a disorder of circadian rhythm, among other factors. It is seen most often in institutionalized demented patients and is characterized by confusion and behavioral problems occurring repetitively in the late afternoon, evening, or night. Behavioral manifestations include confusion, disorientation, anxiety, agitation, aggression, and wandering. Sundowning may be precipitated or exacerbated by changes in routine and/or environment such as experiencing darkness, excess noise, shift change, patient fatigue, or social isolation.[13] As with delirium, medical causes should be sought when sundowning presents acutely.
- A listing of the causes of altered mental status/delirium is presented in Table 30-2. **Often, the cause of delirium is multifactorial**. It is important to note that the elderly are particularly susceptible to the combined effects of multiple causes including seemingly trivial contributors such as reduced visual and auditory acuity and use of physical restraints. Polypharmacy is also a very common cause in the geriatric population.[9,12]

DIAGNOSIS

Clinical Presentation

History

It is imperative to obtain a collateral history, as most delirious patients will not be capable of providing a coherent history. History should be elicited from family members or other

TABLE 30-2 CAUSES OF ALTERED MENTAL STATUS

Infections: UTI, pneumonia, surgical site infection, cellulitis, line infection, meningitis, endocarditis

Medications: anticholinergics (antihistamines, clonidine, tricyclic antidepressants), opioids, benzodiazepines, H_2 blockers, steroids, theophylline, digoxin, antiparkinsonian agents, sulfonylureas, NSAIDs, anticonvulsants, antihypertensives; combined effects of multiple drugs may be particularly important in the elderly (i.e., polypharmacy)

Cardiovascular: myocardial ischemia or MI, hypertensive encephalopathy, severe dehydration, low perfusion states (e.g., shock)

Intoxications: narcotics, hallucinogens, alcohol, toxins/poisons

Withdrawal: ethanol, narcotics, benzodiazepines

Electrolyte abnormalities: hyper- or hyponatremia, hypercalcemia

Metabolic derangements: uremia, hepatic encephalopathy, vitamin B_{12} deficiency, Wernicke-Korsakoff syndrome, hyper- or hypoglycemia, hyper- or hypothyroidism, adrenal crisis, Cushing syndrome, hypoxia, hypercapnia, acidosis or alkalosis

Postoperative: uncontrolled pain, postanesthesia

CNS disorders: sleep deprivation, previously unrecognized dementia, CVA/transient ischemic attack (must involve extensive or crucial areas), subdural hematoma, vasculitis, neoplasia (primary or metastatic), meningitis, encephalitis, neurosyphilis, relative hypotension, postictal state, nonconvulsive status epilepticus

Psychiatric disorders: depression/pseudodementia, mania, psychosis

Environmental: hyperthermia, hypothermia, sensory deprivation.

Trauma: multisystem trauma, burns, fractures

Miscellaneous: fecal impaction, urinary retention

CNS, central nervous system; MI, myocardial infarction; NSAIDs, nonsteroidal anti-inflammatory drugs; UTI, urinary tract infection.

---

caregivers and should focus on several items, as listed in Table 30-3. Attempts should be made to elicit a history of subtle signs of a prior cerebrovascular accident (CVA).[12]

Physical Examination
- The purpose of the physical exam in delirious patients is to identify possible precipitating causes or evidence of a focal neurologic process.
- In a complete physical exam, it is important to look for evidence of infection, hypoxemia, dehydration, and head trauma. Evaluate for both urine and fecal retention as urinary retention is known to be a cause of delirium (cystocerebral syndrome) and patients with delirium are at a higher risk for fecal retention.[10]
- The neurologic exam is important to look for focal changes but may be challenging due to a combination of decreased consciousness, inattention, and lack of cooperation.[12]
- Passive, repeated examinations of patient behaviors are important.
  - Motor activity: Is there psychomotor agitation or retardation?
  - Alertness: What level of stimulus is required to arouse the patient?

TABLE 30-3 KEY HISTORICAL FEATURES OF ALTERED MENTAL STATUS

Baseline mental status (has there been evidence of progressive cognitive decline suggesting dementia?)

Rapidity of development of the change in mental status and consistency of the alteration

Previous history of delirium

Previous history of psychiatric disorders

Previous strokes

History of falls or head injury

Medications (prescription and over-the-counter), especially recent changes

Ethanol or other substance use (especially benzodiazepines)

- Attentiveness: Can the patient maintain focus during a conversation, or is he or she easily distracted? Can the patient shift attention appropriately?
- Speech: Pay attention to content and flow of thought.
- The **Mini Mental State Examination** (MMSE), or Folstein test, is a useful screen for cognitive dysfunction. A score <24 on the MMSE is abnormal, but the test is limited by the fact that biases can occur with advanced age, poor education, and differences in cultural backgrounds.[14]
- The **Short Blessed Test** (SBT) (Table 30-4) is more time-efficient than and nearly as accurate as the MMSE. A score of <9 on the SBT is considered normal.[15] A single normal exam does not exclude cognitive dysfunction because it does not take into account fluctuations. Serial exams are likely to be more useful for identifying and following delirious patients. A baseline exam on admission on all admitted patients with the diagnosis or at high risk for developing delirium is useful.[9]

TABLE 30-4 THE SHORT BLESSED TEST

1. What year is it? Maximum error: 1; weight × 4.
2. What month is it? Maximum error: 1; weight × 3.
3. Repeat this address (three attempts): John Brown, 42 Market Street, Chicago (see item 7 below).
4. Without looking at a watch or clock, what time is it? (Within 1 hour.) Maximum error: 1; weight × 3.
5. Count backwards from 20 to 1. Maximum error: 2; weight × 2.
6. Say the months in reverse order. Maximum error: 2; weight × 2.
7. Repeat the address as above. Maximum error: 5; weight × 2.

Sum of scores (up to maximum error multiplied by weight); 0–8, normal to mild impairment; 9–19, moderate; >19, severe.

Data from Thompson P, Blessed G. Correlation between the 37-item mental test score and abbreviated 10-item mental test score by psychogeriatric day patients. *Br J Psychiatry* 1987;151:206–9.

Diagnostic Testing

- Basic laboratory evaluation includes the following when appropriate:
  - Urinalysis with microscopic analysis (culture if abnormal)
  - Arterial blood gases or pulse oximetry
  - Electrolytes (including calcium, blood urea nitrogen, and creatinine)
  - Blood glucose level
  - Hepatic function panel
  - Complete blood count
  - Further testing such as ethanol level, toxicology screens, thyroid function tests, Venereal Disease Research Laboratory (VDRL) test, and HIV screening should be considered when appropriate.
- **ECG**: The elderly may have delirium as the only symptom of myocardial ischemia or infarction.
- **Lumbar puncture** to exclude meningoencephalitis can be considered for patients with unexplained mental status changes, especially in the face of fever, headache, leukocytosis, or other evidence of sepsis that is not readily attributable to another source.
- **EEG** is not routinely indicated but can be useful in cases where the diagnosis remains in doubt or there is concern for seizure activity.[12]
- Most patients should have a CXR to rule out pneumonia.
- Noncontrast CT of the brain should be performed if there are new focal neurologic deficits (to evaluate for an old CVA or other structural abnormality) or if there is a history of falls (to exclude a subdural hematoma). A CT of the head should also be considered in patients who cannot provide a history or cooperate during a physical exam.[9,12]
- MRI may further identify causes of encephalopathy in patients with a nondiagnostic CT.

TREATMENT

- Preoperative and admission assessment of mental status is critical in applying appropriate interventions and assessing the response. Prevention and early intervention with increasing mobility and activity, reorientation strategies, nonpharmacological prevention of sleep deprivation/interruption, hydration, and reversing hearing and/or visual impairments is effective in decreasing delirium in hospitalized patients.[12,16]
- Treatment is primarily supportive until the underlying precipitants are identified and eliminated if possible.
  - Review medications and give a therapeutic and diagnostic trial of **stopping suspect medications**. Avoid starting new medications that could worsen the problem.
  - Maximize the safety of the surrounding environment. Institute **fall precautions** (e.g., bed alarms, low/floor beds, canopied beds, floor mats, door alarms).
  - **Avoid physical restraints if at all possible**, which can increase agitation, can result in iatrogenic injuries, and can actually precipitate delirium.[10] Do not use bed rails as quasi restraints; at least one foot rail should be down.
  - **Treat pain** adequately with appropriate analgesics, **but avoid excessive doses**, particularly with opioids.
  - Evaluate sensory input.
    - **Avoid sensory extremes**, including darkness during the day, excess light during the night, and excess/unnecessary sensory input at night (e.g., television, radio, conversation).[17]
    - Avoid placing two delirious patients in the same room.
    - Familiar faces: Ask a family member to stay with the patient. Minimally trained so-called sitters unknown to the patient may not be particularly helpful.

- Use windows and a visible clock/calendar to orient the patient to the day–night cycle.
- Get the patient up in the day and in bed at night (hopefully asleep). Provide nutrition at appropriate times (i.e., try to get the patient to eat at breakfast, lunch, and dinner).[12]
- Medications are indicated only for specific clearly disruptive or harmful behaviors.
  - **Neuroleptic agents** may be useful in treating hyperactive patients who represent a real danger to themselves or the staff.
    - Haloperidol may initially be administered IM for prompt control. The starting dose should be low (0.5–1 mg) and given parenterally; it can be repeated every 30–60 minutes until control is achieved. This can be switched to oral administration (dosed every 4–6 hours) if continued maintenance is needed.[9]
    - Newer, atypical antipsychotics (e.g., risperidone, quetiapine, olanzapine) may be preferred in the elderly and those with known Parkinson disease owing to the potentially lower risk of extrapyramidal symptoms compared with higher doses of haloperidol. These drugs also generally cause less sedation.[9,17,18]
    - **The long-term use of atypical antipsychotics in patients with dementia may be associated with a modestly higher mortality rate.**[19]
    - A potential severe side effect of antipsychotics is neuroleptic malignant syndrome although this is rare (<1% for all drugs). In addition, antipsychotics may cause QT prolongation.[18]
  - **Benzodiazepines** can be useful adjuncts to antipsychotic agents for severe agitation and withdrawal syndromes. Lorazepam (0.5–1 mg PO) is the drug of choice. Intravenous use of lorazepam should be limited to emergencies. Of note, there is a risk of excess sedation, confusion, as well as a paradoxical excitation reaction with these medications. These side effects can be prolonged and more pronounced in the elderly population.[9,17]
  - Melatonin agonists have recently been studied for the prevention of delirium. A recent study showed that nightly ramelteon, compared to placebo, decreased the incidence of delirium in an elderly (65–89 years old) hospitalized population. Further studies are needed to validate these results.[20]

REFERENCES

1. Korevaar JC, van Munster BC, de Rooij SE. Risk factors for delirium in acutely admitted elderly patients: a prospective cohort study. *BMC Geriatr* 2005;5:6.
2. Gustafson Y, Berggren D, Brännström B, et al. Acute confusional states in elderly patients treated for femoral neck fracture. *J Am Geriatr Soc* 1988;36:525–30.
3. McNicoll L, Pisani MA, Zhang Y, et al. Delirium in the intensive care unit: occurrence and clinical course in older patients. *J Am Geriatr Soc* 2003;51:591–8.
4. Pitkal KH, Laurila JV, Stranberg TE, Tilvis RS. Prognostic significance of delirium in frail older people. *Dement Geriatr Cogn Disord* 2005;19:158–63.
5. Inouye SK, Rushing JT, Foreman MD, et al. Does delirium contribute to poor hospital outcomes? A three-site epidemiologic study. *J Gen Intern Med* 1998;13:234–42.
6. Leslie DL, Marcantonio ER, Zhang Y, et al. One-year health care costs associated with delirium in the elderly population. *Arch Intern Med* 2008;168:27–32.
7. American Pyschiatric Association *Diagnostic and Statistical Manual of Mental Disorders*, 5th ed. Arlington, VA: American Psychiatric Publishing, 2013.
8. Inouye SK, van Dyck CH, Alessi CA, et al. Clarifying confusion: the confusion assessment method. A new method for detection of delirium. *Ann Intern Med* 1990;113:941–8.
9. Inouye SK. Delirium in older persons. *N Engl J Med* 2006;354:1157–65.
10. Flaherty JH. The evaluation and management of delirium among older persons. *Med Clin North Am* 2011;95:555–77.
11. Fong TG, Tulebaev SR, Inouye SK. Delirium in elderly adults: diagnosis, prevention and treatment. *Nat Rev Neurol* 2009;5:210–20.

12. Inouye SK, Westendorp RG, Saczynski JS. Delirium in elderly people. *Lancet* 2014;383:911–22.
13. Khachiyants N, Trinkle D, Son SJ, Kim KY. Sundown syndrome in persons with dementia: an update. *Psychiatry Invest* 2011;8:275–87.
14. Schultz-Larsen K, Lomholt RK, Kreiner S. Mini-Mental Status Examination: a short form of MMSE was as accurate as the original MMSE in predicting dementia. *J Clin Epidemiol* 2007;60:260–7.
15. Thompson P, Blessed G. Correlation between the 37-item mental test score and abbreviated 10-item mental test score by psychogeriatric day patients. *Br J Psychiatry* 1987;151:206–9.
16. Inouye SK, Bogardus ST Jr, Charpentier PA, et al. A multicomponent intervention to prevent delirium in hospitalized older patients. *N Engl J Med* 1999;340:669–76.
17. Meagher DJ. Delirium: optimising management. *BMJ* 2001;322:144–9.
18. Rea RS, Battistone S, Fong JJ, Devlin JW. Atypical antipsychotics versus haloperidol for treatment of delirium in acutely ill patients. *Pharmacotherapy* 2007;27:588–94.
19. Schneider LS, Dagerman KS, Insel P. Risk of death with atypical antipsychotic drug treatment for dementia: meta-analysis of randomized placebo-controlled trials. *JAMA* 2005;294:1934–43.
20. Hatta K, Kishi Y, Wada K, et al. Preventive effects of ramelteon on delirium: a randomized placebo-controlled trial. *JAMA Psychiatry* 2014;71:397–403.

Approach to the Patient with Vertigo

Yeshika Sharma and Robert J. Mahoney

GENERAL PRINCIPLES

- Vertigo is the sensation of movement or rotation in the absence of actual motion.
- Subjectively and etiologically, it is distinct from presyncope, disequilibrium, and light-headedness.
- The term dizziness may refer to either vertigo or presyncope and is a less-referred clinical term.
- Vertigo generally results from unilateral dysfunction of the vestibular system, which consists of **peripheral** components (semicircular canals, otoliths, and vestibular nerve) and **central** components (particularly the vestibular nuclear cortex, vestibulocerebellum, and brainstem).[1] Differentiating peripheral from central causes of vertigo is of paramount importance in the assessment of the vertiginous patient.
- The true prevalence of vertigo is difficult to determine because of variations in the way vertigo is experienced and described.
- Dizziness ranks among the most common complaints evaluated by physicians. More specifically, vertigo affects between 3% and 10% of individuals over their lifetimes. It is reported more commonly in females, and many specific syndromes become more prevalent with age.[2]

DIAGNOSIS

Clinical Presentation

Vertiginous patients may describe either a sensation of the room spinning around them, or a sensation of **impulsion** (the sensation of being propelled through space). Patients may also describe **unsteady gait**, although such complaints in the absence of the sensation of motion suggest a nonvertiginous etiology. Vertigo can be **episodic** or **continuous**. Episodes of vertigo may be brief, lasting for only a few seconds, or more prolonged (lasting hours or days).

History

- The first objective of the history is to distinguish true vertigo from other syndromes of light-headedness or presyncope. Sensations of impending loss of consciousness, haziness of vision, or disorientation are generally inconsistent with the diagnosis of vertigo and should trigger evaluation for alternative etiologies; however, these features may accompany some forms of central vertigo.
- Once vertigo is confirmed, historical features can help to distinguish peripheral from central causes (Table 31-1).
  - Changes in hearing (such as **tinnitus** or **hearing loss**) suggest a peripheral etiology (e.g., vestibular disease).
  - **Imbalance** or **ataxia** may reflect a central cause (e.g., central nervous system lesion).
  - The presence of recurrent headache may suggest the possibility of **migrainous vertigo** or **malignancy**.

TABLE 31-1 HISTORY AND EXAM FEATURES SUGGESTING PERIPHERAL VERSUS CENTRAL VERTIGO

Suggests Peripheral	Suggests Central
Severe nausea and vomiting	Absent or mild nausea and vomiting
Prominent illusion of movement	Prominent imbalance
Associated hearing loss or tinnitus	Associated neurologic signs
Increased with head movement	Severe oscillopsia
Nystagmus increases with gaze in direction of fast phase; inhibited on gaze fixation	Dysconjugate nystagmus more common
Unilateral impaired caloric testing	

Data from Karatas M. Central vertigo and dizziness: epidemiology, differential diagnosis, and common causes. *Neurologist* 2008;14(6):355–64.

- The differential diagnosis for vertigo is broad, but the diagnosis can often be made by history alone (Tables 31-2 and 31-3).
- The history should include prior head trauma, cerebrovascular accidents, neoplasms, otitis, medication use, ethanol or illicit drug use, diving, air travel, and sinusitis. In addition, asking about timing and duration of symptoms, associated symptoms, and provoking factors can help determine the cause of vertigo.
  - **Benign paroxysmal positional vertigo (BPPV)** is the most common cause of vertigo[3] and causes **recurrent, brief** (<60 seconds) attacks brought on by changes in head position.[4]
  - **Vestibular neuritis** presents with **acute, spontaneous** vertigo. Symptoms are worse with position change and head shaking. Nystagmus is common, and patients frequently fall to the affected side.[5]
  - **Ménière disease** produces a classic triad of episodic **hearing loss, tinnitus**, and **vertigo** lasting **several minutes to several hours**. A sense of fullness in the affected ear is commonly reported. Sudden falls associated with Ménière disease—referred to as **Tumarkin attacks**—can be confused with syncopal episodes, although they are not associated with loss of consciousness.[6]

TABLE 31-2 CAUSES OF PERIPHERAL VERTIGO

Benign paroxysmal positional vertigo	Acoustic neuroma
Ménière disease	Otitis media
Vestibular labyrinthitis/neuritis	Cholesteatoma
Perilymphatic fistula	Mastoiditis
Ramsay Hunt syndrome	Barotrauma
Ototoxic medications: aminoglycosides, furosemide (Lasix)	Otosclerosis
Semicircular canal dehiscence	Otogenic syphilis

TABLE 31-3 CAUSES OF CENTRAL VERTIGO

Cerebrovascular disorders	Migrainous vertigo
Multiple sclerosis	Epilepsy
Craniocervical junction disorders	Malignancy
Inherited ataxias	Neurodegenerative diseases
Trauma	Toxins

- A **perilymphatic fistula** can cause persistent vertigo after head trauma.[7] Vertigo may worsen with **loud or low-frequency sounds** (the **Tullio phenomenon**).[8] In the absence of a history of trauma, the Tullio phenomenon can also be seen in patients with **superior semicircular canal dehiscence**.[9]
- **Acoustic neuroma** frequently presents with **progressive** symptoms of **hearing loss** or **tinnitus**, with later onset of vertigo and ataxia. Other cranial nerve deficits (particularly involving the trigeminal and facial nerves) can be seen as a result of direct tumor extension.[10]
- Although **vertebrobasilar insufficiency** can be associated with other neurologic symptoms (such as diplopia, weakness, or confusion), it commonly presents with isolated vertigo.[11] As many as 20% of patients with **transient ischemic attack** or **cerebral infarction** involving the posterior cerebral circulation also experience vertigo without associated neurologic deficits.[12]

Physical Examination
- An external ear exam may reveal signs of infection or vesicles of **Ramsay Hunt syndrome** (varicella zoster virus [VZV] affecting cranial nerve VII). A detailed neurologic exam focusing on cranial nerves helps to identify focal neurologic findings and further localization (Table 31-1). Other neurologic deficits, particularly **ataxia**, should raise suspicion for a central lesion.
- The **Dix-Hallpike** maneuver helps to distinguish BPPV: With the patient seated on a bed or examination table, the examiner turns the patient's head 45 degrees to the right. In one firm motion, the patient is allowed to fall supine, and the head is allowed to drop ~20 degrees beyond the edge of the bed or table. The patient's eyes are closely observed for rotational nystagmus, and the patient is queried regarding vertigo. The procedure may then be repeated with the head turned to the left. Patients may also develop nystagmus and vertigo when returned quickly to the seated position.[4]
- **Caloric testing** may aid in the diagnosis.
  - **Always establish the integrity of the tympanic membrane before performing caloric testing.**
  - The patient should be positioned supine in bed with the head elevated to 30 degrees. A small amount of warm (not hot) water is instilled into the ear canal. Use cold water only if warm water does not elicit a response.
  - In a normal response, warm water irrigation produces nystagmus with the fast phase **toward** the irrigated ear.
  - Cold water produces nystagmus with the fast phase **away** from the ear. In vestibular disease, the responses are diminished or absent on the affected side.[13]
- The **H.I.N.T.S exam** is a three-step bedside tool that can be used to distinguish a central from a peripheral cause of vertigo based on careful eye examination. It includes a **Head Impulse test**, evaluation of **Nystagmus** type, and a **Test of Skew deviation**. This combination of tests has been shown to have value in detecting central causes of vertigo, such as stroke.[14]

- The Head Impulse Test involves abrupt rotation of the patient's head with his or her vision fixated ahead on an object. In patients with a peripheral cause, this will often be followed by a series of oppositely directed corrective saccades. The absence of corrective saccades is more compatible with central pathology.[15]
- Patients with peripheral vertigo will often demonstrate horizontal nystagmus, beating in only one direction, increasing in amplitude when the gaze is directed toward the beat of the nystagmus. Vertical or torsional nystagmus, or nystagmus that changes direction on eccentric gaze, suggests a central pathology.[14]
- Skew deviation refers to vertical ocular misalignment. This can be elicited via the **alternate cover test**, in which each eye is sequentially covered, then uncovered. Patients with central lesions may exhibit vertical refixation saccades after the eye is uncovered. Patients with peripheral vertigo will tend to maintain their fixation while each eye is covered and uncovered.[14]

Diagnostic Testing

Straightforward diagnoses with characteristic historical features and physical examination findings may not require further evaluation.

- **Electrooculography** and **audiometry** may be useful in unclear cases.
- **Magnetic resonance imaging (MRI)** should be performed for suspected central vertigo or acoustic neuroma. MRI should also be performed when symptoms are accompanied by headache or in patients with risk factors for cerebrovascular accident. Neuroimaging should also be considered in cases of acute peripheral vertigo that worsen after 48 hours.
- **Magnetic resonance angiography** or traditional **cerebral angiography** may identify vertebrobasilar vascular disease.[16]

TREATMENT

- While the treatment options for vertigo are generally directed at the underlying cause, symptomatic pharmacologic therapy can be applied as needed.
- Pharmacologic therapeutic options, with typical adult dosages, include the following:
  - Meclizine, 25–100 mg per day divided into 2–3 doses per day for up to 3 days
  - Diazepam, 2 mg PO two times per day
  - Promethazine, 25 mg PO two times per day for up to 7 days
  - Prochlorperazine, 5–10 mg PO every 6–8 hours for up to 7 days
- More targeted therapy can be useful in particular vertigo syndromes.
  - For patients with benign positional vertigo, a bedside **Epley maneuver** is >70% effective on first attempt and >90% after two attempts. **Brandt-Daroff habituation exercises** involve head and trunk tilts and may be effective for decreasing symptoms when Epley maneuvers fail.[17]
  - Ménière disease can be managed with 2 g sodium restriction or diuretic therapy (acetazolamide or hydrochlorothiazide). Additional symptomatic medications may be given. Surgery may be useful for refractory cases.[17]
  - Vestibular neuritis has traditionally been treated with steroid pulse therapy; however, in studies, the effect on clinical recovery may not be as robust as the effect on normalization of caloric responses.[18,19]
  - Ramsay Hunt syndrome is generally treated with acyclovir (800 mg PO five times per day), famcyclovir (500 mg PO three times per day), or valacyclovir (1000 mg PO three times per day) for 7 days, started within 72 hours of rash onset, often in combination with corticosteroids. However, the effectiveness of therapy is controversial, and there are limited data regarding the impact on vertigo.[20,21]
  - Acoustic neuroma or cerebellar hemorrhage should be managed surgically.

REFERENCES

1. Karatas M. Central vertigo and dizziness: epidemiology, differential diagnosis, and common causes. *Neurologist* 2008;14:355–64.
2. Murdin L, Schilder AG. Epidemiology of balance symptoms and disorders in the community: a systematic review. *Otol Neurotol* 2015;36:387–92.
3. von Brevern M, Radtke A, Lezius F, et al. Epidemiology of benign paroxysmal positional vertigo: a population based study. *J Neurol Neurosurg Psychiatry* 2007;78:710–5.
4. Kim JS, Zee DS. Clinical practice. Benign paroxysmal positional vertigo. *N Engl J Med* 2014;370:1138–47.
5. Jeong SH, Kim HJ, Kim JS. Vestibular neuritis. *Semin Neurol* 2013;33:185–94.
6. Harcourt J, Barraclough K, Bronstein AM. Meniere's disease. *BMJ* 2014;349:g6544.
7. Hornibrook J. Perilymph fistula: fifty years of controversy. *ISRN Otolaryngol* 2012;2012. article ID: 281248.
8. Pyykko I, Ishizaki H, Aalto H, Starck J. Relevance of the Tullio phenomenon in assessing perilymphatic leak in vertiginous patients. *Am J Otol* 1992;13:339–42.
9. Kaski D, Davies R, Luxon L, et al. The Tullio phenomenon: a neurologically neglected presentation. *J Neurol* 2012;259:4–21.
10. Mathew GD, Facer GW, Suh KW, et al. Symptoms, findings, and methods of diagnosis in patients with acoustic neuroma. *Laryngoscope* 1978;88:1893–903, 921.
11. Baloh RW. Vertebrobasilar insufficiency and stroke. *Otolaryngol Head Neck Surg* 1995;112:114–7.
12. Blum CA, Kasner SE. Transient ischemic attacks presenting with dizziness or vertigo. *Neurol Clin* 2015;33:629–42, ix.
13. Goncalves DU, Felipe L, Lima TM. Interpretation and use of caloric testing. *Braz J Otorhinolaryngol* 2008;74:440–6.
14. Kattah JC, Talkad AV, Wang DZ, et al. HINTS to diagnose stroke in the acute vestibular syndrome: three-step bedside oculomotor examination more sensitive than early MRI diffusion-weighted imaging. *Stroke* 2009;40:3504–10.
15. Halmagyi GM, Curthoys IS. A clinical sign of canal paresis. *Arch Neurol* 1988;45:737–9.
16. Labuguen RH. Initial evaluation of vertigo. *Am Fam Physician* 2006;73:244–51.
17. Swartz R, Longwell P. Treatment of vertigo. *Am Fam Physician* 2005;71:1115–22.
18. Goudakos JK, Markou KD, Franco-Vidal V, et al. Corticosteroids in the treatment of vestibular neuritis: a systematic review and meta-analysis. *Otol Neurotol* 2010;3:183–9.
19. Fishman JM, Burgess C, Waddell A. Corticosteroids for the treatment of idiopathic acute vestibular dysfunction (vestibular neuritis). *Cochrane Database Syst Rev* 2011;(5):CD008607.
20. Uscategui T, Doree C, Chamberlain IJ, Burton MJ. Antiviral therapy for Ramsay Hunt syndrome (herpes zoster oticus with facial palsy) in adults. *Cochrane Database Syst Rev* 2008;(4):CD006851.
21. de Ru JA, van Benthem PP. Combination therapy is preferable for patients with Ramsay Hunt syndrome. *Otol Neurotol* 2011;32:852–5.

Approach to the Carotid Bruit

Chien-Jung Lin and Megan E. Wren

GENERAL PRINCIPLES

- Stroke represents the leading cause of functional impairment and the fourth cause of death in the United States.[1] Each year, an estimated 795,000 Americans experience a new or recurrent stroke, among which 87% are ischemic.
- Approximately 4% of strokes are associated with carotid artery stenosis of >60%, the remainder being due to intracranial atherosclerosis, lacunar infarct, cardioembolic, or cryptogenic source.[2]
- Carotid artery stenosis can cause tubulent blood flow, producing audible carotid bruits. Asymptomatic carotid bruits are present in 4.1% of the population 40–96 years old.[3] **Auscultation for carotid bruits has limited utility for diagnosing carotid stenosis**. A sensitivity of 46–77% and a specificity of 71–98% have been reported.[4] Specificity is even lower for severe stenosis, as bruits disappear with decreased blood flow. A positive predictive value of 25% has been reported in an ethnically diverse population.[3]
- While the presence of carotid bruit is associated with a 2.6-fold increase in the incidence of stroke/transient ischemic attack (TIA), less than half of these events map to the carotid artery territory ipsilateral to the bruit.[5] Most ischemic events are contralateral to the bruit, bilateral, or in the vertibrobasilar territory. Furthermore, carotid bruits are associated with an almost twofold increase in myocardial infarction,[5] indicating that the presence of **a carotid bruit should be regarded as a predictor of systemic atherosclerosis and treated accordingly**.
- Carotid bruits in the surgical patient.
  - A medical consultation for carotid bruits usually occurs as part of the preoperative assessment, with the concern being the risk of perioperative stroke.
  - The incidence of perioperative strokes in patients undergoing general surgery with general anesthesia is very low, between 0.08% and 0.7%.[6] The perioperative stroke risk for cardiac and vascular surgeries is higher; for some procedures, it is nearly 10%.[6] Most of these perioperative strokes are embolic in nature. Of note, off-pump coronary artery bypass grafting (CABG) operations do not reduce risk of stroke compared to on-pump operations.[7]
  - The asymptomatic carotid bruit does not increase the risk of perioperative stroke.[8] Even in patients with established carotid stenosis, most perioperative strokes are embolic and are bilateral or contralateral to the stenosis.[6]
  - **A history of TIA or stroke increases the risk, and such patients should be assessed carefully and treated according to guideline recommendations.**

DIAGNOSIS

Clinical Presentation

History
- Most carotid bruits are found in asymptomatic patients during routine or preoperative physical exam.

- **Symptoms of previous stroke or TIA should be sought**, such as aphasia, neglect, visual field deficit, ipsilateral amaurosis fugax, or contralateral weakness or numbness.
- Nonspecific symptoms such as fatigue, dizziness, syncope, blurry vision, or vertigo do not qualify as symptomatic.
- It is also important to ask about risk factors of artherosclerosis: hypertension, hyperlipidemia, smoking, a family history of first-degree relatives with artherosclerosis manifested before age 60, and a family history of ischemic stroke.

Physical Examination
- The carotid bruit should be differentiated from other mimickers, such as a transmitted heart murmur, a venous hum, or a bruit in another artery.
- A bruit at the bifurcation of the common carotid artery is best heard just below the angle of the jaw.[9]
- A bruit heard in the supraclavicular fossa may be from a subclavian or vertebral artery.
- A thorough neurologic exam with a focus on deficits mapping to the anterior circulation is important as the management of asymptomatic patients differs from that of those with prior cerebrovascular accidents.

Diagnostic Testing
- It is critically important to ascertain the presence or absence of symptoms—defined as a history of TIA or stroke in the preceeding 6 months—as the management differs in these two groups.
- In the **asymptomatic** population, recent guideline recommendations have gravitated away from aggressive screening and treatment.
  - While a 2011 multisociety guideline for extracranial carotid artery disease deemed it reasonable to perform duplex ultrasonography to detect hemodynamically significant carotid stenosis in asymptomatic patients with carotid bruit,[10] more recent guidelines recommend against the screening for carotid stenosis in the asymptomatic population despite the presence of bruits.
  - In 2014, the US Preventive Services Task Force (USPSTF) **recommended against screening for asymptomatic carotid stenosis**,[4] citing imperfect sensitivity and the potential of leading to unnecessary surgery and harm.
  - In the same year, the American Heart Association (AHA)/American Stroke Association (ASA) guideline for the primary prevention of stroke did not recommend screening low-risk populations for asymptomatic carotid stenosis.[11]
  - Similar recommendations were also published by the Society for Vascular Surgery and American Academy of Family Physicians as part of the Choosing Wisely initiative.
- **Imaging evaluation for carotid stenosis is strongly indicated in patients with symptoms of TIA or stroke.**
- **Preoperative screening for carotid stenosis in patients who are to undergo elective CABG is still somewhat controversial.** The AHA guideline indicates it reasonable to screen high-risk patients: age >65 years, left main disease, peripheral arterial disease, prior TIA/stroke, smoking, or diabetes mellitus.[7] Similarly, the Society of Thoracic Surgeons recommends against preoperative screening in patients without symptoms or high-risk criteria.

Imaging
- **Duplex ultrasonography** (B-mode ultrasound imaging plus Doppler ultrasound) is the most commonly used test for evaluating carotid stenosis and has estimated sensitivity and specificity of about 85–90%.[10] It is recommended as the first test to diagnose hemodynamically significant carotid stenosis.[10]
- **Computed tomographic angiography (CTA)** and **magnetic resonance angiography (MRA)** are also widely used and have an accuracy similar to that of duplex

ultrasonography.[10] They are particularly useful when ultrasonography is not reliable, such as severe calcification, high bifurcation, or short neck. Their limitations include contrast requirement for CTA and prolonged acquisition time for MRA.

Diagnostic Procedures
Angiography is the gold standard for the diagnosis of carotid stenosis. However, it carries risk of stroke of up to 1%.[9] Due to its invasive nature, angiography has essentially been replaced by the above diagnostic modalities.

TREATMENT

Approaches differ for symptomatic and asymptomatic stenosis.

- **Management of symptomatic carotid stenosis**
  - **Carotid endarterectomy (CEA)**
    - In several randomized controlled trials, CEA has shown benefit in patients with symptomatic (within preceding 6 months), severe (>70%) stenosis. **CEA should be performed for symptomatic patients with >70% stenosis.**[12] The Cochrane Database Review estimates the absolute risk reduction (ARR) of ipsilateral ischemic stroke in these patients to be 16% with a number needed to treat (NNT) of 6 over 5 years.[13] Importantly, however, CEA offers no benefit in patient with carotid total occlusion. The benefit of CEA tapers rapidly with increasing delay of surgery >2 weeks from last ischemic event. These analyses assume a perioperative rate of stroke or death of <6%; thus, if a given surgeon's complication rate is higher than this, the benefit of surgery will be lower.
    - **In patients with moderate (50–69%) stenosis, the benefit of CEA is marginal** with an ARR of 4.6% and NNT of 22. The expertise of the surgeon and coexisting conditions must be carefully considered. CEA should be considered for patients more likely to experience benefit: males, ≥75 years of age and those with hemispheric symptoms (rather than monocular TIA), and stroke within 90 days.
    - **In patients with mild (<50%) stenosis, CEA is not recommended.**
    - In symptomatic patients undergoing CABG, carotid revascularization in conjunction with CABG is reasonable. The decision to perform combined or sequential operation, as well as the sequence of intervention, should be determined by the relative severity of cerebral versus myocardial dysfunction.[7]
  - **Carotid angioplasty and stenting (CAS)**
    - Current data suggest CAS achieves similar long-term outcome compared to CEA.
    - CAS is associated with increased periprocedural stroke or death within 30 days (8.2% vs. 5%, OR 1.72), especially in patients >70 years old.[14] While the overall stroke rate is higher in CAS, it does not differ beyond the periprocedural period. It is reasonable to consider CAS in younger patients as the periprocedural complications and long-term risk for ipsilateral stroke are similar to CEA.
    - CAS may be considered in patients with high surgical risk due to comorbidities, radiation-induced stenosis, or restenosis after CEA.
    - The role of CAS in CABG patients remains to be defined. It is currently reserved for patients with contraindications for CEA.
  - **Medical therapy**: Medical management should be offered regardless of whether the patient is a candidate for CEA/CAS. Medical therapy should focus on modifying the well-documented risk factors of smoking, hypertension, dyslipidemia, and diabetes.
    - Aspirin and other antiplatelet drugs reduce the rate of nonfatal stroke by 25%, nonfatal myocardial infarction by 34%, and vascular death by 17%.[15] On the other hand,

low-dose aspirin doubles the risk of extracranial bleeding in these same patients, but this is clearly outweighed by the benefits.
- □ The recommended dose of **aspirin** is between 75 and 325 mg daily. Higher doses do not provide additional benefit and may be harmful.
- □ Extended-release **dipyridamole** 200 mg bid alone reduces the stroke rate and has an additive benefit in combination with low-dose aspirin (25 mg bid).
- □ **Clopidogrel** 75 mg daily is a reasonable alternative, especially in patients with aspirin allergy.
- Anticoagulation provides no benefit over antiplatelet therapy in the absence of atrial fibrillation or other cardioembolic source and is associated with higher risk of bleeding.
- **High-intensity statin** therapy and other facets of cholesterol management should be provided according to the 2013 American College of Cardiology/American Heart Association guideline.[16]
- **Management of asymptomatic carotid stenosis**
  - **Carotid endarterectomy (CEA)**
    - For **asymptomatic patients with >70% stenosis**, the benefits of CEA are significantly less substantial and are dependent on a low perioperative stroke rate, <3% (a rate not always achieved in routine clinical practice). Benefits may be greater in younger (age <80 years) men. Subgroup analysis suggests that CEA is considerably less effective for asymptomatic women than for asymptomatic men, reflecting a higher perioperative risk and lower risk of vascular events among women with asymptomatic carotid stenosis. Of note, these studies were done in an earlier era; recent advances in medical treatment may have further decreased the benefit margin of revascularization. Decisions must be carefully individualized.
    - **CEA is not indicated for asymptomatic patients with <60% stenosis** and may be harmful.
  - **Carotid angioplasty and stenting** appears to provide similar long-term outcome but higher periprocedural stroke or death rate. Its efficacy compared to medical therapy remains to be defined.
  - Carotid revascularization may be considered in asymptomatic patients scheduled to undergo CABG who have bilateral stenoses >70% or unilateral stenosis >70% with contralateral occlusion.[7]
  - Carotid revascularization prior to elective noncardiac surgery in asymptomatic patients is generally not recommended but may be indicated in selected patients with severe and/or bilateral stenosis.
  - **Medical management** is similar to that for symptomatic carotid stenosis.

REFERENCES

1. Mozaffarian D, Benjamin EJ, Go AS, et al. Heart disease and stroke statistics—2015 update: a report from the American Heart Association. *Circulation* 2015;131:e29–322.
2. White H, Boden-Albala B, Wang C, et al. Ischemic stroke subtype incidence among whites, blacks, and Hispanics: the Northern Manhattan Study. *Circulation* 2005;111:1327–31.
3. Ratchford EV, Jin Z, Di Tullio MR, et al. Carotid bruit for detection of hemodynamically significant carotid stenosis: the Northern Manhattan Study. *Neurol Res* 2009;31:748–52.
4. LeFevre ML. Screening for asymptomatic carotid artery stenosis: U.S. Preventive Services Task Force recommendation statement. *Ann Intern Med* 2014;161:356–62.
5. Wolf PA, Kannel WB, Sorlie P, McNamara P. Asymptomatic carotid bruit and risk of stroke. The Framingham study. *JAMA* 1981;245:1442–5.
6. Selim M. Perioperative stroke. *N Engl J Med* 2007;356:706–13.
7. Hillis LD, Smith PK, Anderson JL, et al. 2011 ACCF/AHA guideline for coronary artery bypass graft surgery: executive summary: a report of the American College of Cardiology Foundation/American Heart Association Task Force on Practice Guidelines. *Circulation* 2011;124:2610–42.

8. Ropper AH, Wechsler LR, Wilson LS. Carotid bruit and the risk of stroke in elective surgery. *N Engl J Med* 1982;307:1388–90.
9. Sandercock PA, Kavvadia E. The carotid bruit. *Pract Neurol* 2002;2:221–4.
10. Brott TG, Halperin JL, Abbara S, et al. 2011 ASA/ACCF/AHA/AANN/AANS/ACR/ASNR/CNS/SAIP/SCAI/SIR/SNIS/SVM/SVS guideline on the management of patients with extracranial carotid and vertebral artery disease. A report of the American College of Cardiology Foundation/American Heart Association Task Force on Practice Guidelines, and the American Stroke Association, American Association of Neuroscience Nurses, American Association of Neurological Surgeons, American College of Radiology, American Society of Neuroradiology, Congress of Neurological Surgeons, Society of Atherosclerosis Imaging and Prevention, Society for Cardiovascular Angiography and Interventions, Society of Interventional Radiology, Society of NeuroInterventional Surgery, Society for Vascular Medicine, and Society for Vascular Surgery. *Circulation* 2011;124:e54–e130.
11. Meschia JF, Bushnell C, Boden-Albala B, et al. Guidelines for the primary prevention of stroke: a statement for healthcare professionals from the American Heart Association/American Stroke Association. *Stroke* 2014;45:3754–832.
12. Kernan WN, Ovbiagele B, Black HR, et al. Guidelines for the prevention of stroke in patients with stroke and transient ischemic attack: a guideline for healthcare professionals from the American Heart Association/American Stroke Association. *Stroke* 2014;45:2160–236.
13. Rerkasem K, Rothwell PM. Carotid endarterectomy for symptomatic carotid stenosis. *Cochrane Database Syst Rev* 2011;CD001081.
14. Bonati LH, Lyrer P, Ederle J, et al. Percutaneous transluminal balloon angioplasty and stenting for carotid artery stenosis. *Cochrane Database Syst Rev* 2012;(9):CD000515.
15. Patrono C, Garcia Rodriguez LA, Landolfi R, Baigent C. Low-dose aspirin for the prevention of atherothrombosis. *N Engl J Med* 2005;353:2373–83.
16. Stone NJ, Robinson JG, Lichtenstein AH, et al. 2013 ACC/AHA guideline on the treatment of blood cholesterol to reduce atherosclerotic cardiovascular risk in adults: a report of the American College of Cardiology/American Heart Association Task Force on Practice Guidelines. *Circulation* 2014;129:S1–S45.

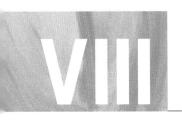

VIII Hematology

Approach to Anemia   33

Devin C. Odom

GENERAL PRINCIPLES

- Anemia is frequently seen in hospitalized patients both as a primary diagnosis and as a comorbidity.
- Anemia is roughly defined as a hemoglobin (Hgb) concentration <13.5 g/dL in men or <12.0 g/dL in women. Normal values may be different in older individuals and different races.[1]
- Anemia can be classified in two general ways:
  - First, anemia can be categorized by the underlying cause. These causes of anemia can be divided into three broad categories:
    - Blood loss
    - Increased destruction of red blood cells (RBCs) (e.g., hemolytic anemia)
    - Decreased production of RBCs (hypoproliferative anemia)
  - The second way categorizes anemia morphologically; anemia may also be classified by RBC size (mean corpuscular volume [MCV]):
    - Microcytic
    - Normocytic
    - Macrocytic
- **Microcytic anemia**: Anemia is considered microcytic when the MCV is <80 fL. See Table 33-1 for the differential diagnosis of microcytic anemia based on laboratory data.
  - Iron (Fe) deficiency is the most common cause of microcytic anemia in adults; it is usually due to chronic blood loss (e.g., gastric ulcer or menorrhagia) but may also be due to malabsorption or excessive phlebotomy.[2]
  - Sideroblastic anemia may be hereditary; idiopathic; or caused by alcohol, lead (microcytic hypochromic anemia), isoniazid, chloramphenicol, malignancy, myelodysplasia, or chronic inflammation.[3]
  - Anemia of chronic disease (or inflammation) is commonly seen as a result of abnormal ferrokinetics and may often be a diagnosis of exclusion.
  - Thalassemias present with varying degrees of anemia. Patients may present with splenomegaly and peripheral smears with varying hypochromia, target cells, or teardrop cells. Diagnosis may require Hgb electrophoresis or chromatography (see next section, "Diagnosis").
- **Normocytic anemias** (MCV between 80 and 100 mL) can be divided into two groups, based on the reticulocyte count to make differential diagnosis more straightforward.
  - **Increased reticulocyte count**: bleeding or hemolytic anemia (see Table 33-2 for the differential diagnosis of hemolytic anemia).
  - **Decreased reticulocyte count**: hypoproliferative disorder.
  - **Anemia of chronic renal failure** generally starts to occur when creatine clearance is <45 mL/min and worsens with increasing renal failure. Classically, this is a hypochromic normocytic anemia owing to decreased renal erythropoietin production, but the causes are multifactorial, and comorbid conditions cause varying presentations.[4]
- **Macrocytic anemias** are classified by an MCV > 100 mL and are divided into megaloblastic or nonmegaloblastic types based on the peripheral smear.

TABLE 33-1 DIFFERENTIAL DIAGNOSIS FOR MICROCYTIC ANEMIA

	Iron Deficiency	Chronic Disease/Inflammation	Thalassemia	Sideroblastic
Serum Fe	↓ or normal	↓	Normal	↑
Total iron-binding capacity	↑	Normal or ↓	Normal	↑
Transferrin saturation	↓	Normal or ↓	Normal	Normal or ↑
Serum ferritin	↓	Normal or ↑	Normal	↑
Bone marrow iron stores	↓ or Absent	Normal or ↓	↑	↑
RBC morphology	Microcytic, hypochromic, anisocytosis	Microcytic or normocytic, normochromic	Microcytic, hypochromic	Microcytic, hypochromic, dimorphic

↑, increased; ↓, decreased; RBC, red blood cell.

TABLE 33-2 DIFFERENTIAL DIAGNOSIS OF HEMOLYTIC ANEMIA

Autoimmune Hemolytic Anemia	Nonimmune Hemolytic Anemia
IgG autoantibody	Microangiopathic/traumatic
IgM autoantibody	DIC, TTP, HUS
Drug induced	Enzyme defects (e.g., G-6-PD deficiency)
Cold agglutinin	Drug induced
Malignancy associated	Paroxysmal nocturnal hemoglobinuria
Systemic lupus	Hemoglobinopathy (e.g., sickle cell disease)
	Malignant HTN
	RBC membrane diseases
	Infections (e.g., malaria)
	Eclampsia
	Transfusion reactions (immune)

DIC, disseminated intravascular coagulation; G-6-PD, glucose-6-phosphate dehydrogenase; HTN, hypertension; HUS, hemolytic–uremic syndrome; RBC, red blood cell; TTP, thrombotic thrombocytopenic purpura.

- Megaloblastic anemia may be caused by the following:
  - Vitamin B_{12} deficiency
  - Folate deficiency
  - Drug-induced (e.g., phenytoin, hydroxyurea, trimethoprim–sulfamethoxazole, azidothymidine, methotrexate)
- Nonmegaloblastic macrocytic anemia may be caused by the following:
  - Reticulocytosis
  - Alcohol
  - Liver disease
  - Hypothyroidism
  - Various bone marrow disorders that interfere with RBC maturation (e.g., acute leukemia or myelodysplastic syndrome)

DIAGNOSIS

Clinical Presentation

History
- General symptoms of anemia may include dyspnea, fatigue, and palpitations.
- Weight loss, night sweats, and fever may point to an underlying malignancy, infection, or inflammatory disorder.
- Vitamin B_{12} deficiency may present with other symptoms including a burning sensation of the tongue, vague abdominal pain, diarrhea, numbness, or paresthesias.
- Bone pain may owe to marrow infiltrating diseases or occlusive crisis in sickle cell disease.
- A careful history concerning blood loss (especially perioperatively or in the stool or menses) is important. Blood loss may be subacute and noted only by occasionally dark or tarry stool or heavy menses and not obvious bleeding.
- Frequency of hemaglobin and hematocrit evaluations and family history of anemia should be sought.
- Past medical history should be reviewed in detail for diseases known to cause or contribute to anemia (e.g., renal failure, autoimmune disease).
- Dark urine may be due to indirect bilirubin in the urine and point to a hemolytic anemia.
- Early cholecystectomy in a family member may be a clue to familial hemolytic anemia.
- A good dietary history should be obtained, including iron intake, B_{12} (deficient in vegans), and folate (from uncooked leafy vegetables), as well as pica symptoms (seen in iron deficiency).

Physical Examination
- Anemia may result in pallor of mucous membranes or the skin, tachycardia, or signs of high-output heart failure.
- In iron deficiency, alopecia, atrophic glossitis, angular cheilosis, koilonychia (spoon nails), or brittle nails may be seen.
- Vitamin B_{12}-deficient patients may have glossitis/smooth tongue, dorsal column findings (decreased vibratory sensation and proprioception), or corticospinal tract findings.
- Assess for jaundice or splenomegaly, which are sometimes present in hemolytic anemias.
- Lymph nodes may be enlarged in hematologic malignancies.
- Evidence of infection, acute or occult, should be investigated.
- **All patients need a stool occult blood test to look for GI blood loss.**

Diagnostic Testing

Laboratories

- Review the full complete blood count (CBC). The presence of leukopenia or thrombocytopenia should raise suspicion for bone marrow failure, infiltration, or severe nutritional deficiency.
- The **peripheral smear** is an important test to obtain. Some pertinent findings include the following:
  - Target cells in iron deficiency, hemoglobinopathies, liver disease, asplenia, and lecithin–cholesterol acyltransferase deficiency.
  - Megaloblastic changes in macrocytic anemia include hypersegmentation of neutrophils, anisocytosis, large ovalocytes, and often pancytopenia.
  - Hemolysis is suggested by acanthocytes, spherocytes, or reticulocytes.
  - Evidence of malignant blood cells, blast cells, sickled cells, or other diagnostic abnormalities.
- **RBC indices** should be noted to aid in the diagnosis. They can be helpful when more than one cause of anemia is present. The following indices should be noted:
  - **MCV** values >115 are almost always owing to vitamin B_{12} or folate deficiency, but can result from the presence of a cold agglutinin that causes RBCs to stick together and thus appear larger.
  - Low **mean corpuscular hemoglobin (MCH)** is seen in iron deficiency while high levels occur in any form of macrocytosis.[5]
  - **Mean corpuscular hemoglobin concentration** can be elevated in spherocytosis and congenital hemolytic anemias.
- The reticulocyte count (normal 0.5–1.5%) should be corrected for anemia, using the following formula:
  Corrected reticulocyte count = uncorrected reticulocyte count × (patient's Hct/45)
  - A stable anemia with a **low reticulocyte count** is evidence of poor marrow RBC production. Renal failure, hypothyroidism, adrenal insufficiency, or gonadal insufficiency are causes to consider.
  - A **high reticulocyte count** may reflect a normal response to bleeding or hemolysis.
- **Macrocytic anemia** should first be evaluated by determining whether it is megaloblastic or nonmegaloblastic based on the peripheral smear.
  - Megaloblastic anemia
    - Measure RBC folate and serum vitamin B_{12}.
    - In cases of borderline low vitamin B_{12} values, one can measure serum methylmalonic acid and homocysteine levels, which are both elevated in vitamin B_{12} deficiency. Only homocysteine is elevated in folate deficiency.
    - When vitamin B_{12} and folate deficiency are excluded, consider one of the drug-induced causes (see the description of macrocytic anemias in the "Etiology" section above).
  - In nonmegaloblastic anemia, first measure the reticulocyte count.
    - If it is elevated, it most likely has a hemolytic cause (see Table 33-2).
    - If the reticulocyte count is inappropriately low, consider one of the other causes of nonmegaloblastic macrocytic anemia (see the description of macrocytic anemias in the "Etiology" section above).
- **Iron deficiency anemia**
  - Obtaining a serum **ferritin** is the most cost-effective way to diagnose iron deficiency. A ferritin of <15 ng/mL almost always indicates iron deficiency. A serum ferritin level >200 ng/mL generally indicates adequate iron stores regardless of other underlying conditions.
  - Because ferritin is an acute phase reactant, intermediate levels can be more challenging to interpret, as normal levels may be seen in inflammatory states, renal disease, liver disease, or malignancy despite low iron stores.

- In these settings, serum iron, total iron binding capacity, and transferrin-saturation iron may be helpful additional labs. Transferrin saturation <20% is usually indicative of absolute iron deficiency in end-stage renal disease, even if the ferritin is within the normal range. Ongoing research seeks to define more sensitive and specific tests for iron deficiency in chronic kidney disease.
- **Thalassemia** may be diagnosed by **hemoglobin electrophoresis.**
  - α-**Thalassemia trait**, the most commonly diagnosed thalassemia, will have a normal Hgb electrophoresis but an MCV that is low, out of proportion to the anemia, and a chronically low hematocrit on review of previous lab data.
  - β-**Thalassemia trait** is associated with mild microcytic anemia and increased Hgb A_2.
- In **hemolytic anemias**, one often sees **signs of increased RBC destruction**. Laboratory information may show increased lactate dehydrogenase (LDH), decreased haptoglobin, increased unconjugated bilirubin, or hemoglobinuria (in intravascular hemolysis or severe extravascular hemolysis). Reticulocytosis should also be seen in patients without other underlying medical problems. If there is evidence of hemolysis, evaluation with an indirect and direct Coombs test is indicated. The direct Coombs test will be positive in autoimmune hemolytic anemias, detecting IgG and C3 antibodies. A false-negative direct Coombs test may occur with IgM-mediated or cold-agglutinin hemolysis.

Diagnostic Procedures

Consider a bone marrow evaluation in difficult cases.

Special Considerations in Postoperative Anemia

- Postoperative bleeding at the site of the surgery should always be considered. Expected bleeding may have occurred intraoperatively with delayed hemodilution or in the perioperative/postoperative period owing to injury or poor hemostasis.
- Other considerations include the following:
  - Patients who experience hypothermia or cold cardioplegia with cardiac surgery may have a shortened RBC life span owing to membrane damage. RBCs recovered with autologous blood recovery systems (e.g., the Cell Saver) also experience significant membrane damage and early hemolysis.
  - Patients with valvular surgery may have a valve-induced hemolytic anemia. Also consider evaluation of the mooring, which, if loosened, can cause significant hemolysis.
  - Bone marrow suppression, iron sequestration, and decreased erythropoietin production may occur owing to inflammatory cytokine production after surgery and may continue for a week or more postoperatively.[6]
  - Perioperative hemodilution owing to aggressive intravenous hydration is common. Review the ins and outs and anesthesiology flow sheets.
  - Consider drug-induced hemolysis and glucose-6-phosphate dehydrogenase deficiency caused by anesthetics or pain medications.
  - Stress gastritis is common perioperatively and can be the source of significant blood loss. This is easier to prevent (with prophylactic histamine-2 [H_2] blockers, proton pump inhibitors, or sucralfate) than it is to treat.

TREATMENT

Treatment will be discussed according to etiology of anemia. First, however, transfusion will be discussed.

- The goal of transfusion is to improve tissue oxygen delivery, not solely to increase serum Hgb.
- Current recommendations do not recommend routine transfusion in patients with Hgb concentration <7.0 g/dL unless there is concern for ongoing or expected bleeding (e.g., surgery).[7]

- There is ongoing debate regarding blood transfusion for patients with acute medical problems caused by poor oxygen delivery (e.g., active cardiac or cerebral infarction). In this population, goal Hgb concentration ranges from 8 to 10 g/dL depending on the literature.
- Massive transfusion of RBCs (>4 units) also requires transfusion of other blood products (e.g., platelets and clotting factors) to prevent dilution, which could exacerbate bleeding.
- Blood transfusions are not without drawbacks. Common complications from blood transfusion are volume overload, transfusion-related acute lung injury (TRALI), and infection. Routine transfusion to Hgb > 10 g/dL has been associated with increased mortality.[7] Transfusions must be approached with caution in individuals with acquired hemolytic anemias or symptoms of heart failure as transfusions could negatively impact these patients.

Iron Deficiency Anemia

- Discover and treat the underlying source of blood loss. Ferrous sulfate ($FeSO_4$), 325 mg PO bid to tid, may be initiated. Parenteral iron may be administered in cases of intolerance or failure to take PO iron, malabsorption, or severe renal failure.[2] The risk of anaphylaxis is significant with iron dextran; a test dose must be administered. The risk is much lower with newer preparations (e.g., ferric gluconate and iron sucrose).
- Expect an increase in the reticulocyte count within 7 to 10 days of therapy. Correction of anemia usually occurs within 6 to 8 weeks, but treatment should continue for ~6 months (if the patient is on oral iron) to fully restore tissue iron stores.
- Men and nonmenstruating women should be considered for endoscopy to evaluate for a potential gastrointestinal source of chronic blood loss.

Vitamin B_{12} Deficiency

- Vitamin B_{12} deficiency should be treated with vitamin B_{12}, 1 mg IM daily for 7 days, and then weekly for 1 to 2 months, followed by monthly doses thereafter.
- High-dose oral vitamin B_{12} (1–2 mg/d) can also provide sufficient long-term replacement.[8]
- An evaluation for the underlying mechanism should be undertaken. Failure to correct or identify the underlying cause of deficiency should result in lifelong therapy.

Folate Deficiency

Folate deficiency should be treated with folic acid 1 mg PO daily, with expected resolution of hematologic abnormalities within 2 months.

Chronic Renal Failure

Anemia of chronic renal failure may respond to erythropoietin, 50 to 100 U/kg IV SC three times a week in dialysis patients and weekly for those not on dialysis. Darbepoetin is dosed at 0.45 mcg/kg SC once a week. Doses can be adjusted when the Hgb is in target range (11–12 g/dL).[9] Ensure adequate iron stores and transfuse only as needed (see the discussion on transfusion above).

Other Medical Conditions

A thorough evaluation of anemia may result in other diagnoses discussed above. Treatment of anemia owing to these conditions are focused on treating the underlying cause and/or close monitoring in stable chronic anemia. For example, causative medications should be reduced or stopped, and hypothyroidism or rheumatoid arthritis should be treated if appropriate.

REFERENCES

1. Price EA, Mehra R, Holmes TH, Schrier SL. Anemia in older persons: etiology and evaluation. *Blood Cells Mol Dis* 2011;46:159.
2. Lopez A, Cacoub P, Macdougall IC, Peyrin-Biroulet L. Iron deficiency anaemia. *Lancet* 2016;387:907–16.
3. Bottomley SS, Fleming MD. Sideroblastic anemia: diagnosis and management. *Hematol Oncol Clin North Am* 2014;28:653–70.
4. Fernández-Rodríguez AM, Guindeo-Casasús MC, Molero-Labarta T, et al. Diagnosis of iron deficiency in chronic renal failure. *Am J Kidney Dis* 1999;34:508–13.
5. Guyatt GH, Oxman AD, Ali M, et al. Laboratory diagnosis of iron-deficiency anemia: an overview. *J Gen Intern Med* 1992;7:145–53.
6. Partridge J, Harari D, Gossage J, Dhesi J. Anaemia in the older surgical patient: a review of prevalence, causes, implications and management. *J R Soc Med* 2013;106:269–77.
7. Goodnough LT, Maggio P. Restrictive blood transfusion practices are associated with improved patient outcomes. *Transfusion* 2014;54:2753–9.
8. Eussen SJ, de Groot LC, Clarke R, et al. Oral cyanocobalamin supplementation in older people with vitamin B_{12} deficiency: a dose-finding trial. *Arch Intern Med* 2005;165:1167–72.
9. National Kidney Foundation. KDOQI Clinical Practice Guidelines for Anemia of Chronic Kidney disease. *Am J Kidney Dis* 2006;47(Suppl 3):S11–S145.

Thrombocytopenia

Scott R. Goldsmith and George Mansour

GENERAL PRINCIPLES

- The normal platelet number is 150,000–450,000/μL of blood. At any given time, approximately one-third of mature platelets are sequestered in the spleen, whereas two-thirds circulate in blood. The lifespan of circulating platelets is 7–10 days.
- In general, thrombocytopenia is caused by decreased production, increased splenic sequestration, or increased destruction of platelets.
- Additionally, certain infectious diseases result in thrombocytopenia from a combination of the previously mentioned mechanisms or due to mechanisms that are not fully understood.
- See Table 34-1[1] for the differential diagnosis of thrombocytopenia.

DIAGNOSIS

Clinical Presentation

History

Symptoms of low platelets vary depending on the platelet count.

- Platelets >100,000/μL should have normal hemostasis.
- Platelets <50,000/μL may stem from a history of prolonged bleeding after a procedure, mucosal bleeding (gingival, gastrointestinal), menorrhagia, or easy bruising.
- Platelets <20,000/μL may be associated with a petechial rash or spontaneous bleeding.
- Platelets <10,000/μL indicate a risk for spontaneous intracerebral hemorrhage.
- These numbers serve as guides; however, the etiology, the presence of mucosal bleeding on presentation, and a history of bleeding at a given platelet count contribute more to the risk of hemorrhage than does the absolute count itself.
- In addition, look for symptoms and risk factors associated with etiologies of decreased platelets (Tables 34-1[1] and 34-2[2]).
  ○ Fatigue, weight loss, or night sweats may be associated with infection or malignancy.
  ○ A medication history and an accurate alcohol history are critical.[2] Identification of heparin or heparin-derivative usage especially in those who are currently or recently hospitalized is important, as a diagnosis of heparin-induced thrombocytopenia (HIT) greatly alters management. HIT occurs after antibodies form and bind to heparin–platelet factor 4 (heparin–PF4). These antibody–heparin–PF4 complexes bind to platelets, leading to both platelet removal and procoagulant release and thus thrombocytopenia and a hypercoagulable state. Establishing the diagnosis of HIT requires both clinical and laboratory features, but a clinical score known as the "4Ts" helps guide one's pretest suspicion and testing, as detailed in Table 34-3.[3]
  ○ Other offending agents include certain antibiotics such as vancomycin, linezolid, and sulfonamides, as well as anticonvulsants such as phenytoin and valproic acid.

TABLE 34-1 ETIOLOGIES OF THROMBOCYTOPENIA

Decreased Platelet Production	Platelet Destruction/Clearance
Marrow Failure Syndromes	**Immune-Mediated Mechanisms**
Congenital: Wiskott-Aldrich syndrome, Fanconi anemia, Bernard-Soulier syndrome	Immune thrombocytopenic purpura
Acquired: Aplastic anemia, paroxysmal nocturnal hemoglobinuria	Thrombotic thrombocytopenic purpura/hemolytic uremic syndrome
Hematologic malignancies	Posttransfusion purpura
Marrow infiltration: Cancer, granulomatous disease	Heparin-induced thrombocytopenia
Myelofibrosis: Primary or secondary	Non–immune-mediated mechanisms
Nutritional deficiencies: Vitamin B_{12}, folate, iron	Disseminated intravascular coagulopathy
Damage to marrow: Radiation, chemotherapy, alcohol	Local consumption: aortic aneurysm, IABP, LVAD, CVVHD
Increased Splenic Sequestration	Acute hemorrhage
Portal hypertension	**Infections Associated with Thrombocytopenia**
Felty syndrome	HIV, HHV-6, ehrlichiosis, rickettsia, malaria, hepatitis C, CMV, EBV, *Helicobacter pylori*, *E. coli* O157
Lysosomal storage disorders	
Infiltrative hematologic malignancies	
Extramedullary hematopoiesis	

IABP, intra-aortic balloon pump; LVAD, left ventricular assist device; CVVHD, continuous venovenous hemodialysis; HIV, human immunodeficiency virus; HHV-6, human herpesvirus 6; CMV, cytomegalovirus; EBV, Epstein-Barr virus.

From Sanfilippo KM, Gage BF, Wang T-F, Yusen RD. Disorders of Hemostasis and Thrombosis. In: Bhat P, Dretler A, Gdowksi M, et al., eds. *The Washington Manual of Medical Therapeutics*. 35th ed. Philadelphia: Wolters Kluwer, 2016.

Also, platelet inhibitors, namely clopidogrel and glycoprotein IIb/IIIa inhibitors (e.g., abciximab), have been reported to cause thrombocytopenia.
- Travel and outdoor exposure may hint at tick-borne or other infectious illnesses, which will help guide further diagnostic testing.
- Try to elicit a history of symptoms suggesting an autoimmune disease.
- The classic pentad of thrombotic thrombocytopenic purpura (TTP) is fever, altered sensorium, renal failure, microangiopathic hemolytic anemia, and thrombocytopenia. Only rarely are all elements present. TTP is similarly related to hemolytic–uremic syndrome (HUS).[4]
- Obtain a transfusion history. **Posttransfusion purpura (PTP)** is a rare disorder caused by the formation of alloantibodies against platelet surface antigens, most commonly human platelet antigen (HPA)-1a. Consider this in the postsurgical patient who has a precipitous drop in platelets 7–10 days after platelet transfusions.

TABLE 34-2	MEDICATIONS COMMONLY ASSOCIATED WITH THROMBOCYTOPENIA
Quinidine	Heparin
H₂ blockers	Vancomycin
Digoxin	Piperacillin
Trimethoprim–sulfamethoxazole	Amiodarone
Quinine	Methyldopa
Rifampin	Valproic acid
Linezolid	Thiazides
GPIIb-IIIa inhibitors	Danazol

Data from Aster R, Bougie D. Drug-induced immune thrombocytopenia. *N Engl J Med* 2007;357:580–7.

TABLE 34-3 FOUR Ts OF HEPARIN-INDUCED THROMBOCYTOPENIA

Clinical Feature	Scoring Criteria
Thrombocytopenia	• Platelet count fall >50% AND nadir ≥20,000/µL (2 points) • Platelet count fall 30–50% OR nadir 10,000–19,000/µL (1 point) • Platelet count fall <30% OR nadir <10,000/µL (0 points)
Timing of platelet fall	• Clear onset between days 5 and 10 of heparin exposure, OR platelet count fall at ≤1 day if prior heparin exposure within the last 30 days (2 points) • Consistent with fall in platelet count at 5–10 days, but unclear (e.g., missing platelet counts), OR onset after day 10, OR fall ≤1 day with prior heparin exposure within 30–100 days (1 point) • Platelet count fall at <4 days without recent heparin exposure (0 points)
Thrombosis or other sequelae	• Confirmed new thrombosis, skin necrosis, or acute systemic reaction after intravenous unfractionated heparin bolus (2 points) • Progressive or recurrent thrombosis, nonnecrotizing (erythematous) skin lesions, or suspected thrombosis that has not been proven (1 point) • None (0 points)
O**T**her causes for thrombocytopenia	• None apparent (2 points) • Possible (1 point) • Definite (0 points)

0–3 points, Low probability; 4–5 points, Intermediate probability; 6–8 points, High probability.
From Lo GK, Juhl D, Warkentin TE, et al. Evaluation of pretest clinical score (4 T's) for the diagnosis of heparin-induced thrombocytopenia in two clinical settings. *J Thromb Haemost* 2006;4:759.

Diagnosis

Physical Examination

Examination should focus on signs and pattern of bleeding as well as signs of the underlying etiology.

- Thrombocytopenia tends to result in mucosal hemorrhage, petechiae and/or small superficial ecchymoses, and it is rare for hemarthroses or muscle hematomas to occur, as compared to coagulopathies in which deep tissue bleeding is more likely to result.
- Vital signs may reveal evidence of sepsis (hypotension, tachycardia, fever), although fever is also frequently present in TTP.
- A thorough lymph node examination is essential to assess for underlying malignancy, infection, or autoimmune condition and can help guide further diagnostics.
- Assessment for hepatosplenomegaly and stigmata of cirrhosis may suggest splenic sequestration from underlying liver disease and portal hypertension, or an infiltrative process within the reticuloendothelial system.
- Signs of superificial and deep thromboses raise the concern of a thrombotic thrombocytopenic disorder such as disseminated intravascular coagulation (DIC), HIT, or TTP and may drastically alter management.

Diagnostic Testing

Laboratories

- Complete blood count with differential: assess for isolated thrombocytopenia or multiple cytopenias.
- Obtain a peripheral blood smear.
  - Look for platelet clumping (spurious thrombocytopenia/pseudothrombocytopenia) in which platelet numbers are normal but clumped by the EDTA and missed by the automated counter. Use collection tubes that lack EDTA (e.g., citrate-coated tube).
  - Look for schistocytes (TTP, DIC).
  - Look for evidence of malignancy or myelofibrosis: these include peripheral blasts, teardrop cells, nucleated RBCs, immature granulocytes.
  - Look for micro- or macrocytosis, which may be associated with a vitamin or iron deficiency: one may see hypersegmented neutrophils in vitamin B_{12}/folate/copper deficiency.
- **Bleeding time (BT)** is an estimate of platelet function (normal is 2–9 minutes).
  - >100,000 platelets, the BT is generally normal.
  - 50,000–100,000 platelets, the BT is mildly prolonged.
  - <50,000 platelets, the BT is significantly prolonged.
  - In general, BT is not usually tested as it provides little diagnostic or prognostic information
- Evaluating prothrombin time/partial thromboplastin time (**PT/PTT**) and **fibrin degradation products/D-dimer** may help identify DIC and distinguish a hemolytic anemia from TTP.
- TTP and HUS may present with hemolytic anemia (decreasing **hemoglobin [Hgb] and hematocrit [Hct]**, elevated **lactate dehydrogenase [LDH]**) and renal failure).
- **Human immunodeficiency virus (HIV) and Hepatitis C virus (HCV) screening** should occur in any patient with new thrombocytopenia.[5]
- Consider checking an antinuclear antibody (**ANA**), as immune thrombocytopenic purpura (ITP) may be the first manifestation of systemic lupus erythematosus (SLE).
- A severely decreased **ferritin, folate, or vitamin B_{12}** level suggests nutritional deficiency.
- If HIT is a consideration based on intermediate or high pretest probability from the 4Ts (Table 34-3),[3] testing begins with ELISA for the **heparin–PF4 antibody**, and the diagnosis is confirmed with the **serotonin-release assay**.

Diagnostic Procedures

- **Consider a bone marrow biopsy** if the etiology is uncertain or to rule out marrow failure or infiltration.
- When other causes are ruled out, then ITP is the most likely diagnosis.

TREATMENT

Etiology-specific treatment will be discussed below; however, platelet transfusions in general will be discussed first.

- Platelet transfusions may be prophylactic or therapeutic.
  - Current evidence supports prophylactic platelet transfusion when the platelet count is <10,000/μL.
  - The evidence also supports therapeutic transfusions to treat or prevent bleeding in trauma or procedures at a level of <100,000/μL for neurosurgical issues and 50,000–100,000/μL for major nonneuroaxial surgeries and with lumbar punctures.
  - A level of <20,000 warrants transfusion prior to central line insertions.[6]
- As previously mentioned, the etiology also holds significant implications in relation to platelet transfusion.
  - For example, platelet transfusion is generally not indicated in cases of immune thrombocytopenia (e.g., ITP and PTP) and thrombotic microangiopathies (e.g., TTP/HUS, or the combination of hemolytic anemia, elevated liver enzymes, and low platelet count [HELLP syndrome]), as these conditions are often less prone to bleeding and also consumptive of platelets.
  - However, in cases of spontaneous life-threatening bleeding, platelet transfusion is appropriate.
- Platelets generally come as single-donor units but may come as pooled random-donor units. A single-donor (apheresis) unit is equal to about six random-donor units and should increase the platelet count by about 30,000/μL.
- In general, ABO, Rh, and human leukocyte antigen (HLA) matching is unneccessary with platelet transfusions, but may be considered in patients refractory to transfusions, which is defined as an increase of <10,000 in platelet count on more than one occasion within an hour of transfusion. In sequestration- or destruction-mediated thrombocytopenia, the platelets may not last long, and administration shortly before procedures is warranted. Otherwise, repeated checks of platelet counts can be done on a daily basis.
- Avoid medications with anticoagulant or antiplatelet effects, such as nonsteroidal anti-inflammatory drugs (NSAIDs) if possible
- Treatment of specific causes of thrombocytopenia includes the following:
  - **TTP**: **Plasmapheresis** is the initial therapy for **TTP** and should be initiated promptly.
  - **Drug-induced thrombocytopenia**: A diagnosis of **drug-induced thrombocytopenia** should prompt **withdrawal of medication** (resolution of thrombocytopenia postwithdrawal also confirms diagnosis).
  - **Heparin-Induced Thrombocytopenia**: If **HIT** is suspected, all heparin products (including flushes and low molecular weight heparins) should be discontinued. Even in the absence of thrombosis, treatment with argatroban, aepirudin, or danaparoid followed by warfarin is indicated, unless there is a strong contraindication, such as high risk of bleeding.[7]
  - **Posttransfusion purpura** may be treated with **IV immunoglobulin**.
  - Most cases of **ITP** can be controlled with **glucocorticoids**. Initial dosage is prednisone 1 mg/kg/d and slowly tapered. If steroids are contraindicated, **IV immunoglobulin or anti-D can be used instead. Refractory and chronic cases may require splenectomy or immunosuppressive therapy with the anti-CD-20 agent, rituximab.** Thrombopoetin recepter agonists are used if splenectomy is contraindicated or ITP relapses after surgery.[5]
  - In cases of infection, malignancy, liver disease, or autoimmune disease, treatment involves supportive care and treatment of underlying disorder.
  - Common etiologies of thrombocytopenia and their management are listed in Table 34-4.

TABLE 34-4 COMMON ETIOLOGIES OF THROMBOCYTOPENIA AND THEIR MANAGEMENT

Clues	Diagnosis	Management
History of alcohol abuse	Alcohol-induced thrombocytopenia	Alcohol abstinence Transient rebound thrombocytosis may occur after quitting.
Fatigue, weight loss with/without fever	Neoplastic or infectious (see infections in Table 34-1)	Diagnose specific infection or neoplasm, then treat accordingly.
Critically ill patient (sepsis, severe pancreatitis, trauma etc.). Oozing from drains and lines sites, Coagulopathy (elevated PT/PTT, low fibrinogen) ± thrombotic events	Disseminated intravascular coagulopathy	Treatment of underlying etiology Transfuse only if <10,000 or if life threatening bleeding.
Exposure to certain drugs (see Table 34-2)	Drug-induced thrombocytopenia	Discontinue the offending agent.
Recent or current exposure to heparin + intermediate or high HIT score.	Heparin-induced thrombocytopenia	Discontinue heparin, and confirm with serotonin assay. Treat with direct thrombin inhibitor and warfarin.
Hemolytic anemia (schistocytes, positive hemolysis labs) with/without fever/neurologic deficits or renal failure	Thrombotic thrombocytopenic purpura	Emergent Plasma exchange ±steroids or rituximab ADAMTS 13 antibodies to confirm (should not delay treatment)
Exposure to transfusion	Posttransfusion purpura	IVIg
Asymptomatic/incidental thrombocytopenia History of SLE.	Immune thrombocytopenic purpura	Start therapy if bleeding or count <30,000/μL. Steroids as initial therapy ± IVIg Splenectomy or rituximab in refractory cases

REFERENCES

1. Eby C, Sanfilippo K, Yusen R, Gage BF. Disorders of Hemostasis and Thrombosis. In: Godara H, Hirbe A, Nassif M, et al., eds. *The Washington Manual of Medical Therapeutics*. 34th ed. Philadelphia: Lippincott Williams & Wilkins, 2014.
2. Aster R, Bougie D. Drug-induced immune thrombocytopenia. *N Engl J Med* 2007;357:580–7.
3. Lo GK, Juhl D, Warkentin TE, et al. Evaluation of pretest clinical score (4 T's) for the diagnosis of heparin-induced thrombocytopenia in two clinical settings. *J Thromb Haemost* 2006;4:759.
4. George JN. Thrombotic thrombocytopenic purpura. *N Engl J Med* 2006;354:1927–35.
5. Neunert C, Lim W, Crowther M, et al. The American Society of Hematology 2011 evidence-based practice guideline for immune thrombocytopenia. *Blood* 2011;117:4190–207.
6. Kaufman RM, Djulbegovic B, Gernsheimer T, et al. Platelet transfusion: a clinical practice guideline from the AABB. *Ann Intern Med* 2015;162:205–13.
7. Linkins LA, Dans AL, Moores LK, et al. Treatment and prevention of heparin-induced thrombocytopenia: Antithrombotic Therapy and Prevention of Thrombosis, 9th ed: American College of Chest Physicians Evidence-Based Clinical Practice Guidelines. *Chest* 2012;141:e495S–e530S.

Approach to a Prolonged Prothrombin Time/Partial Thromboplastin Time

35

Patrick M. Grierson and Natalie C. Battle

GENERAL PRINCIPLES

- Prolongation of the prothrombin time (PT) and partial thromboplastin time (PTT) are common findings in hospitalized patients. Often, the internist is called preoperatively to assess these abnormalities.
- The PT screens the extrinsic or tissue factor–dependent coagulation pathway (including most of the vitamin K–dependent factors).
- The PTT screens the intrinsic pathway (factors VIII, IX, XI, and XII; high molecular weight kininogen; prekallikrein).
- **Both** PT and PTT evaluate the common coagulation pathway.
- There are several points at which the coagulation cascade can be interrupted. See Table 35-1 for some common etiologies and Table 35-2 for differential diagnosis by lab abnormality.

DIAGNOSIS

Clinical Presentation

History
- History should include medications, nutritional status, and any personal or family history of severe bleeding.
- Specifically inquire about prior excessive surgical bleeding or bleeding during childhood tooth extraction, which may be a clue to a long-standing factor deficiency.
- Some "coagulation abnormalities" may be lab artifacts without clinical bleeding. For example, some cephalosporin antibiotics (e.g., ceftriaxone) may cause elevations in international normalized ratio (INR). The new novel oral anticoagulants such as dabigatran, rivaroxaban, and apixaban prolong the PT/INR and PTT, but not in a dose-dependent manner, and do not indicate the degree of anticoagulation.[1]
- The patient should also be assessed for associated conditions, including liver or autoimmune disease.

Physical Examination
Look for evidence of bleeding, bruising, hemarthroses, and hematomas. Also look for stigmata of liver disease or autoimmune disease.

Diagnostic Testing

- In patients who have an elevated PTT as well as an elevated INR while on warfarin (Coumadin), the expected PTT should be approximately $(5 \times INR) + 25$.
- Elevations several points or higher than expected may point to an etiology other than excessive warfarin dosing alone.
- Lupus anticoagulant can prolong the PT and PTT, and different laboratory reagents have varying sensitivities to lupus anticoagulant. In the presence of lupus anticoagulant, escalating coumadin doses magnify the relative variation in PT among different reagents.[2]

TABLE 35-1 DIFFERENTIAL DIAGNOSIS OF PROLONGED PT/PTT

	Etiology	Diagnosis
Liver disease	Decreased production of clotting factors	Signs and symptoms of liver failure Reverses with FFP
Vitamin K deficiency	May be secondary to fat malabsorption, nutritional deficiency, or loss of vitamin storage with liver disease	Reverses with vitamin K supplementation (within 24–48 h)
Medications	Warfarin and cephalosporin antibiotics (primarily leads to elevated PT) Heparin	Medication history/resolution with discontinuation of medication
Circulating coagulation inhibitor	IgG antibodies Nonspecific examples include lupus anticoagulant and anticardiolipin Ab (associated with thrombosis rather than bleeding) Increased risk in postpartum patients, patients with history of frequent plasma transfusions, autoimmune diseases, and reaction to penicillin or streptomycin	Failure of 50:50 mix with plasma to correct elevated PT/PTT
DIC	Accelerated coagulation reactions diminish factor levels Associated with malignancy, bacterial sepsis, trauma	Clinical presentation Thrombocytopenia, decreased fibrinogen, elevated fibrin degradation products
Inherited factor deficiency	Factors VIII and IX, hemophilia A and B Factor VII deficiency: rare autosomal recessive	Bleeding history Assays for factor levels

DIC, disseminated intravascular coagulation; FFP, fresh frozen plasma.

- Elevations of the PT/PTT without an obvious cause should be evaluated by a **50:50 mixing study** of the patient's blood to normal blood.
  - If correction is achieved on a 50:50 mix, then there is a factor deficiency. If a factor deficiency is present, then further evaluation may be performed by assaying specific factors based on the differential listed in Table 35-2.
  - If no correction is achieved, then an inhibitor is likely present.

TREATMENT

- Generally, therapy depends on the underlying disorder.
- **First repeat the PT/PTT** and ensure that enough blood is placed in the tube.

TABLE 35-2 DIFFERENTIAL DIAGNOSIS OF PROLONGED PT/PTT BY COAGULATION ABNORMALITY

Abnormal Lab Result	Etiologies
Prolonged PT only	Deficiency of factor VII
	Vitamin K deficiency or warfarin therapy
	Liver disease
Prolonged PTT only	Deficiency of factors 8, 9, 11, 12; high molecular weight kininogen; or prekallikrein
	von Willebrand disease (± prolonged bleeding time)
	Antiphospholipid syndrome
Prolonged PT and PTT	Deficiency of factors 1 (afibrinogenemia), 2, 5, 10
	Disseminated intravascular coagulation
	Severe vitamin K deficiency or excessive warfarin
	Severe liver disease
	Heparin
	Direct factor Xa or thrombin inhibitor

- Patients with prolonged PTT due to deficiency of factor XII, high molecular weight kininogen, or prekallikrein are not at risk of bleeding. The bleeding risk in factor XI deficiency is very mild. These patients do not need specific preoperative therapy.[3]
- **Vitamin K** (5–20 mg PO) can be administered to patients with vitamin K deficiency or liver disease.
  - Subcutaneous dosing (5–10 mg) is unpredictable, especially in edematous patients.
  - IV vitamin K may cause anaphylactoid reactions (in ~3/10,000 doses). This risk can be minimized by using a formulation without polyethoxylated castor oil and administering over at least 20 minutes.[4]
  - Regardless of route, the response takes 1–2 days and patients with liver disease often have very little response.
  - Patients who are supratherapeutic on warfarin respond well to oral vitamin K, 1 to 2.5 mg.[5]
  - After a few days of vitamin K administration, the body's stores are replenished and additional administration will have little or no effect.
- **Fresh frozen plasma** (FFP) contains all of the coagulation factors at normal serum levels.
  - Administer 2 U before procedures if the PT/PTT is prohibitively prolonged.
  - Patients with severe elevations or who are having life-threatening bleeding should receive 3 to 4 U to start.
  - Frequent monitoring should be done to ensure that the PT and PTT correct to the appropriate range.
- **Cryoprecipitate** contains high levels of fibrinogen (factor I), factor VIII (80 U), and von Willebrand factor. This may be used in bleeding in the volume-overloaded patient and when factor VIII is not available for hemophiliacs. It has also been used topically to stop bleeding from wounds.
- **Prothrombin complex concentrate and recombinant factor VIIa** are not well studied in the reversal of novel oral anticoagulants but remain under investigation.[6] There is presently a reversal agent for one of the novel oral anticoagulants, discussed in Chapter 8.

- Specific **coagulation inhibitors** may resolve in 6–12 months. In cases of severe hemorrhage, plasma transfusion or plasmapheresis to lower antibody titer may be necessary.
- There is no proven benefit to empirically treating the coagulation defects associated with **disseminated intravascular coagulation.** Focus should be on treating the underlying disorder, and factor replacement should be dictated by the occurrence of bleeding.[7]

REFERENCES

1. Pollack CV. Coagulation assessment with the new generation of oral anticoagulants. *Emerg Med J* 2015;0:1–8.
2. Moll S, Ortel T. Monitoring warfarin therapy in patients with lupus anticoagulants. *Ann Intern Med* 1997;127:177–85.
3. Pike GN, Bolton-Maggs PHB. Factor XI-related thrombosis and the role of concentrate treatment in factor XI deficiency. *Haemophilia* 2015;21:477–80.
4. Ageno W, Gallus AS, Wittkowsky A, et al. Antithrombotic therapy and prevention of thrombosis. 9th ed. American College of Chest Physicians evidence-based clinical practice guidelines. *Chest* 2012;141:e44S–e88S.
5. Hanley JP. Warfarin reversal. *J Clin Pathol* 2004;57:1132–39.
6. Suryanarayan D, Schulman S. Potential antidotes for reversal of old and new oral anticoagulants. *Thromb Res* 2014;13:S158–66.
7. Levi M, Toh CH, Thachil J, Watson HG. Guidelines for the diagnosis and management of disseminated intravascular coagulation. *Br J Haematol* 2009;145:24–33.

Venous Thromboembolism 36

Ashish Rastogi and Emily Fondahn

GENERAL PRINCIPLES

- Venous thromboembolism (VTE) refers to a blood clot or thrombus that develops within a vein. Thrombi can be located in superficial veins or deep veins. In the latter case, they form deep venous thrombosis (DVT), which can embolize to the pulmonary arteries and cause pulmonary embolism (PE).
- A DVT can be located either in the distal (calf) veins or in the proximal veins, including the popliteal, femoral, and iliac veins.
- PE can be categorized as central (main pulmonary artery, lobar or segmental) or distal. A massive PE is defined as obstruction of more than half of the pulmonary circulation.
- VTE is a major health care problem, due to difficulties in diagnosis, uncertainties regarding treatment, and strategies to prevent VTE development.
- The incidence of VTE appears to vary based upon ancestry. Annual incidence rates for people of European ancestry range from 104 to 183 per 100,000 person-years.[1] VTE rates appear to be higher among African Americans and lower in Asian, Asian American, and Native American populations.[1,2] An estimated average of 548,000 hospitalizations with VTE occur each year, of which 349,000 are DVT and 278,000 are PE.[3]

Pathophysiology

- **DVT:** The natural history of DVTs is that without any treatment, ~20–25% of calf vein thrombi will extend into the popliteal and femoral veins, causing a proximal DVT.
  - Furthermore, without treatment, ~50% of patients with a proximal DVT will develop a PE.[4]
  - Most PEs are due to DVTs arising from the proximal lower extremities or pelvis.
- **PE:** Pulmonary emboli can lead to several physiologic changes due to obstruction of the pulmonary arteries. This can be categorized into three subgroups: nonmassive, submassive, and massive.
  - **Nonmassive pulmonary emboli** are those that cause symptoms but have no evidence of heart strain or hemodynamic compromise. These patients may exhibit increased respiratory rate, hyperventilation, impaired gas exchange due to impaired perfusion, and hypoxemia from intrapulmonary shunting.
  - In patients with **submassive pulmonary emboli,** the acutely elevated pulmonary vascular resistance causes increased strain on the right ventricle, which may lead to hemodynamic compromise.
  - Patients with **massive pulmonary emboli** will exhibit decreased right ventricular output and hypotension. To maintain pulmonary perfusion and overcome the obstructing thrombus, the right ventricle must produce systolic pressures beyond 50 mm Hg.[5] The normal right ventricle is unable to generate such pressure, thus resulting in right heart failure.

Risk Factors
- The classic teaching for risk factors is Virchow's triad:
  - Alterations in blood flow (stasis) such as prolonged bed rest or immobilization
  - Vascular endothelial injury such as surgery or trauma
  - Hypercoagulable state: either inherited (genetic tendency to form VTEs) or acquired (malignancy, nephrotic syndrome, pregnancy or use of estrogen)
- The majority of hospitalized patients have at least one risk factor for a DVT,[6] and hospitalization for an acute medical illness is associated with an eightfold increased risk of VTE.[7]

DIAGNOSIS

Clinical Presentation
History
- Typical symptoms of DVT include unilateral lower or upper extremity pain, tenderness, and swelling.
- Typical symptoms of a PE include dyspnea, pleuritic chest pain, hemoptysis, or syncope.[8] Syncope is more common in a massive PE. Between 33% and 42% of patients with a PE report calf or thigh pain,[9] and symptoms that increase the probability of PE are sudden dyspnea, syncope, and hemoptysis.[9]

Physical Examination
- Signs on physical exam indicating possible DVT include increased warmth, edema, and/or erythema. Physical examination findings associated with a probability of finding a DVT are asymmetric calf swelling with at least a 2-cm difference between calves, superficial vein dilation, swelling of the entire length, and asymmetrical skin warmth.[9]
- Homans sign is pain in the calf with forceful abrupt dorsiflexion of the patient's foot while the knee is extended. Unfortunately, this test has fallen out of favor as it is estimated to have a low sensitivity and specificity.[10]
- The individual physical findings that increase the probability of a PE are left parasternal heave, unilateral calf pain or swelling, respiratory rate >30 breaths/min, and systolic blood pressure of 100 mm Hg or less.[9]

Diagnostic Criteria
- **Wells Criteria for DVT**: The Wells Criteria are a risk stratification tool to help assess the pretest probability of a patient having a DVT and can guide the need for further diagnostic testing (Table 36-1).[11] This test has a sensitivity of 75–98% and a specificity of 40–60%.[11]
- **Wells Criteria for PE**: Similar to the Wells Criteria for DVT, there exists another risk stratification tool to help assess the pretest probability of a patient having a PE (Table 36-2).[12]

Diagnostic Testing
Laboratories
D-Dimer is a fibrin degradation product that is present in blood as a blood clot gets broken down by intrinsic anticoagulant factors. It has a very high sensitivity (99%) and negative predictive value, but low specificity (40–60%) for diagnosis of DVT/PE, and thus is best used as a test to rule out disease in cases of low-moderate pretest probability. Due to the low specificity, there is a high false-positive rate typically in patients with malignancy, trauma, infection, recent surgery, pregnancy, or active bleeding.[13]

TABLE 36-1 WELLS CRITERIA FOR DVT

Criteria	Points
Malignancy w/ treatment in last 6 months or palliative	+1
Calf swelling ≥ 3 cm compared to other calf	+1
Swollen unilateral superficial veins	+1
Unilateral pitting edema	+1
Previous DVT	+1
Swelling of entire leg	+1
Paralysis, paresis, or recent cast immobilization	+1
Recently bedridden ≥ 3 days or surgery in last 3 months	+1
Localized tenderness along deep venous system	+1
Alternative diagnosis possible	−2
Score	**Category**
≤0 points	Low probability
1–2 points	Intermediate probability
≥3 points	High probability

TABLE 36-2 WELLS CRITERIA FOR PE

Criteria	Points
Clinical signs and symptoms of a DVT	3
PE is most likely diagnosis	3
Tachycardia > 100 bpm	1.5
Surgery within last month or immobilization	1.5
Previous PE/DVT	1.5
Hemoptysis	1
Malignancy w/ treatment in last 6 months or palliative	1
Score	**Category**
<2 points	Low probability
2–6 points	Moderate probability
>6 points	High probability

Adapted from Wells PS, Anderson DR, Rodger M, et al. Derivation of a simple clinical model to categorize patients probability of pulmonary embolism: increasing the models utility with the SimpliRED D-dimer. *Thromb Haemost* 2000;83:416–20.

Electrocardiography

ECG can be used to assess for evidence of right heart strain. Signs of right heart strain on ECG include right axis deviation, early R-wave progression in precordial leads with persistent S wave in V6, new right bundle branch block, T-wave inversions in V1–V4 and/or II/III/aVF, and evidence of right atrial enlargement with peaked P wave in lead II > 2.5 mm in height. The most common finding in PE, however, is sinus tachycardia. The S1Q3T3 finding, which is an S wave in lead I and both a Q-wave and a T-wave inversion in lead III, is classically taught but is not very common and is neither sensitive nor specific for PE.[14]

Imaging
- **Imaging modalities for diagnosing DVT**
  - **Duplex ultrasound** is the test of choice for the diagnosis of DVT. Depending on the operator, the sensitivity is about 95% and specificity is about 98% in detecting DVT in symptomatic patients.[15]
  - **Contrast venography** is the gold standard test for diagnosis of DVT and involves injecting contrast dye to assess for the presence of an intraluminal filling defect. It is not commonly done and has been replaced by the noninvasive Duplex ultrasound.
- **Imaging modalities for diagnosing PE**
  - **Computed tomography pulmonary angiography (CTPA):** this is the test of choice for the diagnosis of PE due to its wide availability and the ability to visualize the thrombus directly. The sensitivity is 83% and specificity is 96%.[16] CTPA also allows for direct imaging of both the heart (assess for right ventricular [RV] strain) and inferior vena cava (IVC) (alternative source for venous thrombosis). The major disadvantages of this test are radiation exposure, high cost, and nephrotoxicity.[17]
  - **Ventilation–perfusion (V/Q) scan:** V/Q scanning is the second-line imaging test of choice for the diagnosis of PE useful in patients with a normal chest radiograph and who are unable to receive contrast. A normal scan has a specificity of 97% and can rule out PE, whereas a high probability PE finding has a sensitivity of about 80%, similar to that of contrast CT. The majority of V/Q scans are nondiagnostic with intermediate or low probability findings, which necessitate further workup.[18]
  - **Pulmonary angiography** is the gold standard test for PE, though it is infrequently used due to being invasive with higher risk for complications.
  - **Magnetic resonance angiography (MRA)** may be an alternative to CTPA for the diagnosis of PE, especially in those patients with contrast allergy or who need avoidance of radiation. MRA is less used than V/Q scans due cost and variability. This test is best done at experienced centers, and when technically adequate, MRA has a sensitivity of 92% and specificity of 96%.[19]
  - **Echocardiography:** Both transthoracic echocardiography (TTE) and transesophageal echocardiography (TEE) can be helpful in differentiating nonmassive PE from submissive and massive.
    - Findings include RV dilation, hypokinesis, tricuspid regurgitation, septal flattening, paradoxical septal motion leading to impaired left ventricular filling, elevated RV systolic pressure, and lack of inspiratory collapse of the IVC due to elevated right-sided pressures.
    - **McConnell sign** is a specific finding of RV free wall akinesia with relative sparing and/or hyperkinesis of the apex and has a specificity of at least 95% and positive predictive value (PPV) of 71% for acute PE.
    - Another important sign is the **60/60 sign**, which is present when the right ventricular outflow tract (RVOT) acceleration time is <60 ms and the tricuspid insufficiency pressure gradient is <60 mm Hg, thus suggesting impairment in RV outflow in the absence of significant pulmonary hypertension. This sign is 94% specific.[17]

TREATMENT

Medications

- Anticoagulation is the mainstay of treatment for DVT/PE. This section will discuss various anticoagulation strategies. It should be noted that warfarin historically was the first-line treatment; however, new guidelines recommend the use of non–vitamin K–dependent oral anticoagulants (NOACs) to be used over warfarin (Grade 2B) for oral anticoagulation in non–malignancy-related DVT/PE.[20]
- **Warfarin** inhibits the synthesis of vitamin K–dependent clotting factors, including factors II, VII, IX, and X. Warfarin should be overlapped with heparin for a minimum of 5 days and until the INR has been within the therapeutic range (2–3) for at least 24 hours.[20]
    - Dosing of warfarin is variable and must be tailored to each individual patient with a goal INR of 2–3. Several dosing strategies exist, however, in general starting with an initial dose of 5–10 mg followed by a daily dose of 5 mg leads to a decreased incidence of a supratherapeutic INR. The INR should be checked 2 days after the initial dose and then daily thereafter until therapeutic.[21]
    - Benefits of warfarin include low cost and long half-life.
    - There are many disadvantages including[13] narrow therapeutic range (goal INR 2–3), slow onset/offset of action, delaying invasive procedures when weaning off, bleeding when a patient is supratherapeutic, many drug–drug/drug–food interactions, and requiring frequent monitoring and INR checks, which can decrease quality of life.
- **NOACs:** There are currently four FDA-approved NOACs available to treat DVT/PE: dabigatran, rivaroxaban, apixaban, and edoxaban. When compared to warfarin, all four of these medications have less food/drug interactions, quicker half-life/time to maximum level of activity, and fixed dosing, thus eliminating the need for monitoring. They each also have slightly different dosing and pharmacokinetics when compared to one another (Table 36-3).
    - There were four major trials done, each comparing one of these medications to warfarin in patients with acute DVT and PE. In general, all four medications were found to be noninferior to warfarin with regard to efficacy in preventing recurrent VTE or acute PE at up to 1-year follow-up. With regard to safety (major bleeding), dabigatran, rivaroxaban, and edoxaban all were noninferior to warfarin; however, apixaban was the only NOAC found to be superior.[22–25]
    - There are several disadvantages of NOACs.
        - No good way to monitor therapeutic level if desired (difficult to determine poor compliance vs. failure of the medication).
        - Short half-life causes anticoagulation effect to decline quickly if compliance is poor.
        - Dose needs to be adjusted for liver/renal dysfunction.
        - Higher cost compared to warfarin.
        - Lack of a FDA-approved reversal agent, except for the idarucizumab for reversal of dabigatran.
    - When picking which NOAC to use, the choice should be tailored to the patient based on his or her ability to afford the medication, manage taking a once-daily medication versus twice-daily medication, and level of renal or hepatic dysfunction. Of the NOACs, **only** dabigatran and edoxaban require a 7–10-day bridge.[22,25]
- Options for parenteral anticoagulation for VTE include intravenous unfractionated heparin (UFH), subcutaneous UFH, low molecular weight heparin (LMWH), or subcutaneous fondaparinux, These agents are used to treat patients empirically when there is

TABLE 36-3 PHARMACOKINETICS AND DOSING OF ANTICOAGULANTS

	Warfarin	Dabigatran	Rivaroxaban	Apixaban	Edoxaban
Mechanism	Vitamin K Antagonist	Direct Thrombin Inhibitor	Factor Xa Inhibitor	Factor Xa Inhibitor	Factor Xa Inhibitor
Dosing	Variable, goal INR 2-3	150 mg bid	3 weeks 5 mg bid, then 20 mg Daily	7 days of 10 mg bid, then 5 mg bid	60 mg Daily
Half-life	40 h	7-17 h	3-9 h	8-15 h	10-14 h
Max Activity	72-96 h	2-3 h	2-4 h	3 h	1-2 h
Bioavailability	80-100%	3-7%	80-100%	60%	60%
Renal excretion	n/a	80%	36%	25%	50%
Reversal	Vitamin K, PCC, FFP	Dialyzable, PCC, Idarucizumab	PCC	PCC	PCC

a high clinical suspicion for PE while the workup is being performed and once a DVT/PE has been confirmed.[20]
- **UFH** produces its anticoagulation effect by inactivating thrombin and factor Xa. UFH is given either intravenously or subcutaneous. UFH is generally given either as a weight-based regimen or as a bolus followed by an infusion.[26] Monitoring is done with the activated partial thromboplastin time (aPTT) levels. UFH can be reserved with IV protamine sulfate.
- **LMWH** (e.g., enoxaparin) has a similar mechanism of action as UFH.
  - LMWH has been shown to have decreased mortality, fewer recurrent thromboembolic events and less major bleeding than UFH.[27]
  - Additionally, LMWH has greater bioavailability, predictable pharmacokinetics, once- or twice-daily administration, fixed dosing regimen that does not require adjustment, and a decreased likelihood of thrombocytopenia.[28]
  - Disadvantages to LMWH include a contraindication for patients with a creatinine clearance ≤30 mL/min, longer time for reversal if patient is bleeding, and possible concerns about subcutaneous absorption (e.g., morbid obesity).[26]
  - LMWH can be used as a subcutaneous injection twice a day for long-term treatment.
  - Generally, monitoring is not performed, though factor Xa levels may be useful in particular clinical situations (renal dysfunction, obesity, pregnancy).[26]
  - Patients with malignancy may have reduced VTE recurrence when treated with LMWH rather than warfarin for long-term therapy.[29]
- Subcutaneous fondaparinux is a synthetic pentasaccharide factor Xa inhibitor that can be used in hemodynamically stable PE patients. Studies have shown that fondaparinux has similar clinical outcomes as UFH for treatment of acute PE and has similar clinical outcomes as LMWH for patients with DVT.[20,30]
- Use of **thrombolytics**, such as tissue plasminogen activator (tPA, alteplase), is reserved for patients with either significant submassive or massive PEs. Evidence from randomized control trials and retrospective observational studies indicates that use of thrombolytics leads to early hemodynamic improvement at the risk of increased major bleeding.
  - Dosing of tPA typically is 100 mg IV over 2 hours.
  - The only widely accepted indication for thrombolysis is in a patient with massive PE and persistent hypotension and/or shock.
  - In patients with submassive PE, there is no consensus on when to use thrombolytics.[31–33] In general, clinicians should consider thrombolysis in the absence of persistent hypotension in the following situations: significant right ventricular dysfunction or strain on echo or CT, extensive clot burden on CT scan or V/Q scan, cardiopulmonary resuscitation, or severe hypoxemia.
  - Absolute contraindications to thrombolysis include prior intracranial hemorrhage, ischemic stroke within last 3 months, known primary intracranial neoplasm, known structural intracranial cerebrovascular disease (e.g., arteriovenous malformation), intracranial surgery or head trauma within last month, or active internal bleeding.
  - Relative contraindications to thrombolysis include thrombocytopenia, current use of anticoagulation, pregnancy, brain metastasis, recent internal bleeding in last month, remote ischemic stroke > 3 months ago, and severe hypertension (systolic blood pressure > 180 mm Hg, diastolic blood pressure > 110 mm Hg).

Interventional Management

- **Surgical embolectomy** involves removing the thrombus. It is usually reserved for the unstable patient who has failed thrombolysis or has a contraindication to it. There is

decreased recurrent PE with surgical embolectomy but higher mortality, specifically in unstable patients.[34]
- **Catheter-directed therapies** include suction embolectomy, rotational embolectomy, rheolytic embolectomy, or ultrasound-assisted thrombolysis. Each form of catheter-directed embolectomy uses a different method to fragment clot followed by aspiration.
- **IVC filters** should be placed in patients who have contraindications to anticoagulation or who have a high bleeding risk. Additionally, IVC filters may be beneficial as an adjunct to anticoagulation in patients with DVTs who would not tolerate an embolic event if one were to happen.
    - There are both retrievable and nonretrievable filters depending on if the indication for filter is permanent. Typically retrievable filters should be removed within 6 months after placement.
    - Complications of IVC filters include those associated with placement (bleeding, infection, contrast reaction, etc.) as well as filter erosion, migration, embolization, or filter-related thrombosis (occurs in 10–30% of patients).[35]

SPECIAL CONSIDERATIONS

- **Duration of therapy** depends on if DVT or PE was provoked or recurrent[20].
    - In patients with leg DVT/PE **provoked** by surgery or nonsurgical transient risk factor, the American College of Chest Physicians (ACCP) recommends 3 months of anticoagulation over either a shorter (Grade 1B if proximal leg or PE, 2C if distal leg) or longer period (Grade 1B).
    - If leg DVT/PE was **provoked** by nonsurgical transient risk factor, they further support the above recommendation despite bleeding risk (Grade 2B if low-moderate bleeding risk and Grade 1B if high bleeding risk).
    - In patients with **first unprovoked** leg DVT/PE, the ACCP recommends 3 months of therapy over a longer time-limited period (Grade 1B, regardless of location). If proximal leg DVT or PE and patient has low-moderate bleeding risk, then >3 months of therapy (no scheduled stop date) is reasonable (Grade 2B).
    - In patients with a **second unprovoked** VTE they recommend 3 months of therapy if high bleeding risk (Grade 2B) and extended therapy (no scheduled stop date) if low bleeding risk (Grade 1B) or moderate bleeding risk (Grade 2B).
    - In patients receiving extended therapy, the continuation of treatment should be reassessed annually.[20]
- **Hypercoagulable workup:** routine evaluation for hypercoagulable disorders in patients with unprovoked VTE is unwarranted and should be limited to select populations.
    - Evaluating for occult malignancy should also not be done unless patient has risk factors for cancer.[36]
    - Those who may benefit from a hypercoagulable workup include those who are young (age < 45), have recurrent thrombosis, have thrombosis in multiple venous sites or unusual locations (splenic vein, hepatic vein, etc.), or have a family history of VTE at young age (age < 45).
    - A typical hypercoagulable workup includes testing for all five inherited thrombophilias (protein C, protein S, and thrombin, factor V Leiden, or prothombin gene mutations) and for antiphospholipid syndrome (APS).
- **Prevention VTE in hospitalized patients:** Every patient admitted to the hospital should have an assessment for VTE prevention. The ACCP has published guidelines for VTE prophylaxis in nonsurgery patients,[6] orthopedic surgery patients,[37] and nonorthopedic surgery patients.[38] Table 36-4 highlights VTE prophylaxis for medical patients.

TABLE 36-4 GUIDELINES FOR VTE PREVENTIONS

Group	Recommendation
Acutely ill medical patients at increased risk of thrombosis	[a]Low molecular weight heparin (LMWH), low-dose unfractionated heparin (LDUH) bid or tid, or fondaparinux
Acutely ill medical patients at low risk of thrombosis	[a]Recommend against the use of pharmacopropylaxis or mechanical prophylaxis
Acutely ill medical patients who are bleeding or at high risk for bleeding	[a]Recommend against anticoagulant thromboprophylaxis. If they are at high risk of thrombosis, recommend for mechanical prophylaxis. Reassessment of prophylaxis based upon VTE risk when bleeding risk decreases
Nonorthopedic surgery patients	[b]For specific type of surgery and patient risk, please consult the 2009 antithrombotic guidelines for VTE prevention in Nonorthopedic surgery patients published in *Chest* for recommendation
Orthopedic surgery patients	[c]For specific type of surgery/joint please consult the 2009 antithrombotic guidelines for VTE prevention in Orthopedic surgery patients published in *Chest* for recommendation

[a]From Kahn SR, Lim W, Dunn AS, et al. Prevention of VTE in nonsurgical patients: Antithrombotic therapy and prevention of thrombosis, 9th ed: American college of chest physicians evidence-based clinical practice guidelines. *Chest* 2012;141:e195S–e226S.
[b]Gould MK, Garcia DA, Wren SM, et al. Prevention of VTE in nonorthopedic surgical patients: antithrombotic Therapy and Prevention of Thrombosis, 9th ed: American College of Chest Physicians Evidence-Based Clinical Practice Guidelines. *Chest* 2012;141:e227S–77S.
[c]Falck-Ytter Y, Francis CW, Johanson NA, et al. Prevention of vte in orthopedic surgery patients: Antithrombotic therapy and prevention of thrombosis, 9th ed: American college of chest physicians evidence-based clinical practice guidelines. *Chest* 2012;141:e278S–e325S.

REFERENCES

1. Heit JA. Epidemiology of venous thromboembolism. *Nat Rev Cardiol* 2015;12:464–74.
2. Zakai NA, McClure LA, Judd SE, et al. Racial and regional differences in venous thromboembolism in the United States in 3 cohorts. *Circulation* 2014;129:1502–9.
3. Centers for Disease Control. Venous thromboembolism in adult hospitalizations—United States, 2007–2009. *Morbidity and Mortality Weekly Report* 2012;61:401–4.
4. Dalen JE. Pulmonary embolism: what have we learned since Virchow? Natural history, pathophysiology, and diagnosis. *Chest* 2002;122:1440–56.
5. Reissig A, Richartz B, Kroegel C. Diagnosis of pulmonary arterial embolism. *Dtsch Med Wochenschr* 2001;126:857–63.
6. Kahn SR, Lim W, Dunn AS, et al. Prevention of VTE in nonsurgical patients: antithrombotic therapy and prevention of thrombosis, 9th ed: American College of Chest Physicians evidence-based clinical practice guidelines. *Chest* 2012;141:e195S–e226S.
7. Heit JA, Silverstein MD, Mohr DN, et al. Risk factors for deep vein thrombosis and pulmonary embolism: A population-based case–control study. *Arch Intern Med* 2000;160:809–15.
8. Piazza G, Goldhaber SZ. Acute pulmonary embolism: Part I: epidemiology and diagnosis. *Circulation* 2006;114:e28–e32.

9. McGee S. *Evidence-Based Physical Diagnosis.* Philadelphia: Elsevier Saunders, 2012.
10. Joshua AM, Celermajer DS, Stockler MR. Beauty is in the eye of the examiner: reaching agreement about physical signs and their value. *Intern Med J* 2005;35:178–87.
11. Wells PS, Anderson DR, Bormanis J, et al. F. Value of assessment of pretest probability of deep-vein thrombosis in clinical management. *Lancet* 1997;350:1795–98.
12. Wells PS, Anderson DR, Rodger M, et al. Derivation of a simple clinical model to categorize patients probability of pulmonary embolism: increasing the models utility with the SimpliRED D-dimer. *Thromb Haemost* 2000;83:416–20.
13. Goldhaber SZ, Bounameaux H. Pulmonary embolism and deep vein thrombosis. *Lancet* 2012;379:1835–46.
14. Harrigan RA, Jones K. ABC of clinical electrocardiography. Conditions affecting the right side of the heart. *BMJ* 2002;324:1201–4.
15. Lensing AW, Prandoni P, Brandjes D, et al. Detection of deep-vein thrombosis by real-time B-mode ultrasonography. *N Engl J Med* 1989;320:342–45.
16. Stein PD, Fowler SE, Goodman LR, et al. Multidetector computed tomography for acute pulmonary embolism. *N Engl J Med* 2006;354(22):2317–27.
17. Ramzi DW, Leeper KV. DVT and pulmonary embolism: Part I. Diagnosis. *Am Fam Physician* 2004;69:2829–36.
18. PIOPED Investigators. Value of the ventilation/perfusion scan in acute pulmonary embolism. Results of the prospective investigation of pulmonary embolism diagnosis (PIOPED). *JAMA* 1990;263:2753–59.
19. Stein PD, Chenevert TL, Fowler SE, et al. Gadolinium-enhanced magnetic resonance angiography for pulmonary embolism: a multicenter prospective study (PIOPED III). *Ann Intern Med* 2010;52:434–43.
20. Kearon CE, Akl A, Ornelas J, et al. Antithrombotic therapy for VTE disease: American College of Chest Physicians Evidence-Based Clinical Practice Guidelines. *Chest* 2016;149(2):315–52.
21. Garcia P, Ruiz W, Loza Munarriz C. Warfarin initiation nomograms for venous thromboembolism. *Cochrane Database Syst Rev* 2013;(7):CD007699.
22. Schulman SC, Kearon A, Kakkar K, et al. Dabigatran versus warfarin in the treatment of acute venous thromboembolism. *N Engl J Med* 2009;361:2342–52.
23. EINSTEIN Investigators; Bauersachs R, Berkowitz SD, et al. Oral rivaroxaban for symptomatic venous thromboembolism. *N Engl J Med* 2010;363:2499–10.
24. Agnelli G, Buller HR, Cohen A, et al. Oral apixaban for the treatment of acute venous thromboembolism. *N Engl J Med* 2013;369:799–808.
25. Hokusai-VTE Investigators; Büller HR, Décousus H, et al. Edoxaban versus warfarin for the treatment of symptomatic venous thromboembolism. *N Engl J Med* 2013;369:1406–15.
26. Garcia DA, Baglin TP, Weitz JI, Samama MM. Parenteral anticoagulants: antithrombotic therapy and prevention of thrombosis, 9th ed: American College of Chest Physicians Evidence-Based Clinical Practice Guidelines. *Chest* 2012;141:e24S–e43S.
27. van Dongen CJ, van den Belt AG, Prins MH, Lensing AW. Fixed dose subcutaneous low molecular weight heparins versus adjusted dose unfractionated heparin for venous thromboembolism. *Cochrane Database Syst Rev* 2004;(4):CD001100.
28. Weitz JI. Low-molecular-weight heparins. *N Engl J Med* 1997;337(10):688–99.
29. Lee AYY, Levine MN, Baker RI, et al. Low-molecular-weight heparin versus a coumarin for the prevention of recurrent venous thromboembolism in patients with cancer. *N Engl J Med* 2003;349:146–53.
30. Buller HR, Davidson BL, Décousus H, et al. Fondaparinux or enoxaparin for the initial treatment of symptomatic deep venous thrombosis: a randomized trial. *Ann Intern Med* 2004;140:867–73.
31. Konstantinides S, Geibel A, Heusel G, et al. Heparin plus alteplase compared with heparin alone in patients with submassive pulmonary embolism. *N Engl J Med* 2002;347:1143–50.
32. Sharifi M, Bay C, Skrocki L, et al. Moderate pulmonary embolism treated with thrombolysis (from the "MOPETT" Trial). *Am J Cardiol* 2013;111:273–77.
33. Meyer G, Vicaut E, Danays T, et al. Fibrinolysis for patients with intermediate-risk pulmonary embolism. *N Engl J Med* 2014;370:1402–11.
34. Meneveau N, Séronde M-F, Blonde M-C, et al. Management of unsuccessful thrombolysis in acute massive pulmonary embolism. *Chest* 2006;129:1043–50.

35. Becker DM, Philbrick JT, Selby JB. Inferior vena cava filters. Indications, safety, effectiveness. *Arch Intern Med* 1992;152:1985–94.
36. Carrier M, Lazo-Langner A, Shivakumar S, et al. Screening for Occult Cancer in Unprovoked Venous Thromboembolism. *N Engl J Med* 2015;373:697–704.
37. Gould MK, Garcia DA, Wren SM, et al. Prevention of VTE in nonorthopedic surgical patients: Antithrombotic Therapy and Prevention of Thrombosis, 9th ed: American College of Chest Physicians Evidence-Based Clinical Practice Guidelines. *Chest* 2012;141:e227S–77S.
38. Falck-Ytter Y, Francis CW, Johanson NA, et al. Prevention of VTE in orthopedic surgery patients: antithrombotic therapy and prevention of thrombosis, 9th ed: American College of Chest Physicians evidence-based clinical practice guidelines. *Chest* 2012;141:e278S–e325S.

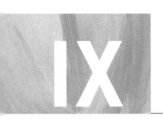

Oncology

Pain Control in the Cancer Patient

37

Eileen M. Lee

GENERAL PRINCIPLES

- Pain is a debilitating symptom that is frequently experienced by patients with cancer. It is reported by approximately one-quarter of patients with newly diagnosed malignancy, one-third of patients undergoing treatment for cancer, and at least three-quarters of patients with advanced disease. Over one-third of patients with metastatic disease report pain severe enough to impair function.
- Progressive pain leads to progressive disability and adversely affects quality of life. A patient's role in his/her family may be significantly altered. Loss of routine duties or employment can erode a patient's sense of identity, self-worth, and self-esteem.
- Cancer patients with pain are more likely to have high levels of depression, fatigue, anxiety, and mood disturbance. Disability related to pain can ultimately force patients into institutionalization when they can no longer be managed at home.

ASSESSMENT

- The most common way of assessing pain intensity is with a numeric scale of 0–10 (1–3 = mild pain, 4–7 = moderate pain, 8–10 = severe pain).
- Other scales, including the visual analog scale (Fig. 37-1)[1] and a verbal rating scale, are available. Pain scales can be used to track pain over time.
- Patients with cognitive impairment or altered mental status may be unable to rate their pain, and it may be necessary to instead monitor for behavior that might indicate pain. This may include mood swings, agitation, restlessness, and increased fatigue. Currently there exists no valid and reliable method of objectively quantifying pain.
- The most important aspect of pain management is thorough and frequent reassessment:
  - Assessing pain at every visit emphasizes the physician's commitment to patient comfort, and giving patients the opportunity to discuss the emotional and practical implications of their pain in their lives is also important
  - Information regarding pain levels, location, intensity, radiation, aggravating factors, timing, and quality of the pain should be obtained with each assessment as well as interference with daily activities. Furthermore, current medications and treatments need to be reviewed, including the frequency of use of breakthrough medications.
  - In patients receiving chemotherapy, watching for signs and symptoms of chemotherapy-induced peripheral neuropathy (CIPN) can facilitate early recognition and intervention.
  - For patients being started on opioids, reassessment within the first 24 hours is recommended to ensure effectiveness of treatment and preempt adverse sequelae.
  - Patients receiving palliative care often have rapidly changing symptoms requiring frequent escalations in pain medication dosage to achieve good symptom control.
- When assessing acute pain in a patient with a previous history of cancer, recurrence or progression of disease should be on the differential diagnosis. In patients with active cancer and new pain, oncologic emergencies must be ruled out. The characteristics of the pain are can help differentiate the pathophysiology. Patients may have more than one pain syndrome.

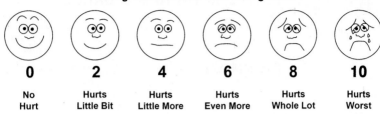

FIGURE 37-1 Wong-Baker FACES Pain Rating Scale. (From Wong-Baker FACES Foundation. (2016). Wong-Baker FACES® Pain Rating Scale. Retrieved June 28, 2016, with permission from http://www.WongBakerFACES.org. Originally published in *Whaley & Wong's Nursing Care of Infants and Children*. © Elsevier Inc.)

- **Bone and other musculoskeletal/somatic pain** is one of the most common types of pain in cancer patients. It is sharp, is well localized, does not radiate, and may increase with movement of the involved area. **Bone pain emergencies include unstable pathologic fractures**, which may present with pain on movement and localized tenderness, and **epidural spinal cord compression**, which may present with progressive, central back pain radiating bilaterally, often worse with recumbency or intra-abdominal pressure and with bilateral sensory or motor changes in the lower extremities.
- New or different **headache** in the setting of malignancy may be related to brain metastases. Associated signs and symptoms can include nausea, vomiting, lethargy, photophobia, and personality or mental status changes. Progressive neurologic symptoms in the setting of headache is considered a medical emergency until proven otherwise. Metastatic disease to the base of the skull can present as facial pain or headache or dysfunction of specific cranial nerves affected by the tumor; consultation with a pain specialist and a surgeon is indicated.
- **Visceral pain** is poorly localized and deep and may also be lancinating, episodic, and colicky. In some patients, visceral pain may be related to direct tumor infiltration, constipation, radiation, or chemotherapy. Obstruction of a hollow viscus may represent an emergency if it leads to perforation, ischemic necrosis, or organ failure. Intestinal obstruction can present with continuous or colicky pain with associated nausea, vomiting, constipation, diarrhea, or abdominal distension. Surgical evaluation should be considered, and fecal impaction should be ruled out.
- **Neuropathic pain** is often described as burning, shooting, electrical, or "pins and needles" and is generally constant. Radiculopathy may cause pain in a dermatomal distribution and may also be characterized by allodynia (pain worse with light touch). Neuropathic pain is often related to neuronal injury by tumor invasion or cancer therapies, but nerve injury by compression must be ruled out. CIPN is a common treatment-related adverse event and is more likely to occur with regimens that include platinum drugs, vinca alkaloids, bortezomib, and/or taxanes. African Americans are at significantly increased risk of taxane-induced neuropathy.[2] CIPN usually presents with symmetric, distal, in a glove and stocking distribution that tends to be sensory more than motor. Symptoms develop gradually and may progress 2–6 months after discontinuation of chemotherapy. Some neuropathy-inducing chemotherapy drugs, like taxanes and oxaliplatin, can also cause an acute neurotoxicity (separate from CIPN) that occurs hours to days after infusion.

TREATMENT

- The underlying cause of pain should be identified and addressed when possible (e.g., with antitumor therapy using radiation, chemotherapy, or palliative tumor debulking surgery when appropriate), but treatment of the pain should not be delayed by the diagnostic process. Though the evidence demonstrating its efficacy is limited, the three-step World Health Organization (WHO) analgesic ladder has been accepted as a framework for the initiation and titration of analgesics (Table 37-1).[3,4]
  - For mild pain (Step I), acetaminophen and nonsteroidal anti-inflammatory drugs (NSAIDs) are first-line therapy, barring contraindications.

TABLE 37-1 SELECTED AGENTS IN THE THREE-STEP ANALGESIC LADDER

Agent	Oral	Parenteral
Step I. Mild pain: nonopioid (± adjuvant)		
Acetaminophen	650 mg q4–6h PRN or 1000 mg q6h PRN	—
Aspirin	650 mg q4–6h PRN or 1000 mg q6h PRN	—
Ibuprofen	400–800 mg q6–8h PRN	—
Step II. Moderate pain: opioid formulated for mild/moderate pain (± nonopioid; ± adjuvant)		
Hydrocodone 5 mg + acetaminophen 325 mg	1–2 tablets PO q4–6h PRN	—
Oxycodone 5 mg + acetaminophen 325 mg	1–2 tablets PO q4h PRN	—
Oxycodone	5 mg q4–6h	—
Tramadol	50–100 mg q4–6h (maximum, 400 mg/d)	—
Step III. Severe pain: opioid formulated for moderate/severe pain (± nonopioid; ± adjuvant)		
Morphine	10–30 mg q3–4h (around-the-clock or intermittent dosing)	0.1–0.2 mg/kg (up to 15 mg) q4h
Morphine (controlled release)	Can start 30 mg q8–12h and increase PRN to 90–120 mg q12h	
Fentanyl[a]	—	0.1 mg q1–3h
Hydromorphone	2–4 mg q4–6h	1–4 mg q4–6h

[a]Transdermal fentanyl: 100 mcg/h = 315–404 mg/d of oral morphine and 53–67 mg/d of IM morphine.

Adapted from Jaycox A, Carr DB, Payne R. New clinical practice guidelines for the management of pain in patients with cancer. *N Engl J Med* 1994;330:651–5; World Health Organization. *WHO's cancer pain ladder for adults.* 2016. Available at: http://www.who.int/cancer/palliative/painladder/en/ (last accessed March 15, 2016).

- Opioids can be started if these are not effective or if pain is moderate-to-severe (Step II). "Weak" opioids such as codeine, hydrocodone, and low-dose oxycodone are often used initially.
- If these are not adequate, stronger opioids like high-dose oxycodone, morphine, or hydromorphone are indicated (Step III).

Medications

Nonopioid Medications

- **Nonopioid analgesics**: NSAIDs and acetaminophen are commonly used for the treatment of mild cancer pain as part of Step I. When scheduled in moderate-to-severe pain, they may also decrease concurrent opioid doses. NSAIDs and cyclooxygenase-2 (COX-2) inhibitors may be helpful for bone pain. NSAIDs may also reduce peritumoral edema, which may decrease pain (e.g., in hepatic tumors that cause stretching of the liver capsule).
  - NSAID use requires consideration of major side effects (gastrointestinal [GI] bleed, renal toxicity, hepatic dysfunction) and minor side effects (nausea, vomiting, dyspepsia, bloating, and constipation). There is no evidence that one NSAID is more effective than another, and switching to another NSAID may be worthwhile when one is not providing relief. Naproxen has a higher risk of GI side effects but is preferred for patients with cardiovascular risk, whereas ibuprofen has a lower risk of GI side effects at low doses but a higher cardiovascular and stroke risk.
  - Acetaminophen must be used with caution in patients with hepatic dysfunction, generally at a reduced maximum dose of 2–3 g/d, if at all. Note all acetaminophen-containing medications to avoid inadvertent acetaminophen overdose.
- **Adjuvant pain therapies**: Nonopioid medications and adjuvant pain therapies may be introduced at any point in the WHO analgesic ladder and may help decrease the amount of opioid required. Agents include the following:
- **Antidepressants**
  - **Tricyclic antidepressants** (TCAs) are first-line agents to treat neuropathic pain. They should be initiated at a low dose and can be titrated up every 3–14 days depending on the medication and side effects. Amitriptyline tends to have the greatest incidence of side effects. Nortriptyline and desipramine are minimally sedating and anticholinergic and only have a modest effect on orthostasis and weight gain. Trazodone is sedating but without the anticholinergic activity and has minimal orthostasis and weight gain. TCAs should be used with caution in patients with arrhythmias and ischemic heart disease.
  - If the dose is limited by side effects, or if TCAs are ineffective, **selective serotonin reuptake inhibitors (SSRIs)** can be added. Citalopram and escitalopram are the preferred SSRIs to use with TCAs because they do not interfere with their metabolism. Duloxetine is the only recommended treatment for patients with CIPN, and there is no established agent recommended to prevent CIPN.
- **Antiepileptic drugs** (AEDs) like gabapentin and pregabalin are also used for neuropathic pain. Phenytoin, carbamazepine, and valproic acid are also used. Side effects of AEDs include diplopia, headache, nystagmus, and ataxias. Some AEDs require serum level monitoring. These drugs also tend to be more sedating in elderly patients and must be used with caution.
- **Corticosteroids** can be considered to treat bone pain in patients who fail NSAIDs; the usual dose of prednisone for this indication is 20 mg PO bid followed by a taper.[5] Steroids may also be helpful in reducing peritumoral edema, which may be causing pain. In patients with spinal cord compression, early dexamethasone burst and taper has been shown to improve outcomes.[6] Steroids may also benefit patients with neuropathic pain that is refractory to antidepressants and AEDs. Mild side effects of corticosteroids include euphoria and increased appetite. Serious side effects include increased risk of GI bleeding, increased risk of infection, hyperglycemia/diabetes, and psychosis.

- **Local or topical agents** offer short-term relief for well-localized pain with little or no systemic effects. Useful agents include capsaicin cream and local anesthetics, such as transdermal or topical lidocaine (available in patch, gel, or liquid form). Topical lidocaine may alleviate pain related to mucositis or esophagitis (in a swish-and-swallow preparation) or for treating pain from wounds or other skin irritation (e.g., radiation dermatitis). A pain specialist can offer subcutaneous local anesthetics like lidocaine and mexiletine for neuropathic pain that has failed antidepressants and AEDs.
- **Bisphosphonates** like pamidronate and zoledronate have been used to treat bone pain, most commonly in breast cancer, prostate cancer, and multiple myeloma. Their use is best managed in consultation with a medical oncologist.
- **Antispasmodic agents** (e.g., hyoscyamine) may be considered to treat colicky visceral pain.
- **Muscle relaxants** (e.g., cyclobenzaprine, baclofen, and methocarbamol) may be helpful in relieving somatic pain. These medications may cause sedation and must be used with some caution in patients already on other sedating medications.

Opioid Analgesics
- Opioids remain the mainstay for pain control in moderate-to-severe pain.
- When starting oral therapy for severe pain, a short-acting drug should be given.
  - Depending on the severity of the pain and the desired speed of onset of analgesia, parenteral medication (e.g., morphine 2–4 mg or hydromorphone 0.5–1 mg) **OR** oral opioid (e.g., immediate-release morphine sulfate 5–15 mg or oxycodone 5–15 mg) may be selected.
  - Efficacy and side effects should be assessed at 60 minutes and after two or three dosing cycles to consider further dose titration.
  - If bolus parenteral therapy is inadequate, even at frequencies of every 2–3 hours, a switch to patient-controlled analgesia can be considered, which provides rapid means to titrate the analgesic dose. For patients who urgently require parenteral opioids but lack ready intravenous access, subcutaneous preparations are preferred over intramuscular preparations.
- After five or six half-lives (24 hours for morphine) of adequate pain control, the daily requirement can be determined and a scheduled long-acting preparation can be started at approximately an equivalent dose, though some practitioners prefer to start at half or two-thirds the daily opioid requirement.
  - Short-acting agents, at 10–20% of the daily dose, should also be offered q3–8h as needed for breakthrough pain (defined as transient exacerbations of pain occurring on stable pain otherwise controlled by around-the-clock therapy).
  - Oral immediate-release opioids, buccal/sublingual, or intranasal preparations (where available) are all appropriate for breakthrough pain. On reassessment, patient reliance on breakthrough medication (i.e., use of the short-acting opioid more than three times per day) should be taken as a sign that the pain regimen may need to be adjusted.
  - Opioids can be further up-titrated by adding the equivalent of the total amount of required breakthrough medication to the long-acting preparation or by increasing the dose of the long-acting preparation by 25–50%, depending on the severity of the pain.[5]
  - Regimens should be titrated to minimize pain and the need for breakthrough medication. However, all patients need continued access to breakthrough medication.
- Transdermal fentanyl patches are the long-acting opioids of choice in many cancer patients, but they are generally not recommended as first-line opioids given the long latent period to steady state (36–48 hours) and difficulty/delay of titration (3 days). Despite wide variability in the pharmacokinetics for this product and concern for impaired absorption in cases of decreased body fat, it is a valid option when oral medications are problematic (e.g., dysphagia). Dosage should be based on the daily dose of breakthrough opioid, with 50–75 mg/24 h of oral morphine converted to a 25 μg/h increase in fentanyl patch dose.[5] An alternate conversion: oral morphine mg/100 = transdermal

fentanyl mg/24 h (manufacturer-recommended dosing ratio of 150:1).[7] Despite the variable pharmacokinetics, the potency of transdermal fentanyl should not be underestimated.

- **Opioids in renal insufficiency**: Some medications will have increased half-life as metabolites accumulate. These include codeine, oxycodone, tramadol, and the active metabolites of meperidine (normeperidine), propoxyphene, and morphine (morphine-6-glucoronide). Tramadol and normeperidine lower seizure threshold. In general, propoxyphene, meperidine, and mixed agonist–antagonists agents are not recommended for cancer patients.
- Converting between opioids: Incomplete cross-resistance may lead to unanticipated potency with a new agent. In converting between opioid agents for a patient with adequate pain control, practitioners should consider calculating the initial dose as half of the total daily oral morphine equivalent to account for this reduced cross-resistance. If inadequate analgesia has led to the change in agents, then the new drug may be started at a nearly equivalent dose (Table 37-2).
  - When using codeine, practitioners should be aware that there is wide variation in the ability of individual patients to covert codeine to morphine due to the genetic polymorphism of the CYP2D6 enzyme involved. Current guidelines recommend converting between oral codeine and oral morphine with a ratio of 10:1. Because codeine converts to morphine, the same caution for use in renal patients applies.
  - When using oxycodone, it is important to note that oral oxycodone has a bioavailability of 60–87%, whereas the bioavailability of oral morphine is 15–64%.[7] Therefore, many guidelines give the potency ratio for oral oxycodone to oral morphine as 1.5:1 (i.e., a lower dose of oxycodone is theoretically needed to have comparable analgesic effect).

TABLE 37-2 EQUIPOTENT ANALGESIC DOSES (MORPHINE, 10 mg IV/IM = 1 U)

Drug	Onset (min)	Dose Interval (h)	PO Equivalent Dose (mg)	IM/IV Equivalent Dose (mg)
Codeine	10–30	4	200	130
Hydrocodone	15–30	4	30	—
Hydromorphone (Dilaudid)	15–30 (PO)	2–4 (IV) 4–6 (PO)	7.5	1.5
Morphine sulfate	15–60 (PO)	4 (PO) 2–4 (IV)	30	10
Morphine sulfate, sustained release	60	12	90	—
Oxycodone	15–30	6	30	—
Oxycodone, sustained release	15–30	12	30	—
Methadone[a]	30–60	6	20	10

[a] A dose ratio of 1:4 of oral methadone to oral morphine is used for oral morphine doses <90 mg/d. For doses of 90 to 300 mg, a ratio of 1:8 and >300 mg should use a ratio of 1:12 of oral methadone to oral morphine.

- **Side effects:** Patients should be monitored closely for analgesic-related side effects; they often do not report side effects unless specifically asked. For patients on opioids, routine inquiries should be made about sedation, constipation, nausea/vomiting, and pruritus. For patients who are having negative side effects from pain medications, there are five main strategies:
  - **Change the medication dose or dosing frequency** (e.g., changing to long-acting formulations promotes a more constant serum level of the medication and may ameliorate the side effect experienced with short-acting formulas).
  - **Rotate to another opioid**. Pruritus may trigger switching to fentanyl, which tends to be less pruritic.
  - **Change the route of administration.**
    - Subcutaneous, intravenous, and transdermal routes may have fewer GI side effects than the oral route.
    - Administering opioids intrathecally allows for dramatic dose reduction, which often eliminates CNS side effects like sedation, nausea, and vomiting. However, its use is usually limited to patients who have failed a more conservative approach and who are not homebound.
    - Not all patients have easily obtainable venous access; central or peripherally inserted central venous catheter (PICC) line placement may be required. This requires fastidious line care; line infection is a continuous risk.
  - **Add nonopioid analgesics** or coanalgesics and nondrug methods of pain control in order to reduce the total opioid requirement.
    - Acetaminophen, NSAIDs, and caffeine can act synergistically with opioids.
    - Coanalgesics are agents that enhance analgesics and are themselves at either least partially analgesic or counteract the side effects of analgesics. These include caffeine, TCAs, AEDs, and corticosteroids. Physical, psychological, and/or complementary modalities may also be opioid sparing and thus may also be considered coanalgesics.
  - **Add a medication specifically to counteract** the unwanted opioid side effect. The most common opioid side effects and their targeted treatments are described below.
    - **Nausea and vomiting** can result from opioid effects on the chemoreceptor trigger zone and the vestibular apparatus (producing vertigo) or as a consequence of their constipating effects. Other causes of nausea in the cancer patient should be excluded (e.g., bowel obstruction, fecal impaction, chemotherapy, radiation therapy, hypercalcemia, and intracranial pathology). Antiemetic therapy options include prochlorperazine, metoclopramide, and ondansetron. Lorazepam can also be very effective. If one antiemetic is prescribed as needed and nausea persists, that antiemetic can be changed to scheduled dosing and/or additional antiemetics can be added.
    - Constipation and stool impaction must be diagnosed and treated. **Constipation** prophylaxis should always be started with initiation of opioid therapy, including, a stool softener (e.g., docusate 100 mg PO bid) and a stimulant laxative (e.g., senna 2 tablets PO qam or bid). Impaction and bowel obstruction and other causes of constipation must be ruled out. After other causes have been excluded, osmotic laxatives (e.g., polyethylene glycol 17 g PO daily, lactulose 30–60 mL PO daily, magnesium citrate 1.745 g/30 mL, 8 oz PO daily, bisacodyl 2–3 tablets PO daily or 1 rectal suppository daily, or sorbitol 30 mL PO every 2 hours × 3 and then PRN) may be initiated. Subcutaneous methylnaltrexone may be utilized in acute constipation once obstruction has been ruled out. Oral naloxone can be considered for refractory cases. Patients may require disimpaction (glycerin suppositories, enemas, or manual disimpaction).
    - **Respiratory depression** may occur with any of the systemic pure opioid agonists. For symptomatic respiratory depression, naloxone may be given (0.04 mg q30–60 seconds PRN for respiratory depression, 0.4–1 mg for apnea, and 2 mg for

cardiopulmonary arrest). The half-life of naloxone is shorter than that of most opioid medications and redosing or continuous infusion may be necessary.
- **Sedation:** stimulants such as caffeine, dextroamphetamine 2.5–10 mg PO, or methylphenidate 2.5–10 mg PO 1–3×/day are an option to treat opioid-related sedation.
- **Pruritus** can be addressed with diphenhydramine 25–50 mg PO/IV q12h, dexamethasone 1 mg PO daily, or topical preparations such as Sarna lotion or 1% hydrocortisone cream q6h.
- Additional complications
  - **Tolerance** is defined as the progressive decline of opioid potency with continued use. All patients who use an opioid for an extended period of time usually develop physiological dependence. **Addiction** is a psychological behavioral syndrome characterized by drug-seeking behavior; it is very rare among cancer patients. Opioids should never be abruptly discontinued in patients on chronic opioids, but rather tapered under the supervision of a physician in order to prevent acute withdrawal. See Chapter 48 for opioid withdrawal.
  - **Opioid-induced hyperalgesia** (OIH) is a state of nociceptive sensitization caused by opioid use. It may manifest as rapid tolerance to opioids, increasing pain despite increasing opioid doses, and pain which extends beyond the distribution of the preexisting pain. The mechanism is not well understood. Care needs to be taken to differentiate between OIH and increased pain related to disease progression or opioid tolerance. Treatment for OIH involves reducing the causal opioid and/or switching to an opioid that is less likely to cause OIH (such as methadone or buprenorphine), maximizing nonopioid analgesics, and considering the use of ketamine.[7]

Other Nonpharmacologic Therapies

Patients also may choose to pursue complementary or alternative therapies, including massage, acupuncture, heat therapy, transcutaneous electrical nerve stimulation, and immobilization. Those who value physical activity may find relief with exercise, stretching, yoga, or physical therapy. Some may find comfort in relaxation techniques, imagery, support groups, family or individual counseling, biofeedback, and psychotherapy. Advance care planning, patient education, and emotional support are important and are considered modalities for pain relief.

Interventional Therapies

- **Radiation and radionuclide therapies**: Focal pain and referred pain that are related to bony metastases will generally respond to external-beam radiation; almost half of patients will get complete relief while up to 90% will get at least partial relief.[7] Patients with evidence of spinal cord compression should also be urgently referred to a radiation oncologist for palliative radiation. When radiation therapy has been maximized or metastases are too widespread for local treatments to be effective, bone pain may be treated with radionuclides like Strontium-89. As with radiation, it can take 2–3 weeks to see full effect of treatment.
- Interventional therapies, performed by anesthesiologists, interventional radiologists, and occasionally surgeons, may be beneficial for cancer-related pain. These include nerve blocks, spinal anesthetics, and surgical procedures. They may be indicated when systemic medications are inadequate to control pain or when pain control requires medication doses high enough to create unacceptable side effects.
  - Celiac plexus block is probably the most useful nerve block used for tumor-related pain; it is indicated for pain from pancreatic and other upper abdominal cancers. It is effective in up to 90% of cases and can produce analgesia for 2–6 months.[7] Other plexus blocks are also done, though none are generally considered first-line therapy for pain.

- Intrathecal infusion of anesthetics allows reduction in dosing of oral and transdermal medications and must be performed by an anesthesiologist. In 2011, an expert panel at the Polyanalgesic Consensus Conference created updated, evidence-based algorithms for the rational use of intrathecal medications for the treatment of neuropathic and nociceptive pain. Morphine and ziconotide are the only agents that are approved for intrathecal analgesia, but the use of other agents is still common.[8]
- Neurosurgical and neuroablative techniques are only seen as a last resort as they have the highest morbidity and mortality of the interventional pain therapies.

SPECIAL CONSIDERATIONS

- **Patient and caregiver education:** The patient and family members are generally responsible for providing much or most of the care in the patient's home setting. Because the patient is frequently dependent on family members for care, good communication between the family and the health care team is essential. It is essential to evaluate a patient's support system and living environment.
- Interventions that analyze and improve the ability of a patient's home caretakers to assist them in pain management have been shown to be effective in decreasing patient pain, improving quality of life for patients and caregivers, increasing caregiver feelings of self-efficacy in helping the patient control pain and other symptoms, and decreasing levels of caregiver strain.[9] Goals should be set with the patient and family regarding pain management. The health care team's ideal objectives should include educating the patient and caregiver about cancer pain and its management along with teaching a variety of pain coping skills and strategies.

REFERENCES

1. Wong DL, Baker CM. Pain in children: comparison of assessment scales. *Pediatr Nurs* 1988;14:9–17.
2. Hershman DL, Lacchetti C, Dworkin RH, et al. Prevention and management of chemotherapy-induced peripheral neuropathy in survivors of adult cancers: American Society of Clinical Oncology clinical practice guideline. *J Clin Oncol* 2014;32:1941–67.
3. Jaycox A, Carr DB, Payne R. New clinical practice guidelines for the management of pain in patients with cancer. *N Engl J Med* 1994;330:651–5.
4. World Health Organization. *WHO's Cancer Pain Ladder for Adults.* 2016. Available at: http://www.who.int/cancer/palliative/painladder/en/ (last accessed March 15, 2016).
5. Perron V, Schonwetter RS. Assessment and management of pain in palliative care patients. *Cancer Control* 2001;8:15–24.
6. Rainone F. Treating adult cancer pain in primary care. *J Am Board Fam Pract* 2004;17:S48–S56.
7. Harris DG. Management of pain in advanced disease. *Br Med Bull* 2014;110:117–28.
8. Deer TR, Prager J, Levy R, et al. Polyanalgesic Consensus Conference 2012: recommendations for the management of pain by intrathecal (intraspinal) drug delivery: report of an interdisciplinary expert panel. *Neuromodulation* 2012;15:436–64.
9. Keefe FJ, Ahles TA, Sutton L, et al. Partner-guided cancer pain management at the end of life: a preliminary study. *J Pain Symptom Manage* 2005;29:263–72.

Neutropenic Fever

38

Merilda O. Blanco-Guzman and
Erik R. Dubberke

GENERAL PRINCIPLES

- Neutropenic fever is defined as a single temperature ≥38.3°C or a temperature ≥38°C for >1 hour in a patient with an absolute neutrophil count (ANC) <500/µL or <1000/µL with a predicted decline to ≤500/µL.
- The onset of fever should be dated from the first day of the last cycle of chemotherapy, which allows estimation of the duration of neutropenia.
- Ten to fifty percent of patients with solid malignancies and >80% of patients with hematologic malignancies will develop neutropenic fever during treatment.[1]
- Only in 20–30% of these cases will a source of infection be documented.[2]
- Common etiologic agents include various *Staphylococcus* species, *Streptococcus* species, *Enterococcus* species, *Escherichia coli*, *Klebsiella* species, *Pseudomonas* species, and anaerobes. The gastrointestinal tract is a common source of bacterial entry owing to chemotherapy-induced mucosal damage.

DIAGNOSIS

Clinical Presentation

History

The history should focus on the following:

- Subtle symptoms of infection. Even with a severe bacterial infection, a neutropenic patient may have minimal symptoms.
- Recent hospitalizations, HIV status and other comorbid conditions, prior infections, exposures and travel, recent antimicrobial therapy or prophylaxis, as well as the date of last chemotherapy.[2]
- Determination of the exact chemotherapeutic agents and doses can help in predicting the severity and duration of neutropenia and likelihood that the fever may be a manifestation of a noninfectious chemotherapy-induced adverse event (e.g., bleomycin-induced pneumonitis).

Physical Examination

- Inflammation may be subtle to nonexistent because of the neutropenia.[2]
- Examine for signs of infection at commonly affected sites, including the periodontium, pharynx, lower esophagus, lungs, perineum and anus, eyes, and skin; include intravascular access device sites, bone marrow aspiration sites, and tissue around the nails.
- Many physicians recommend against performing a digital rectal exam as it may induce more mucosal damage and allow further bacterial translocation.
- Sinus tenderness or ulcers may be indicative of mucormycosis or aspergillosis.
- Right lower quadrant tenderness may suggest typhlitis (neutropenic enterocolitis).

Diagnostic Testing

Laboratories
- Obtain a complete blood count including differential, hepatic function panel, electrolytes, and renal function tests at fever onset and at least every 3 days thereafter.[2]
- Two sets of **blood cultures** should be obtained from different sites (at least one, preferably both, from a peripheral blood draw).
- Also obtain a **urinalysis** (and **urine culture** in the presence of pyuria or symptoms).
- Gram stain and culture should be taken from any suspicious site.
- Biopsy with microscopic evaluation should be considered for any new or undiagnosed skin lesions. If there are chronic mucosal or soft tissue lesions, samples should be sent for fungal and atypical mycobacterial cultures. Vesicular or ulcerated lesions of the skin or mucosa should be sent for herpes simplex virus (HSV) and varicella zoster virus (VZV) testing if the clinical presentation is appropriate.
- If the patient has clinically significant diarrhea, stool should be tested for *Clostridium difficile* toxin. Stool culture, ova and parasites, bacterial pathogens, viruses, and protozoa can be considered in travelers, patients from endemic regions, or patients with specific exposures.[2]
- Nasopharyngeal swabs for viral diagnostic testing should be obtained in patients with symptoms of an upper respiratory infection in the winter or at times of local viral outbreak.[2]
- Cerebrospinal fluid should be obtained if there are signs or symptoms of central nervous system infection.[2]

Imaging
A chest radiograph should be obtained in all patients with respiratory symptoms. Further imaging should be guided by clinical judgment. Many clinicians have a low threshold for obtaining computed tomography scans of the sinuses, chest, and/or abdomen.[2]

TREATMENT

- Risk assessment is important to determine if the patient needs to be hospitalized, as well as the duration and choice of antimicrobial treatment.
- High-risk patients are those with anticipated prolonged neutropenia (>7 days duration), significant clinical instability, recent exposure to antimicrobials, renal or hepatic insufficiency, inpatient status at fever onset, recent use of alemtuzumab, grade 3 or 4 mucositis, pneumonia, new-onset abdominal pain, or neurologic changes. High-risk patients should be admitted to the hospital for empiric IV antimicrobials.[3]
- Low-risk patients have an anticipated brief (≤7 days) duration of severe neutropenia (≤100 cells/μL), no recent antimicrobial exposures, no acute comorbid illness, good performance status (Eastern Cooperative Oncology Group [ECOG] score of 0–1), and no renal or hepatic impairment and live in close proximity to a hospital. These patients may initially be managed in the outpatient setting with oral antimicrobial agents.[3]
- **Empiric antimicrobial management:** Empiric antimicrobials should be given promptly to neutropenic patients because overwhelming sepsis can occur in a short period of time.
  - **High-risk patients** can be initially treated with monotherapy with an antipseudomonal β-lactam agent, such as a carbapenem (imipenem/cilastatin or meropenem), an antipseudomonal cephalosporin (cefepime or ceftazidime), or piperacillin–tazobactam.[2,3]
    - No study has demonstrated differences in efficacy between monotherapy and multidrug combinations. However, if antimicrobial resistance is suspected or if the patient has pneumonia or hemodynamic instability, other antimicrobials such as aminoglycosides or fluoroquinolones may be added to the β-lactam agent.[2]

- Fluoroquinolone monotherapy is not recommended[2]
- Vancomycin (or other active agent against β-lactam–resistant gram-positive organisms) is not recommended as a standard part of the initial empiric regimen.[2] It should be considered in patients with suspected catheter-related infection, known colonization with methicillin-resistant *Staphylococcus aureus* (MRSA) or β-lactam–resistant *Streptococcus*, mucositis, skin and soft tissue infection, pneumonia, hemodynamic instability, or a recent history of fluoroquinolone or trimethoprim–sulfamethoxazole prophylaxis.
- Patients who remain hemodynamically unstable after initial doses of standard treatment regimens should have their antimicrobials broadened to include resistant organisms as follows (and based on local resistance patterns)[2]:
  - MRSA: vancomycin, linezolid or daptomycin (not if pneumonia)
  - Vancomycin-resistant *Enterococcus* (VRE): linezolid or daptomycin (not if pneumonia)
  - Extended spectrum β-lactamase (ESBL)-producing organisms: initial use of carbapenem
  - Carbapenemase-producing organisms: aminoglycoside, colistin, or tigecycline
- **Low-risk patients** can receive either PO or IV empiric antimicrobial regimens.[2] For oral empiric treatment, a combination of ciprofloxacin plus amoxicillin–clavulanate is recommended. Other combinations such as ciprofloxacin and clindamycin are commonly used but less well studied. For patients receiving fluoroquinolone prophylaxis, oral therapy is not appropriate.
- **Subsequent antimicrobial management:** After 2–4 days of treatment, the course is determined by the clinical response and culture results. Persistent fever in itself is not a clinical indicator of nonresponse, as median time to defervescence in responsive patients is 2 (solid tumors) to 4 (leukemia/stem cell transplants) days.[2] Instead, hemodynamic and overall stability, improvement in the initial symptoms and signs of infection, and culture results should be used for guidance.
  - **If pathogen or site of infection identified**, therapy should be directed according to the site of infection and susceptibilities of the isolated organism(s).
    - If the patient defervesces and the site of infection improves, antimicrobials are continued for 7–14 days (or as appropriate for the documented infection) or until the ANC is >500 cells/μL and rising, whichever is longer.[2,3]
    - If the patient does not defervesce or the site of infection does not clinically improve, the patient should be reevaluated and additional cultures should be obtained. If the patient is unstable, infectious diseases consultation should be considered.[2] If the patient is stable, continued monitoring and continuation of the initial antimicrobial regimen are appropriate. The antimicrobial regimen should be adjusted as indicated based on culture results, a worsening in clinical site of infection, or if the patient becomes hemodynamically unstable.
    - If vancomycin (or other gram-positive agent) was started, it can be stopped if cultures do not grow a β-lactam–resistant gram positive and there is no clinical site of infection concerning for a β-lactam–resistant gram positive (e.g., cellulitis).[2,3]
  - **If pathogen or site of infection not identified:**
    - If the patient responds to empiric treatment, antimicrobials are continued for 7–14 days or until ANC is >500 cells/μL and rising, whichever is longer.[2]
    - Low-risk patients initially treated in the outpatient setting who become unstable or are not responding to empiric treatment should be hospitalized for intravenous antimicrobials and monitoring.[3]
    - High-risk patients with persistent fever but otherwise clinically stable should be assessed daily, and cultures should be obtained. It is not necessary to empirically change antimicrobials in stable patients unless cultures become positive or a clinical site of infection becomes apparent indicating a change is needed.

- Adding vancomycin in the absence of culture results or a clinical site of infection concerning for the presence of a β-lactam–resistant gram-positive organism is **not** associated with more rapid defervescence and is **not** indicated.[2]
  - **Persistent fever:** Once fever has persisted for ≥4–7 days of antimicrobials in patients with anticipated duration of neutropenia for an additional ≥7 days, antifungal therapy with activity against molds should be considered.[2]
    - High-risk patients with unexplained fever, who have not responded to 2–4 days of treatment, should be assessed for a nonbacterial infection, a resistant bacterial infection, emergence of a secondary infection, inadequate tissue levels of antimicrobials, drug fever, or infection at an avascular site.
    - In addition to a thorough physical exam with vascular catheter inspection (this should be performed daily), consider chest or sinus radiographs, repeat cultures of blood and specific sites of infection, and imaging of any organ suspected of infection. If clinical features suggest any of the following disease processes, special studies may be done for fungal infections, *Toxoplasma gondii*, HSV, cytomegalovirus (CMV), Epstein-Barr virus, Enterovirus, enteric protozoa, *Mycobacterium tuberculosis*, nontuberculous mycobacteria, and *Chlamydia pneumoniae*.

SPECIAL CONSIDERATIONS

- Available agents for **antifungal therapy** include amphotericin B in liposomal (L-AMB), colloidal dispersion (ABCD) or lipid complex (ABLC) formulation; the azoles, such as fluconazole (limited by lack of activity against molds and frequent use as antifungal prophylaxis), itraconazole, voriconazole, posaconazole, and isavuconazole; and the echinocandins caspofungin, anidulafungin, and micafungin (which are limited by unreliable activity against opportunistic fungi other than *Candida* or *Aspergillus* species).[3] For patients already receiving prophylaxis with fluconazole, switching to an agent with antimold activity is recommended. In patients receiving prophylaxis with an antimold agent such as voriconazole or posaconazole, it is recommended to switch to a different drug class or from the PO to IV formulation to ensure therapeutic drug levels.
- Routine use of **antivirals** is not indicated. If skin or mucous membrane lesions are suggestive of HSV or VZV, treatment with acyclovir (5 mg/kg IV q8h) is indicated even in patients who are afebrile. All patients with suspected VZV infection should be placed in negative pressure and on contact precautions.
- The routine use of granulocyte colony-stimulating factor (G-CSF) or **granulocyte–macrophage colony-stimulating factor** (GM-CSF) as secondary prophylaxis (after neutropenia has developed) is not recommended because it has not been demonstrated to affect mortality.[2] It may decrease hospitalization time and decrease the duration of neutropenia. Consider use of G-CSF or GM-CSF in patients with pulmonary infiltrates, invasive fungal infections, severe deterioration, expected prolonged neutropenia, or no bone marrow recovery after 5 days.

REFERENCES

1. Klastersky J. Management of fever in neutropenic patients with different risks of complications. *Clin Infect Dis* 2004;39:S32–7.
2. Freifeld AG, Bow EJ, Sepkowitz KA, et al. Clinical practice guideline for the use of antimicrobial agents in neutropenic patients with cancer: 2010 update by the Infectious Diseases Society of America. *Clin Infect Dis* 2011;52(4):e56–93.
3. National Comprehensive Cancer Network. NCCN practice guidelines in oncology: prevention and treatment of cancer-related infections. Version 2:2015. Available at: http://www.nccn.org/ (last accessed 27/07/15).

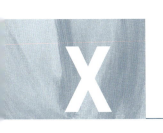

X Endocrinology

Inpatient Diabetes Management

Sushma Jonna and Michael Y. Lin

GENERAL PRINCIPLES

- The increasing prevalence of glucose intolerance and diabetes in the United States translates into rising numbers of hospitalized patients requiring hyperglycemic management.
- Hospitalized patients are faced with many unique factors that affect glycemic control.
  - Some of these include stress-induced epinephrine and cortisol release, medication use such as glucocorticoids and vasopressors, altered activity levels, and caloric intake changes.[1]
  - Dietary intake changes may result from surgery, procedures, or tests.
  - The use of parenteral nutrition or continuous enteral nutrition can also affect blood glucose (BG) control.
- This chapter will be organized into management of diabetes in specific patient populations (i.e., critically ill patients, noncritically ill patients, patients with acute myocardial infarction [AMI], etc.)

CRITICALLY ILL PATIENTS

- Glycemic targets in critically ill patients remain controversial as interventions to control hyperglycemia have had mixed results.
- Early randomized control trials showed that intensive insulin therapy with target BGs of 80–100 mg/dL improved survival.[2]
- In patients with sepsis, one trial found that intense insulin therapy resulted in risk of hypoglycemia and no changes in mortality.[3]
- The Normoglycemia in Intensive Care Evaluation–Survival Using Glucose Algorithm Regulation (NICE-SUGAR) trial challenged previous studies supporting tight glycemic control in critically ill patients. This study showed an increase in mortality in the intensive glycemic control group as well as a greater risk of the serious adverse effects from hypoglycemia.[4]
- Taking into account these variable trials, the American Association of Clinical Endocrinologists (AACE) and the American Diabetes Association (ADA) formed a consensus statement on inpatient glycemic control.[5] The goals of hyperglycemic treatment in critically ill patients are outlined as follows:
  - Insulin therapy should begin at BG levels above 180 mg/dL.
  - BG levels should be maintained between 140–180 mg/dL.
  - BG levels below 110 mg/dL should be avoided.
  - The preferred route of administration is IV infusion.
- When **transitioning care from the critical care unit to the medicine floor**, IV insulin can be replaced with subcutaneous basal–bolus insulin.
  - Continue IV insulin for at least 4 hours after long-acting insulin is given.
  - The basal dose should be 20–30% less than patient's daily requirement as stress of critical illness increases insulin requirements. Preprandial insulin should be initiated at 10% of the basal dose.[6]

NONCRITICALLY ILL PATIENTS

- Tight glycemic control for patients not in critical care units is not well studied. However, hyperglycemia has been associated with increased risk of infection and prolonged hospitalization.[7]
- The current consensus on goals of hyperglycemic treatment in noncritically ill patients per the AACE/ADA guidelines is as follows:
  - Insulin therapy should begin at BG levels above 180 mg/dL.
  - Pre-meal BG target is below 140 mg/dL.
  - Random BG values should be maintained below 180 mg/dL.
  - Reevaluate regimen if BG levels fall below 100 mg/dL.
- The preferred route of administration is subcutaneous including basal and correctional elements.
- Sliding scale insulin (SSI) or correction dosing insulin regimens are commonly ordered to supplement scheduled diabetic therapies. Be aware that sliding scale is given in response to existing hyperglycemia and requires reevaluation of basal insulin dosing.
  - The Randomized Study of Basal–Bolus Insulin Therapy in the Inpatient Management of Patients with Type 2 Diabetes (RABBIT 2) trial showed that retreatment with basal–bolus insulin was more effective than SSI alone.[8]
  - More optimal management is to anticipate hyperglycemia and increase longer-acting insulin analogs or preprandial short-acting analogs.

Management of Patients Tolerating PO

- BG monitoring through point-of-care meters should occur before meals and at bedtime.
- Patients who are managed on diet therapy alone at home should be continued on a diabetic diet with regular BG monitoring while in hospital.
  - A sliding scale/supplemental insulin regimen may be used for elevated BG glucose levels above 180 mg/dL.
  - If persistent hyperglycemia occurs, initiation of basal insulin may be required.
- Oral agents should typically be discontinued during hospitalization especially in patients experiencing renal failure, hemodynamic instability, or contrast requiring imaging.
- Patients requiring insulin at home should continue with an insulin regimen when hospitalized.
  - One method is to use weight-based insulin dosing. The basal insulin dose is calculated as 0.2–0.3 units/kg/d of insulin glargine every 24 hours or neutral protamine Hagedorn (NPH) insulin every 12 hours. This should be combined with preprandial insulin dosing at 0.05–0.1 units/kg per meal of short-acting insulin lispro, aspart, or regular insulin.[9]
  - The other method is to reduce a patient's home insulin regimen by 20%.
  - To minimize risk of hypoglycemia, a patient's daily insulin dose can be calculated using both methods and initiating the one with the lower insulin requirement.
  - Sliding scale or correctional insulin can be used in addition and dosing depends on insulin sensitivity. The 1700 rule, calculated by dividing 1700 by the total daily insulin requirement, approximates the decrease in glucose with 1 unit of insulin. This can be used to choose between low, medium, and high sliding scales.[10]
- Adjustments to insulin regimens may need to be made regularly.
  - Basal insulin dose should be adjusted based on fasting glucose.
  - BG measurements prior to meals represent the efficacy of mealtime insulin given before the prior meal. For example, the BG level prior to dinner is reflective of the lunchtime insulin dose.

Management of Patients Who Will Be NPO

- Patients with type II diabetes mellitus will still require basal insulin while being NPO. Glargine or detemir is preferred over NPH in NPO patients given their relative stable effects. Pre-meal insulin should be discontinued.

- Type 1 diabetic patients sometimes require both glucose and basal insulin to prevent catabolism and ketogenesis.
  - Long-acting basal insulin should be continued to avoid development of diabetic ketoacidosis.
  - Ketogenesis can be avoided by using two primary infusion types.
    - Fixed-rate infusion uses glucose/insulin/potassium (GIK) solution. This consists of 500 mL D5W, 10 mmol KCl, and 15 units of short-acting insulin run at a rate of 100–150 mL/hour. The amount of insulin in the solution is adjusted depending on BG levels. However, GIK fixed-rate infusion is limited by the need to replace the entire solution bag for any change in amount of insulin.
    - Variable-rate infusion uses dextrose fluid and insulin in separate solution bags. D5W is set at a rate of 150 mL/hour, and short-acting insulin infusion would be set at 0.5–1 units/hour. Insulin infusion can be adjusted by 0.3–0.5 units/hour as needed for a target BG range of 120–180 mg/dL. If ketonuria develops, it is treated by increasing the glucose rate.

PATIENTS WITH ACUTE MYOCARDIAL INFARCTION

- Recommendations for glycemic control in patients with AMI are difficult to delineate because of varying study designs and outcomes.
- Although the Diabetes and Insulin-Glucose Infusion in Acute Myocardial Infarction (DIGAMI 1) study showed a mortality reduction with intensive insulin therapy, the DIGAMI 2 trial failed to show the same result.[11,12] In the later study, however, recruitment goals and the primary treatment goal were not met.
- The Hyperglycemia Intensive Insulin Infusion in Infarction (Hi-5) study and the Clinical Trial of Metabolic Modulation in Acute Myocardial Infarction Treatment Evaluation—Estudios Cardiologicos Latinoamerica (CREATE-ECLA) study failed to show a mortality benefit with intensive glucose control in patients with AMI. The Hi-5 study did demonstrate a lower rate of heart failure and reinfarction in patients with tighter glucose control.[13,14]

MANAGEMENT OF DIABETES IN THE PERIOPERATIVE PERIOD

The primary goal of BG management in the perioperative setting is to avoid hypoglycemia, excessive hyperglycemia, ketogenesis, catabolism, and electrolyte abnormalities.

- Key factors must be known that will affect the timing and type of hyperglycemic treatment needed. Some of these include the duration of surgery, the type of anesthesia planned, anticipated resumption time of caloric intake, and activity level.[15] Please see Table 39-1 for the management of diabetes in the setting of short procedures.
- It is also important to evaluate the potential long-term complications of diabetes (microvascular, macrovascular, and neuropathic) that may potentiate surgical risk.
  - Cardiovascular risk assessment must be given special priority, as undiagnosed coronary artery disease and silent ischemia are more prevalent among diabetics.[16]
  - Renal dysfunction from diabetic nephropathy may also be undiagnosed; hence, assessment is needed.
  - Diabetic autonomic neuropathy may adversely affect the postoperative phase and has been associated with excess nonsurgical mortality.
- Studies to evaluate metabolic, renal, and cardiac status should include electrolytes, renal function, BG levels, urinalysis for ketones/proteinuria, and an electrocardiogram. It is essential to correct any underlying hypoglycemia; excessive hyperglycemia; and electrolyte, metabolic, and volume abnormalities prior to surgery.

TABLE 39-1 MANAGEMENT OF DIABETES MELLITUS FOR SHORT PROCEDURES

Timing of Procedure	Diabetic Regimen	Recommended Management Strategy
Early morning	Any	Delay diabetic agent dosing.
Late morning	Oral agents	Hold oral agent on day of surgery. Supplemental insulin (short-acting) may be used to achieve tighter control.
Late morning	Single-dose insulin (Ultralente/Lantus)	Give two-thirds of total daily dose preoperatively.
Late morning	2–3 doses of insulin daily	Give one-half of the total morning dose of long-acting insulin.
Late morning	Multiple doses of short-acting insulin	Give one-third of morning dose.
Afternoon	Oral agents	Hold oral agent.
Afternoon	Single-dose insulin	Give one-half of daily dose.
Afternoon	2–3 doses of insulin daily	One-third of total morning dose
Afternoon	Multiple doses of short-acting insulin	Give one-third of the morning and lunchtime doses.
Any	Insulin pump	Continue basal rate only.

- Further cardiac risk stratification may also be warranted. One study showed that an elevated preoperative BG level ≥200 mg/dL was associated with deep sternal wound infection following coronary artery bypass grafting.[17] However, in patients with chronically poor diabetic control, the effect on patient outcome of rapid normalization of BG levels preoperatively is not well established.[18–20]

MANAGEMENT OF GLUCOCORTICOID-INDUCED DIABETES MELLITUS

- Many patients with mild glucose intolerance may develop hyperglycemia with the initiation of glucocorticoid therapy.[21]
- Nondiabetics who experience BG levels between 140–200 mg/dL shortly after initiation of high-dose glucocorticoids may be observed, because β-cell adaptation may correct the metabolic derangement in 1–2 weeks. If normoglycemia is not obtained, therapy is indicated. Therapy should be initiated in patients with glucose levels >200.
- Typically, mealtime insulin will need to be adjusted as postprandial levels are most affected.
- Poorly controlled diabetics starting glucocorticoid therapy should have anticipatory increases in diabetic therapy. Even well-controlled diabetics receiving more than the equivalent of 20 mg of prednisone daily should have a 20% increase in their insulin doses or advancement of their oral therapy.
- The hyperglycemic effects of oral glucocorticoids should remit 48 hours after cessation of therapy. IM and intra-articular glucocorticoids may have effects lasting <10 days.

MANAGEMENT OF INPATIENTS ON ALIMENTARY FEEDINGS

- Patients on total parental nutrition (TPN) also require appropriate insulin therapy especially given their higher risk for hyperglycemia.
  - Regular insulin as calculated as 0.1 unit for every gram of carbohydrate or from the daily insulin requirement can be added directly into the TPN solution. Titration of insulin in the TPN can be done as needed.
  - Patients previously on insulin can receive 40% of their total daily insulin as basal dose given subcutaneously and the remainder in TPN.
- Patients on continuous enteral feedings also require insulin therapy. The use of a basal insulin dosing regimen and sliding scale is useful in most cases. However, if there is concern for feeding limitations or possible feeding interruptions, the use of only a sliding scale regimen may be needed. Or, if basal insulin is used, substitute IV dextrose solution with a similar carbohydrate amount as the missing enteral feeds.

TRANSITION TO OUTPATIENT MANAGEMENT

- Insulin regimens should be reviewed with patients with written and verbal instructions prior to discharge to prevent medication error.
- Patients should follow with a primary care physician or endocrinologist within 1 month of discharge from the hospital.

REFERENCES

1. Bloomgarden ZT. Inpatient diabetes control: approaches to treatment. *Diabetes Care* 2004;27(9):2272–7.
2. van den Berghe G, Wouters P, Weekers F, et al. Intensive insulin therapy in critically ill patients. *N Engl J Med* 2001;345:1359–67.
3. Brunkhorst FM, Engel C, Bloos F, et al. Intensive insulin therapy and pentastarch resuscitation in severe sepsis. *N Engl J Med* 2008;358:125–39.
4. Investigators N-SS; Finfer S, Chittock DR, et al. Intensive versus conventional glucose control in critically ill patients. *N Engl J Med* 2009;360:1283–97.
5. Moghissi ES, Korytkowski MT, DiNardo M, et al. American Association of Clinical Endocrinologists and American Diabetes Association consensus statement on inpatient glycemic control. *Diabetes Care* 2009;32:1119–31.
6. Magaji V, Johnston, JM. Inpatient management of hyperglycemia and diabetes. *Clin Diabetes* 2011;29:3–9.
7. Clement S, Braithwaite SS, Magee MF, et al. Management of diabetes and hyperglycemia in hospitals. *Diabetes Care* 2004;27:553–91.
8. Umpierrez GE, Smiley D, Zisman A, et al. Randomized study of basal-bolus insulin therapy in the inpatient management of patients with type 2 diabetes (RABBIT 2 trial). *Diabetes Care* 2007;30:2181–6.
9. Inzucchi SE, Bergenstal RM, Buse JB, et al. Management of hyperglycemia in type 2 diabetes, 2015: a patient-centered approach: update to a position statement of the American Diabetes Association and the European Association for the Study of Diabetes. *Diabetes Care* 2015;38:140–9.
10. Davidson PC, Hebblewhite HR, Bode BW, et al. Statistically based CSII parameters: correction factor (CF) (1700 rule), carbohydrate-insulin ratio (CIR) (2.8 rule), and basal-to-total ratio. *Diabetes Technol Ther* 2003;5:237.
11. Malmberg K, Ryden L, Efendic S, et al. Randomized trial of insulin-glucose infusion followed by subcutaneous insulin treatment in diabetic patients with acute myocardial infarction (DIGAMI study): effects on mortality at 1 year. *J Am Coll Cardiol* 1995;26:57–65.
12. Malmberg K, Ryden L, Wedel H, et al. Intense metabolic control by means of insulin in patients with diabetes mellitus and acute myocardial infarction (DIGAMI 2): effects on mortality and morbidity. *Eur Heart J* 2005;26:650–61.

13. Cheung NW, Wong VW, McLean M. The Hyperglycemia: Intensive Insulin Infusion in Infarction (HI-5) study: a randomized controlled trial of insulin infusion therapy for myocardial infarction. *Diabetes Care* 2006;29:765–70.
14. Mehta SR, Yusuf S, Diaz R, et al. Effect of glucose-insulin-potassium infusion on mortality in patients with acute ST-segment elevation myocardial infarction: the CREATE-ECLA randomized controlled trial. *JAMA* 2005;293:437–46.
15. Jacober SJ, Sowers JR. An update on perioperative management of diabetes. *Arch Intern Med* 1999;159:2405–11.
16. Lee TH, Marcantonio ER, Mangione CM, et al. Derivation and prospective validation of a simple index for prediction of cardiac risk of major noncardiac surgery. *Circulation* 1999;100:1043–9.
17. Trick WE, Scheckler WE, Tokars JI, et al. Modifiable risk factors associated with deep sternal site infection after coronary artery bypass grafting. *J Thorac Cardiovasc Surg* 2000;119:108–14.
18. Gandhi GY, Nuttall GA, Abel MD, et al. Intensive intraoperative insulin therapy versus conventional glucose management during cardiac surgery: a randomized trial. *Ann Intern Med* 2007;146:233–43.
19. Schmeltz LR, DeSantis AJ, Thiyagarajan V, et al. Reduction of surgical mortality and morbidity in diabetic patients undergoing cardiac surgery with a combined intravenous and subcutaneous insulin glucose management strategy. *Diabetes Care* 2007;30:823–8.
20. Furnary AP, Gao G, Grunkemeier GL, et al. Continuous insulin infusion reduces mortality in patients with diabetes undergoing coronary artery bypass grafting. *J Thorac Cardiovasc Surg* 2003;125:1007–21.
21. Donihi AC, Raval D, Saul M, et al. Prevalence and predictors of corticosteroid-related hyperglycemia in hospitalized patients. *Endocr Pract* 2006;12:358–62.

Thyroid Diseases

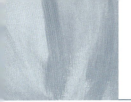

Monalisa Mullick

Hyperthyroidism

GENERAL PRINCIPLES

- Hyperthyroidism is defined by increased circulating levels of T4 and/or T3. T4 is a prohormone that is peripherally monodeiodinated to the active hormone, T3.
- Hyperthyroidism can be up to 10 times more common in women than in men.[1]
- Excess thyroid hormone has been associated with osteoporosis, cardiac arrhythmias (especially atrial fibrillation), angina, and heart failure.[2]
- Subclinical hyperthyroidism (thyroid-stimulating hormones [TSH] below the lower limit but normal T4 and T3) can solely be a laboratory diagnosis, with no definite signs or symptoms of hyperthyroidism.[3,4]
- Under normal circumstances, the pulsatile secretion of hypothalamic thyrotropin releasing hormone (TRH), which stimulates the pituitary TSH, is maintained in balance by feedback from the thyroid gland end product, T3 and T4.[4]
- The etiologies of increased circulating thyroid hormone can be broken down into disorders that involve heightened production of T4 (Table 40-1), augmented release of preformed hormone from the thyroid gland (Table 40-2), and exogenous sources.
- Graves disease (GD) is the most common cause of hyperthyroidism especially in young patients. Incidence of toxic multinodular goiter increases with age. Secondary hyperthyroidism is extremely rare.[5]

DIAGNOSIS

Clinical Presentation

History
- Symptoms may include weight loss, heat intolerance, increased sweating, anxiety, insomnia, palpitations, dyspnea, diarrhea, tremor, and oligomenorrhea.[6]
- They are often less pronounced in the elderly (apathetic hyperthyroidism).[7]
- A thorough medication history is important because several medications alter thyroid hormone physiology (Table 40-3).[8]
- **Thyroid storm** is an overwhelming manifestation of thyrotoxicosis, with fever, tachycardia, delirium, and systemic symptoms such as nausea and vomiting.[5] It often presents in patients with underlying hyperthyroidism in whom additional T4 release is precipitated by severe stress such as surgery, infection, stroke, diabetic ketoacidosis, parturition, administration of iodine contrast, or withdrawal of thyroid medication. It may also be seen in patients being treated for hyperthyroidism who are noncompliant with their antithyroid medications or are on an inadequate regimen.[4]

TABLE 40-1 DISORDER OF INCREASED THYROXINE PRODUCTION

Disorder	Prevalence	Mechanism	Clinical Course
Graves disease	Up to 80% of cases in United States	Antibodies to TSH receptor	Chronic, waxing and waning, some remissions
Toxic adenoma or multinodular goiter	Higher in middle-aged and elderly	Increased production of hormone independent of TSH	Chronic, unremitting
Iodine induced	—	Secondary to iodine load or amiodarone	Self-limiting
Central/ secondary	Rare (<5% of total cases)	Hypersecretion of TSH by pituitary adenoma	Chronic
Molar pregnancy or hyperemesis gravidarum	Rare	Hypersecretion of hCG	Self-limiting

Physical Examination
- Exam may reveal tachycardia, sometimes consistent with atrial fibrillation, or hypertension. Fever, hypotension, or delirium suggest thyroid storm.
- Assess the thyroid for tenderness, nodules, or enlargement. Size can range from normal in an elderly with GD or with exogenous source of thyroid hormone to massive with diffuse or nodular goiter.
- Listen for bruit over the thyroid, which may occur in GD.

TABLE 40-2 DISORDERS OF INCREASED PREFORMED HORMONE RELEASE

Disorder	Epidemiology	Mechanism	Course
Painful subacute thyroiditis (de Quervain thyroiditis)	Female to male ratio: 3–6:1; average age at onset: 20–60 y	Immune-mediated, potentially postviral	**Up to half have transient increase in T4 for several weeks**; subsequent hypothyroidism for several months; almost all have full recovery in 6–12 mo
Hashimoto thyroiditis (chronic lymphocytic thyroiditis)	Female to male ratio: 8–9:1; 30–50 y	Autoimmune, associated with antithyroid antibodies	**May have transient increase in T4**; most progress to chronic hypothyroidism

TABLE 40-3 DRUGS AFFECTING THYROID FUNCTION

Mechanism	Drugs
Decreased TSH secretion	Dopamine, glucocorticoids, octreotide
Altered thyroid hormone secretion	
Decreased secretion	Lithium, iodide, amiodarone, aminoglutethimide
Increased secretion	Iodide, amiodarone
Decreased T4 absorption	Colestipol, cholestyramine, aluminum hydroxide, ferrous sulfate, sucralfate
Altered T4 and T3 transport in serum	
Increased serum TBG	Estrogens, tamoxifen, heroin, methadone, mitotane, fluorouracil
Decreased serum TBG	Androgens, anabolic steroids, slow-release nicotinic acid, glucocorticoids
Displacement from protein	Furosemide, fenclofenac, salicylates binding sites
Altered T4 and T3 metabolism	
Increased hepatic metabolism	Phenobarbital, rifampin, phenytoin, carbamazepine
Decreased conversion of T4 to T3	Propylthiouracil, amiodarone, β-blockers, glucocorticoids
Associated with transient thyroiditis	Interleukin-2
Development of antiperoxidase Ab	Interferon alpha

TBG, thyroid-binding globulin.
Data from Surks M, Sievert R. Drugs and thyroid function. *N Engl J Med* 1995;333:1688–94.

- Other findings may include proptosis (due to Graves ophthalmopathy), lid lag, smooth/warm skin, infiltrative dermopathy (pretibial myxedema specific to GD), onycholysis, proximal muscle weakness, and tremor.[5] A brisk uptake and release of the deep tendon reflexes are commonly found and may be best examined at the Achilles tendon.

Diagnostic Testing

Laboratories
- **The thyroid-stimulating hormones (TSH) are used for initial screening**, followed by free T4 (FT4) with or without free T3 (FT3) if TSH is abnormal or if there is high suspicion of hyperthyroidism. At steady state, a normal TSH excludes hyperthyroidism. See Table 40-4 for patterns.
- Hyperthyroidism may be due to elevated FT3 alone, so it should be measured if the TSH is suppressed but the FT4 is normal.[5]
- TSH may be suppressed in severe nonthyroidal illnesses.[1]

TABLE 40-4 PATTERNS OF THYROID FUNCTION TESTS IN THYROID DISORDERS

TSH	Free T4	Free T3	Thyroid Function
↔	↔	↔	Euthyroid
↑	↑	↑	Central hyperthyroidism
↓	↑	↑	Primary hyperthyroidism
↓	↔	↔	Subclinical hyperthyroidism
↓	↓	↓	Central hypothyroidism
↑	↓	↓	Primary hypothyroidism
↑	↔	↔	Subclinical hypothyroidism

↑, increased; ↓, decreased; ↔, unchanged.

- Associated lab abnormalities in hyperthyroidism could show an elevated alkaline phosphatase, normochromic normocytic anemia, decreased high-density lipoprotein and total cholesterol, hypercalcemia, and elevated transaminases.[1,4,9]
- In thyroid storm, there may be an elevated white blood cell (WBC) count and associated adrenal insufficiency.[5] Consider cosyntropin stimulation test to evaluate the adrenal axis (see Chapter 41).
- Thyroid receptor antibody can be tested in ambiguous circumstances of elevated thyroid hormones as management may vary (i.e., symptoms preceded by viral illness resulting in viral thyroiditis is managed differently than GD). Positive thyroid receptor antibody has sensitivity/specificity of >90% for GD; normal levels may be present in early or mild cases. Up to 50% of those with GD may also be positive for thyroid peroxidase antibody.[10]

Imaging

- Radioactive iodine (RAI) uptake nuclear scan may prove most useful with nodular thyroid disease.
- Functioning or hyperproducing areas of the thyroid are seen on the scan, whereas nonfunctioning or "cold" areas are not visualized. The pattern may suggest diffuse uptake (GD) or hyperfunctioning nodules (toxic multinodular goiter).
- Low uptake is seen with preformed release or exogenous sources of T4.
- RAI is contraindicated in pregnancy.[5]

TREATMENT

Medications

- **β-Blockers** provide symptomatic relief of tachycardia and tremor. Titrate to effect or heart rate of 80–90 starting at a low dose (e.g., propranolol 20 mg PO tid or atenolol 25 mg PO qd). Verapamil may be used to control tachycardia in patients with contraindication to β-blockers.[5]
- Graves hyperthyroidism can be treated with thionamide drugs, RAI, or thyroidectomy, and benefits and risks of each should be fully considered.
- For toxic adenoma or toxic multinodular goiter, RAI or surgery is the treatment of choice.[2]

- The antithyroid thionamide drugs, **propylthiouracil (PTU) and methimazole,** inhibit the synthesis of thyroid hormone by interfering with iodination of thyroglobulin and may have immunosuppressive effects.[5]
  - PTU also blocks the peripheral conversion of T4 to T3.[11] It is dosed 100 mg PO tid.
  - Methimazole is typically dosed 10–30 mg PO daily. Except in pregnancy, methimazole is preferable to PTU, owing to its once-daily dosing, fewer side effects, and more rapid onset of action.[5]
  - Thionamides may be used as primary treatment in GD or in preparation for radioactive or surgical ablation. Pretreatment may be particularly important in the elderly and those with cardiac disease because of the potential for exacerbation of hyperthyroidism with radioiodine or surgery.[2]
  - **Agranulocytosis**, while infrequent, can occur with either drug at any time during therapy, usually early on. Although routine monitoring is generally not recommended, WBC count with differential should be obtained with febrile illnesses.
  - PTU infrequently causes **severe hepatitis;** methimazole rarely causes **cholestasis**.
  - Follow-up should be monthly with monitoring of thyroid function until the patient is euthyroid; thereafter, monitoring can be less frequent. Of note, TSH levels may be suppressed for weeks to months; therefore, T3 and T4 are better early measures of treatment success. T3 sometimes remains elevated longer that T4.
  - Once control is achieved, dosages may be decreased to avoid hypothyroidism.
  - Remission of GD may be achieved in some patients after 12–18 months of being on the antithyroid drug. Tapering and discontinuation of the medication can be attempted at this point. Patients should be monitored for relapse, which usually occurs in the initial 3–6 months after stopping treatment.[5]

Other Nonpharmacologic Therapies
Radioactive iodine (^{131}I) ablation is a definitive therapy for multinodular toxic goiter and GD.[5] Recurrence rate can be high, and follow-up for return of symptoms of hyperthyroidism and posttherapy hypothyroidism is important.[2]

Surgical Management
- **Total or subtotal thyroidectomy** may be performed if the previously mentioned therapies are contraindicated or have failed, there is significant mass effect from the goiter, or if it is needed for coexisting reasons like malignancy.[12]
- The surgery itself may trigger a perioperative exacerbation of hyperthyroidism.[6] Patients should be prepared for the procedure by one of two methods:
  - A thionamide until the patient is nearly euthyroid and supersaturated potassium iodide (SSKI) added 1–2 weeks before surgery (SSKI reduces vascularity of the thyroid in GD but is not used in multinodular toxic goiter where the gland tends to be less vascular[5])
  - β-Blocker and SSKI for 1–2 weeks before surgery

SPECIAL CONSIDERATIONS

- **Preoperative management**
  - Patients with well-controlled hyperthyroidism have no significant increase in operative morbidity or mortality.
  - Those with uncontrolled disease are at high risk for perioperative thyroid storm. Elective surgery should be postponed until they are euthyroid. If surgery cannot be delayed, many clinicians consult endocrinology and treat preoperatively with a loading dose of antithyroid medication, stress-dose steroids, SSKI, and β-blocker.[13]

- **Thyroid storm**
  - Thyroid storm and hyperthyroidism exacerbating congestive heart failure and acute coronary syndromes require urgent therapy.
  - To decrease T4 levels, thionamides (e.g., **PTU 500 mg load and then 250 mg q4h PO**) followed 1 hour later by **SSKI (250 mg q6h PO)** are used to block the release of T4 and T3 from the thyroid.
  - Stress-dose steroid (e.g., **hydrocortisone 100 mg q8h IV**) is often administered, which may treat an underlying adrenal insufficiency as well as decrease peripheral conversion of T4 to T3.
  - β-Blockers should be strongly considered (e.g., **propranolol, 60–80 mg PO q4h**).[5]
- **Subclinical hyperthyroidism**
  - Subclinical hyperthyroidism has been associated with progression to overt hyperthyroidism, atrial fibrillation, reduced bone mineral density, and possibly increased cardiovascular mortality.[7,14] The data, however, are of variable strength and sometimes conflicting.
  - Treatment is recommended when the TSH is <0.1, particularly for those >60 years of age and those with or at increased risk for heart disease and/or reduced bone mineral density.[1]

Hypothyroidism

GENERAL PRINCIPLES

- **Hypothyroidism** is defined as deficient secretion of T4 by the thyroid. The majority of the cases occur in women.
- **Subclinical hypothyroidism** is a laboratory diagnosis (TSH above the upper limit but FT4 and T3 within normal limits); theoretically, symptoms should be absent, although some studies suggest an increase in nonspecific findings. Also, median TSH is higher in the elderly; however, there is no age-based standard reference.
- Subclinical hypothyroidism may progress to overt hypothyroidism and therefore should be monitored.[14]
- Deficient secretion of T4 can result from impaired TSH stimulation of the thyroid gland or reduction of T4 production or release.[6]
- The vast majority of cases are primary in origin (Table 40-5).
- Hashimoto thyroiditis (chronic lymphocytic thyroiditis) is the most prevalent form of hypothyroidism with goiter in the United States and in other iodine-sufficient areas.
- Iatrogenic hypothyroidism from thyroidectomy or ^{131}I treatment is also very common.[6]
- Painful subacute thyroiditis due to a preceding viral illness or postpartum thyroiditis can cause transient hypothyroidism.[5]
- Secondary and tertiary causes are rare and include pituitary macroadenoma, empty sella syndrome, pituitary infarction (Sheehan syndrome), radiation, or surgery and often occur with other evidence of pituitary disease.[6]

DIAGNOSIS

Clinical Presentation

History

- Symptoms may include fatigue, somnolence, poor memory, weight gain (usually mild), depression, cold intolerance, hoarseness (with a compressive goiter), constipation, and menorrhagia.[6]
- Most signs and symptoms have an insidious onset. Inquire about anginal symptoms or coronary artery disease as therapy for hypothyroidism may worsen cardiac ischemia.[11]

TABLE 40-5 CAUSES OF PRIMARY HYPOTHYROIDISM

Disorder	Prevalence	Mechanism	Clinical Course
Hashimoto thyroiditis (chronic lymphocytic thyroiditis)	Most common cause in iodine-sufficient areas	Antithyroid Ab (antithyroglobulin and antiperoxidase)	May have transient increase in T4 (preformed release of the hormone); most cases progress to chronic subclinical or overt hypothyroidism
Iatrogenic hypothyroidism	Second most common cause in United States	Destruction or removal of thyroid follicular cells after treatment for hyperthyroidism	Chronic
Iodine deficiency	Most common cause worldwide; rare in the United States	Inhibition of hormone synthesis	Chronic if iodine deficiency not corrected
Painful subacute thyroiditis (de Quervain thyroiditis)	Exact prevalence not known	Postviral immune-mediated	Self-limiting; painful thyroid; may include transient increase in T4 for several weeks followed by decrease in T4 for several months; almost all patients recover fully in 6–12 mo.
Postpartum thyroiditis	5–9% of postpartum women	Associated with antiperoxidase Ab	Usually, decrease in T4 is transient but may be permanent in up to 25–30%.

- A medication history is essential, because thyroid hormone physiology may be altered by several drugs (Table 40-3).
- In its most severe form, hypothyroidism is called **myxedema coma**, often presenting with hypotension, heart failure, and altered mental status. Precipitating factors include severe infection, surgery, trauma, stroke, and medications.[6]

Physical Examination
- Findings may include slight bradycardia, goiter (painful in subacute thyroiditis), lateral eyebrow thinning, dry skin, myxedema skin changes (with severe disease), muscle weakness, pericardial or pleural effusions, and slowed relaxation of deep tendon reflexes.[11,13]
- Hypothermia, bradypnea, depressed mental status, and ileus may all be seen with myxedema coma. Notably, myxedema and coma per se are not requirements for the clinical diagnosis of myxedema coma, but some alteration in mental status is expected.[6]

Diagnostic Testing
- TSH is used for initial screening. At steady state, a normal TSH excludes primary hypothyroidism.[11]
- FT4 should be obtained next if the TSH is high or there is suspicion of central hypothyroidism.[15]
- TSH is elevated in primary hypothyroidism. A combination of low TSH and low FT4 is seen in central hypothyroidism (Table 40-4).
- Antithyroid antibodies (antiperoxidase being most specific) can help confirm the diagnosis of Hashimoto thyroiditis but does not need to be checked routinely.[9]
- High erythrocyte sedimentation rate and C-reactive protein are seen in subacute thyroiditis.[5]
- Associated abnormalities in hypothyroidism may include hypercholesterolemia (increased low-density lipoprotein and total cholesterol, reduction in high-density lipoprotein), mild normochromic normocytic anemia, hyponatremia, increased creatine kinase, and increased lactate dehydrogenase.[6]
- Consider testing adrenal axis in selected cases to rule out other pituitary hormone deficiencies.

TREATMENT

- **Levothyroxine is the drug of choice.**[11]
  - The therapeutic dose is generally **1.6–1.7 mcg/kg PO daily. Start therapy at 50–100 mcg/d,** with the lower dose used for the elderly.
  - In patients with coronary artery disease, a starting dose of 25 mcg/d PO is recommended, as replacement of T4 can precipitate cardiac ischemia.
  - Doses often need to be increased during pregnancy.
  - TSH should be monitored and dose changed by **12.5–25 mcg increments at 6-week intervals** until the patient is euthyroid.
  - Changing formulation of levothyroxine may result in alteration in the control of hypothyroidism.
- There is a lack of well-controlled research showing that combination of levothyroxine plus liothyronine is any more efficacious than levothyroxine alone, although in certain circumstances such as myxedema, expert opinions may vary.
- Treatment with desiccated thyroid is not recommended owing to its variable potency and bioavailability.
- In central hypothyroidism, thyroid hormone replacement should be based on normalization of T4 level; concomitant glucocorticoid therapy should be started if adrenal insufficiency is present.
- The discomfort of painful subacute thyroiditis may be treated with nonsteroidal anti-inflammatory drugs (NSAIDs) or, in severe cases, glucocorticoids. Levothyroxine is often not necessary for the mild, transient hypothyroidism seen in painful subacute thyroiditis.[16]

SPECIAL CONSIDERATIONS

- **Perioperative management**
  - Patients with mild hypothyroidism do well perioperatively.
  - Those with severe hypothyroidism should have elective surgery delayed until they are symptomatically improved.
  - If surgery cannot be delayed, patients may be treated preoperatively with a loading dose of T3 and T4 intravenously, along with stress dose of steroids if the status of the pituitary adrenal axis is uncertain. Afterwards, they may be switched to a maintenance dose of thyroid hormone. Symptoms of hypothyroidism and the magnitude of TSH

elevation should help guide selection of the loading dose. The effects of levothyroxine last for several days and cumulative levels can build up rapidly.[13]
- **Myxedema coma**
  - Provide urgent supportive measures, including intensive care unit monitoring. Hemodynamic assessment and mechanical ventilation may be necessary.
  - Check a random cortisol to evaluate for associated adrenal insufficiency. Stress-dose steroids are generally given.
  - Thyroid hormone is replaced with **levothyroxine, 50–100 mcg IV q6–8h for 24 hours initially, and then 75–100 mcg IV daily** until the patient is able to take medications PO reliably.
  - Some favor prescribing both levothyroxine and liothyronine during acute situation. **Loading dose of liothyronine at 5–20 mcg is followed by 2.5–10 mcg IV every 8 hours,** with care to avoid high serum T3 level as that is associated with increased mortality.
  - T3 and T4 should be measured every 1–2 days to follow treatment progress.[11]
- **Subclinical hypothyroidism**
  - Treatment of subclinical hypothyroidism is controversial and based on limited data.
  - Some advocate treatment when the TSH is >10 mIU/L; most patients, however, will have minor TSH elevations between 5 and 10 mIU/L.[1]
  - Treatment may also be tried in those individuals with lesser elevations of TSH with symptoms potentially referable to hypothyroidism or hypercholesterolemia.[17]
  - Care should be taken to avoid inducing subclinical hyperthyroidism.[11]
  - Treatment is recommended in pregnancy.[18]

Euthyroid Sick Syndrome

GENERAL PRINCIPLES

- Euthyroid sick syndrome is defined as changes in thyroid function tests associated with systemic illness, surgery, or fasting.[19] Signs and symptoms of thyroid dysfunction are absent.
- There is some controversy regarding this term, since whether or not these patients are truly euthyroid is unclear.
- This is one of the most common causes of thyroid test abnormalities in inpatients.

DIAGNOSIS

Typical changes in thyroid function tests seen with nonthyroidal illness may include the following[20]:

- **TSH levels may be low,** although undetectable levels usually indicate primary thyroid disease. A transient increase may be seen during recovery from illness.
- **Low serum T3** is seen in up to 70% of hospitalized patients. The serum free T3 is usually decreased by ~40%.
- **Low serum T4,** usually with a **normal free T4.**

TREATMENT

- Studies have not consistently indicated a benefit from thyroid hormone supplementation in this patient population; in fact, it may increase mortality.[11]
- Follow-up (preferably after recovery from acute illness) to confirm abnormal values before initiating any treatment.[19]

REFERENCES

1. Boelaert K. Thyroid dysfunction in the elderly. *Nat Rev Endocrinol* 2013;9:194–204.
2. Ross DS. Radioiodine therapy for hyperthyroidism. *N Engl J Med* 2011;364:542–50.
3. Blum MR, Bauer DC, Collet TH, et al. Subclinical thyroid dysfunction and fracture risk: a meta-analysis. *JAMA* 2015;313:2055–65.
4. Gan EH, Pearce SH. Clinical review: the thyroid in mind: cognitive function and low thyrotropin in older people. *J Clin Endocrinol Metab* 2012;97:3438–49.
5. Bahn RS, Burch HB, Cooper DS, et al. Hyperthyroidism and other causes of thyrotoxicosis: management guidelines of the American Thyroid Association and American Association of Clinical Endocrinologists. *Thyroid* 2011;21:593–646.
6. Hampton J. Thyroid gland disorder emergencies: thyroid storm and myxedema coma. *AACN Adv Crit Care* 2013;24:325–32.
7. Papaleontiou M, Haymart MR. Approach to and treatment of thyroid disorders in the elderly. *Med Clin N Am* 2012;96:297–310.
8. Surks M, Sievert R. Drugs and thyroid function. *N Engl J Med* 1995;333: 1688–94.
9. Abrams JJ, Grundy SM. Cholesterol metabolism in hypothyroidism and hyperthyroidism in man. *J Lipid Res* 1981;22:323–38.
10. Matthews DC, Syed AA. The role of TSH receptor antibodies in the management of Graves' disease. *Clin Interv Aging* 2012;7:97–111.
11. Jonklaas J, Bianco AC, Bauer AJ, et al. Guidelines for the treatment of hypothyroidism: prepared by the American Thyroid Association Task Force on Thyroid Hormone Replacement. *Thyroid* 2014;24:1670–751.
12. Hoang JK, Sosa JA, Nguyen XV, et al. Imaging thyroid disease. *Radiol Clin North Am* 2015;53:145–61.
13. Mehta V, Savino JA. Surgical management of the patient with a thyroid disorder. In: Gambert SR, ed. *Clin Geriatr Med* 1995;11:291–309.
14. Gencer B, Collet TH, Virgini V, et al. Subclinical thyroid dysfunction and the risk of heart failure events: an individual participant data analysis from 6 prospective cohorts. *Circulation* 2012;126:1040–9.
15. Bensenor IM, Olmos RD, Lotufo PA. Hypothyroidism in the elderly: diagnosis and management. *Clin Interv Aging* 2012;7:97–111.
16. Benbassat CA, Olchovsky D, Tsvetov G, Shimon I. Subacute thyroiditis: clinical characteristics and treatment outcome in fifty-six consecutive patients diagnosed between 1995 and 2005. *J Endocrinol Invest* 2007;30:631–5.
17. Tabatabaie V, Surks MI. The aging thyroid. *Curr Opin Endocrinol Diabetes Obes* 2013;20:455–9.
18. Esteves-Villar H, Saconato H, Valente O, Atallah AN. Thyroid hormone replacement for subclinical hypothyroidism. *Cochrane Database Syst Rev* 2007;CD003419.
19. Pantalone KM, Nasr C. Approach to a low TSH: patience is a virtue. *Cleve Clin J Med* 2010;77: 803–11.
20. Chopra IJ. Euthyroid sick syndrome: is it a misnomer? *J Clin Endocrinol Metab* 1997;82:329–33.

Adrenal Insufficiency

M. Phillip Fejleh and Mark S. Thoelke

GENERAL PRINCIPLES

- Adrenal insufficiency (AI) is defined as inadequate production of cortisol ± aldosterone by the adrenal gland.
- Primary AI refers to decreased production due to dysfunction of the adrenal gland.
- Secondary insufficiency occurs secondary to interruption of hypothalamic–pituitary–adrenal (HPA) axis, leading to decreased adrenal gland function.
- "Tertiary insufficiency" is sometimes used to describe patients with iatrogenic adrenal suppression from chronic steroid supplementation.
- The various etiologies of AI are presented in Table 41-1.

DIAGNOSIS

Clinical Presentation

History
- Acute AI often presents in inpatients as a result of undiagnosed chronic insufficiency with decompensation secondary to physiologic stressors.
- **It is essential to obtain a thorough medication history** to rule out recent (up to 1 year) or chronic steroid use. Patients taking 20 mg of prednisone for 3 weeks or more are presumed to have some degree of suppression. Conversely, patients on ≤5 mg of prednisone per day are presumed to have an intact HPA axis. Those in the middle ground must undergo testing to be properly assessed.
- Patients with acquired immunodeficiency syndrome (AIDS) are at high risk for adrenal failure.
- **Symptoms** occur as a consequence of decreased levels of cortisol ± aldosterone and may include fatigue/weakness/light-headedness/fever, anorexia/weight loss, myalgias/joint pain, nausea/vomiting/abdominal pain, and salt craving.
- Autoimmune AI is frequently associated with other autoimmune disorders, such as type I diabetes mellitus, Hashimoto thyroiditis, vitiligo, and others. Additional symptoms in rarer cases of pituitary dysfunction or mass may include amenorrhea, cold intolerance, headache, or visual field loss.
- History of recent abdominal surgery or anticoagulation should increase suspicion of adrenal hemorrhage. Overwhelming infection with ***Pseudomonas* species, meningococcus, or pneumococcus** may result in hemorrhagic necrosis of the adrenal gland (Waterhouse-Friderichsen syndrome).
- Inquire about a history of malignancy (metastases to the pituitary or adrenals), B-symptoms (AI secondary to lymphoma), pulmonary symptoms (sarcoidosis), visual changes (pituitary mass), and irradiation to the head and neck.

Physical Examination
- Orthostatic hypotension, shock, fever, or hypothermia may be evident.
- Auricular cartilage calcifications may be present in chronic AI.

TABLE 41-1 CAUSES OF ADRENAL INSUFFICIENCY

Primary	Secondary
Autoimmune adrenalitis[a]	Suppression of gland secondary to chronic glucocorticoid use[a]
Adrenal hemorrhage (meningococcal sepsis)	Pituitary infection (cytomegalovirus, toxoplasmosis)
Infiltrative disease (amyloidosis, malignancy, sarcoidosis, hemochromatosis)	Pituitary tumor or infarction (Sheehan syndrome)
Adrenal infection (tuberculosis, fungal, cytomegalovirus)	Pituitary irradiation
Medications[b]	
Acquired immunodeficiency syndrome	

[a]Most common etiologies.

[b]Several medications may interrupt adrenal function or change cortisol metabolism, including ketoconazole, rifampin, phenytoin, opiates, and megestrol.

- Abdominal tenderness may be present.
- There may be hyperpigmentation (in primary adrenal failure secondary to increased adrenocorticotropic hormone [ACTH]), loss of axillary or pubic hair (especially in women), and signs of volume depletion.
- Classic signs of AI may be present but are nonspecific; therefore, a high level of clinical suspicion is critical.

Diagnostic Testing

Laboratories

- Primary and secondary failure (due to glucocorticoid deficiency) may present with hyponatremia, fasting hypoglycemia, normocytic anemia, hypercalcemia, lymphocytosis, and/or eosinophilia. Primary adrenal failure (secondary to concomitant aldosterone deficiency) may also present with hyperkalemia, urine Na >20 mEq/L, and a non–anion gap metabolic acidosis.
- **Morning cortisol level**: A morning cortisol level is useful in diagnosing insufficiency only if levels are very low (<3 mcg/dL). **The sensitivity of morning cortisol levels in diagnosing AI is very low.** Levels are frequently elevated in acutely ill patients, although the patient still may be unable to mount an appropriate response to increased stress. It is recommended to proceed directly to "dynamic testing" with the cosyntropin stimulation test.
- The **cosyntropin stimulation test** assesses the ability of the adrenal gland to respond to ACTH. This test can be performed any time of day, but time of day and illness will affect basal levels. After 250 mcg of cosyntropin is given IV or IM, cortisol levels are traditionally measured at baseline and at 30 and 60 minutes after injection. However, drawing cortisol levels at only the 30-minute mark is likely to be adequate, reducing confusion and patient discomfort.[1,2] The 250-mcg dose is supraphysiologic and simply represents the amount contained in a standard vial.
  - **Peak cortisol levels of >20 mcg/dL are normal and essentially rule out AI.**
  - One limitation of the cosyntropin stimulation test is in patients with recent-onset secondary AI, where the adrenals will still respond normally to the exogenous ACTH.[3]
  - Another note of caution is that low protein may lead to low total cortisol levels in the face of normal free cortisol levels.[4]

- An **ACTH level** is useful in **differentiating primary from secondary causes**. ACTH should be elevated in primary causes and may be decreased in secondary causes.
- **Pituitary function tests** are useful if there is suspicion of pituitary dysfunction. Consider serum T_4, TSH, or testosterone (in men).

Imaging
A computed tomography (CT) scan of the abdomen may be obtained to rule out adrenal hemorrhage. CT of the head or magnetic resonance imaging (MRI) of the brain may be obtained if there is suspicion of a pituitary mass or infarction.

TREATMENT

- **Acute adrenal crisis is a medical emergency; therapy should be initiated immediately if clinical suspicion is high**. Therapy should include the following:
  - Aggressive IV fluid hydration with D5NS to support blood pressure and correct hypoglycemia and/or hyponatremia
  - Hydrocortisone, 100 mg IV q8h slowly tapered over several days
  - If the diagnosis of AI is not yet established, hydrocortisone may be replaced with dexamethasone (which does not interfere with cortisol measurements) until cosyntropin testing has been completed.
- **Long-term maintenance therapy** for primary adrenal sufficiency should include prednisone (2.5–5 mg PO bid) or hydrocortisone (20–25 mg/d PO divided bid) along with mineralocorticoid repletion with fludrocortisone (0.05–0.3 mg PO qd). Doses are adjusted based on correction of symptoms and electrolyte abnormalities.
- **Patients with known primary or secondary AI should be treated empirically in situations of stress** (acute illness, perioperatively, injury) with high-dose hydrocortisone. Stress doses depend on the stressor. A long taper after surgery is not necessary and may retard wound healing.
- **Contrary to past dogma, patients with AI secondary to chronic steroid use likely do not require stress dosing for acute illness or for surgery**. Past recommendations were based on an untested proposal by the authors of an early case report of operative death in a patient on steroids. The best studies available show that there is little benefit in offering stress-dose steroids (in addition to maintenance dosing) for mild- to moderate-risk surgery or acute illness.[5] This obviates the need for testing the HPA axis. On a practical level, changing to an IV form of steroids the day of surgery may be beneficial, as it is less likely to be held in patients taking nothing by mouth. If there is any concern, supplemental replacement may be given (see below).
- Additionally, the relative AI and physiologic dose steroids in sepsis concept have been largely abandoned.[6] Septic shock patients who are not responding to conventional therapies should be offered empiric steroids without testing the HPA axis. Dosage recommendations for stress-dose steroids are relatively imprecise and should be individualized. Coursin et al. recommend the following:[7]
  - **Minor stress** (e.g., hernia repair, mild febrile illness): a single dose of hydrocortisone 25 mg
  - **Moderate stress** (e.g., open cholecystectomy, significant febrile illness): hydrocortisone 50–75 mg/d tapered quickly over the next 1–2 days
  - **Major stress** (e.g., coronary artery bypass grafting): hydrocortisone 100–150 mg/d tapered quickly over the next 1–2 days
  - **Critical illness** (e.g., sepsis/shock): 50–100 mg hydrocortisone IV q6–8h plus fludrocortisone 0.5 mg/d[8]
- Patients with established AI should be provided with medical alert bracelets identifying their diagnosis.

REFERENCES

1. Lindholm J, Kehlet H. Re-evaluation of the clinical value of the 30 min ACTH test in assessing the hypothalamic-pituitary-adrenocortical function. *Clin Endocrinol (Oxf)* 1987;26:53–9.
2. Hurel SJ, Thompson CJ, Watson MJ, et al. The short Synacthen and insulin stress tests in the assessment of the hypothalamic-pituitary-adrenal axis. *Clin Endocrinol (Oxf)* 1996;44:141–6.
3. Dorin RI, Qualls CR, Crapo LM. Diagnosis of adrenal insufficiency. *Ann Intern Med* 2003;139:194–204.
4. Hamrahian AH, Oseni TS, Arafah BM. Measurements of serum free cortisol in critically ill patients. *N Engl J Med* 2004;350:1629–38.
5. Brown CJ, Buie WD. Perioperative stress dose steroids: do they make a difference? *J Am Coll Surg* 2001;193:678–86.
6. Dellinger RP, Levy MM, Rhodes A, et al. Surviving sepsis campaign: international guidelines for management of severe sepsis and septic shock, 2012. *Intensive Care Med* 2013;39:165–228.
7. Coursin DB, Wood KE. Corticosteroid supplementation for adrenal insufficiency. *JAMA* 2002;287:236–40.
8. Annane D, Sébille V, Charpentier C, et al. Effect of treatment with low doses of hydrocortisone and fludrocortisone on mortality in patients with septic shock. *JAMA* 2002;288:862–71.

Approach to the Adrenal Incidentaloma

Lauren S. Levine and William E. Clutter

GENERAL PRINCIPLES

- The likelihood of discovering an adrenal incidentaloma on computed tomography (CT) scanning performed for other reasons excluding the staging and workup of a known malignancy depends on the patient's age and probably varies from 0.4% up to 10% in those >70 years old.[1]
- The prevalence is about 2% of patients at autopsy with a range of 1–9% and higher prevalence in obese, diabetic, and hypertensive patients.[2]
- The distribution of resultant pathologic diagnoses varies widely among studies, but the majority are benign. The medical consultant is often called to evaluate an adrenal mass found on abdominal imaging on the surgical service.
- The large majority of adrenal incidentalomas are nonfunctioning adenomas.
- Those that are functional adenomas include the following:
  - Subclinical Cushing syndrome
  - Conn syndrome (primary hyperaldosteronism)
- Other etiologies include the following:
  - Subclinical pheochromocytoma
  - Metastatic lesions (usually lung cancer; less commonly renal cell, breast, and melanoma)
  - Primary adrenocortical cancers are very rare. They may be functional or nonfunctional. The possibility of malignancy increases with mass size.
  - Myelolipoma
  - Ganglioneuroma
  - Adrenal cyst
- Approximately 10% of adrenal masses are bilateral. The etiology of bilateral adrenal masses includes metastatic disease, cortical adenomas, congenital adrenal hyperplasia, lymphoma, fungal or tubercular infection, and infiltrative disease (amyloidosis, sarcoidosis), among others.[3]

DIAGNOSIS

Clinical Presentation

- Subtle indicators of cortisol excess may be present in "early Cushing syndrome" presenting as an incidentaloma without overt symptoms.
- The presence of the triad of hypertension (HTN), headache, and sweating favors the diagnosis of pheochromocytoma. Its absence renders it an exceedingly unlikely diagnosis.
- The association of drug-resistant refractory HTN requiring >3 antihypertensive agents and hypokalemia increases the likelihood of hyperaldosteronism (Conn syndrome).
- Evidence of another primary malignancy should be sought from the history. Inquire about family history of adrenal tumors, multiple endocrine neoplasia (MEN) syndromes, or other familial pheochromocytoma syndromes.

- Also look for evidence of nonclassic congenital adrenal hyperplasia (21-hydroxylase deficiency), which sometimes presents as an adrenal mass in adulthood. Hirsutism, oligomenorrhea, acne, and frontal balding (in females) are the most common symptoms in adults.[4]

Diagnostic Testing

Laboratories

- Characteristically, **subclinical Cushing syndrome** (SCS) will be associated with normal 24-hour urine and 8 a.m. serum cortisol but without circadian rhythms. The 10 p.m. cortisol may be elevated and 1-mg overnight **dexamethasone suppression tests** will be positive, as defined by a serum cortisol level exceeding 2.0 μg/dL.[2] Since pituitary Cushing disease is not a consideration, some physicians have skipped directly to the high-dose dexamethasone test. The diagnosis of SCS is further supported by a suppressed adrenocorticotropic hormone (ACTH) level or low dehydroepiandrosterone sulfate (DHEA-S) concentration.
- Biochemical assessment for **pheochromocytoma** is reasonable for all patients. The **24-hour urine fractionated metanephrine and normetanephrine** have high sensitivity and specificity. If they are normal and suspicion still high, fractionated free metanephrines may be done, but the specificity is low. Pheochromocytoma should be ruled out before surgical or fine-needle manipulation of the adrenal is considered.[5]
- **Primary hyperaldosteronism** is associated with hypokalemia, but potassium can be normal. The **morning aldosterone-to-renin ratio** can be used as a screen and should probably be done in all hypertensive patients with an incidentaloma.[6] An aldosterone-to-renin ratio >20 in the absence of spironolactone or mineralocorticoid receptor blockers is highly suggestive of primary hyperaldosteronism. Other biochemical tests will be needed for confirmation.
- Increased adrenal androgens are seen in nonclassic congenital adrenal hyperplasia. The definitive test is 17-hyroxyprogesterone before and 60 minutes after cosyntropin administration. Routine testing is probably not necessary unless there are clinical signs of androgen excess.[7]
- Adrenocortical carcinoma may result in Cushing syndrome and/or virilization or be nonfunctional; testing for both may be indicated. Plasma DHEA-S should be measured since it may be the only biochemical abnormality in this disease.

Imaging

Imaging characteristics of various adrenal tumors are presented in Table 42-1.[6] **Nearly all lesions <4 cm are benign**.

Diagnostic Procedures

Pheochromocytoma should be ruled out prior to needle biopsy, as it may precipitate a hypertensive crisis or hemorrhage. Fine needle biopsy may be used to confirm metastatic disease; however, it cannot distinguish a benign adrenal adenoma from adrenal adenocarcinoma. Because of the risk of seeding cancer cells if a primary adrenal malignancy is suspected, surgical exploration is indicated. Negative cytology does not rule out malignancy.[8]

TREATMENT

The appropriate management of adrenal masses is not precisely defined.

- Functional adrenal masses: Surgical excision should generally be performed when there are symptoms related to and biochemical evidence of glucocorticoid, catecholamine, adrenal sex hormone, or mineralocorticoid excess. The long-term benefit of adrenalectomy for SCS remains unclear. Therefore, surgical resection should only be considered in cases of worsening HTN, glucose intolerance, hyperlipidemia, or osteoporosis.

TABLE 42-1 IMAGING CHARACTERISTICS OF ADRENAL TUMORS

	Benign Adenoma	Pheochromocytoma	Metastases	Adrenocortical Carcinoma
Size	<4 cm	Variable	Variable	>4 cm
Shape/border	Round, smooth, sharp	Round, smooth, sharp	Irregular, ill-defined	Irregular, ill-defined
Texture	Homogeneous	Inhomogeneous	Inhomogeneous	Inhomogeneous
CT appearance	<10 HU, limited enhancement with contrast	>10 HU, vascular enhancement with contrast, delayed contrast washout	>10 HU, vascular enhancement with contrast, delayed contrast washout	>10 HU, vascular enhancement with contrast, delayed contrast washout
MRI appearance	Isointensity with liver, signal drop on chemical shift imaging.	High T2 signal intensity	High T2 signal intensity	High T2 signal intensity
Other	Usually unilateral, very slow growth	Sometimes bilateral, slow growth, cystic. Hemorrhagic changes may be seen.	Often bilateral, variable growth	Usually unilateral, fast growth, necrosis, hemorrhage, and calcification common. Evidence of metastasis may be seen.

CT, computed tomography; HU, Hounsfield units; MRI, magnetic resonance imaging.

Data from Young WF Jr. Clinical practice. The incidentally discovered adrenal mass. *N Engl J Med* 2007;356:601–10.

- Large adrenal masses (>6 cm): It is recommended that **all adrenal lesions >6 cm be excised** owing to the much increased risk of malignancy. Open adrenalectomy should be performed if adrenocortical carcinoma is suspected, particularly in the case of masses >10 cm.[9]
- Intermediate adrenal masses (4–6 cm): Adrenalectomy should be strongly considered for lesions that have malignant imaging characteristics (Table 42-1). If not, close follow-up with repeat imaging is reasonable, but the appropriate frequency is unclear. Annual overnight dexamethasone suppression test for 4 years has also been recommended in light of the fact that novel glucocorticoid autonomous function may be detected during follow-up in some cases. However, the yield from this strategy remains unclear. The selection of appropriate serial imaging interval and imaging modality should be based on individual circumstance and clinical judgment.[2]
- Small nonfunctional masses (<4 cm): Presuming that the imaging appearance of such lesion is not suggestive of malignancy, the utility and frequency of follow-up imaging are currently unclear.

REFERENCES

1. Bovio S, Cataldi A, Reimondo G, et al. Prevalence of adrenal incidentaloma in a contemporary computerized tomography series. *J Endocrinol Invest* 2006;29:298–302.
2. Terzolo M, Stigliano A, Chiodini I, et al. AME Position Statement on adrenal incidentaloma. *Eur J Endocrinol* 2011;164:851–70.
3. Barzon L, Scaroni C, Sonino N. Incidentally discovered adrenal tumors: endocrine and scintigraphic correlates. *J Clin Endocrinol Metab* 1998;83:55–62.
4. Allolio B, Fassnacht M. Clinical review: adrenocortical carcinoma: clinical update. *J Clin Endocrinol Metab* 2006;91:2027–37.
5. Vanderveen K, Thompson S, Callstrom M, et al. Biopsy of pheochromocytomas and paragangliomas: potential for disaster. *Surgery* 2009;146:1158–66.
6. Young WF Jr. Clinical practice. The incidentally discovered adrenal mass. *N Engl J Med* 2007;356:601–10.
7. Speiser PW, White PC. Congenital adrenal hyperplasia. *N Engl J Med* 2003;349:776–88.
8. Mazzaglia P. Limited value of adrenal biopsy in the evaluation of adrenal neoplasm. *Arch Surg* 2009;144:465.
9. Gonzalez R, Shapiro S, Sarlis N, et al. Laparoscopic resection of adrenal cortical carcinoma: a cautionary note. *Surgery* 2005;138:1078–86.

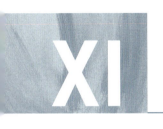

XI Rheumatology

Approach to the Patient with Positive Antinuclear Antibodies

Adam Littich

GENERAL PRINCIPLES

- Antinuclear antibodies (ANA) are autoantibodies that target normal nuclear constituents such as DNA, RNA, and nuclear proteins.
- These autoantibodies are produced in a variety of normal and inflammatory states and are nonspecific. Therefore, they are most useful when ordered to confirm a diagnosis that has been made on clinical grounds, such as that of systemic lupus erythematosus (SLE).
- Greater than 95% of SLE patients have a positive ANA with a titer of >1:160.[1] Thus, a negative ANA is usually helpful in excluding the diagnosis of SLE. The same cannot be said of other autoimmune connective tissue diseases, as only approximately half have a positive ANA.[2] Therefore, due to its lower sensitivity in other connective tissue diseases, ANA is not recommended to broadly rule out connective tissue diseases or autoimmunity and **should not** be ordered unless strong clinical suspicion of disease exists.
- Furthermore, ANA **should not** be ordered in patients with fibromyalgia or nonspecific symptoms such as fatigue or generalized myalgia.[3] Unfortunately, the most common reason for nonrheumatologists to order ANA is widespread pain.[4]

Definition

- The ANA test is performed by incubating control human cells derived from a cell line of human epithelial tumor cells (HEp2 cells) with a patient's serum and developing with anti–human immunoglobulin that is fluorescein tagged.
- A positive result is determined using indirect immunofluorescence microscopy and often reported along with the staining pattern—see classification below.
- Traditionally, ANA testing detected antinuclear antibodies; however, the term is somewhat of a misnomer as most laboratories now report both nuclear and cytoplasmic results.
- Newer methods rely on an enzyme-linked immunosorbent assay (ELISA), which is more sensitive, but may be less specific.[5]

Classification

- The reporting of staining pattern can aid in determining the type of autoantibodies present and disease association (see Table 43-1).[1,6–11]
- It is important to note that this is a relatively subjective process and open to significant laboratory or individual variation. In addition, labs may use different terminology to describe the staining pattern, though an attempt is being made at standardization.[6]
- The following are some of the more useful staining patterns:
  - Nuclear homogenous: associated with anti-dsDNA, antihistone, and antinucleosome and suggest SLE or drug-induced SLE.[12] **Never** found in the healthy.[13]
  - Nuclear large/coarse speckled: associated with anti-RNP and suggest MCTD or SLE.[12] **Never** found in the healthy.[13]
  - Nuclear fine speckled: most common pattern, but nonspecific. Most common pattern found in both healthy and those with true disease.[13]

TABLE 43-1 AUTOANTIBODIES AND DISEASE ASSOCIATIONS

Disease	ANA[1]	Pattern[6]	dsDNA[7]	Sm[8]	SS-A/Ro[9]	SS-B/La[9]	Scl-70[10]	Centromere[10]	Jo-1[11]	RNP[8]
Systemic lupus erythematosus	>95%	P,H,S	50–60%	20–30%	10–35%	5–15%	—	—	—	25–50%
Rheumatoid arthritis	30–45	H,Cy	—[a]	—	10	—	—	—	—	5–10
Sjögren syndrome	40–50	S,N	—	—	30–50	20–40	—	—	—	10
Diffuse systemic sclerosis	>85	S,N,H,Cy	—	—	—	—	20–40	25–35	—	10–15
Limited systemic sclerosis	>85	S,N,H,C	—	—	—	—	<15	45–65	—	10–15
Polymyositis and dermatomyositis	60–75	Cy	—	—	—	—	—	—	20–30	—
Mixed connective tissue disease	>95	S,Cy	—	—	—	—	—	—	—	>95

ANA, antinuclear antibody; Jo-1, anti-Jo-1 antibody; RNP, antiribonucleoprotein; Sm, anti-Smith; SS-A/Ro, anti-Sjögren syndrome A/Ro; SS-B/La, anti-Sjögren syndrome-B/La; S, nuclear **s**peckled; H, nuclear **h**omogenous; P, nuclear **p**eripheral or rim; N, **n**ucleolar; C, **c**entromere; Cy, **cy**toplasmic.

[a]Note: Dash (—) indicates antibody found rarely (0–5%), but exceptions may occur.

- Nuclear dense fine speckled: **only** occurs in healthy individuals.[13] Associated with anti-DFS70 antibody, which is also nearly exclusively found in the healthy.[14]
- Nuclear centromere: anticentromere and suggests limited systemic sclerosis (also known as CREST syndrome).[12] **Never** found in the healthy.[13]
- Nuclear peripheral or rim pattern: specific and suggests SLE.[12]
- Nucleolar: anti-Scl-70 (also known as anti–topoisomerase I) and anti-PM/SCL; often seen in systemic sclerosis.[12]
- Cytoplasmic diffuse: anti–Jo-1; can be associated with inflammatory myopathies.[12]
- Cytoplasmic fine speckled: anti–Jo-1; inflammatory myopathies.[12]

Epidemiology

- The incidence of a positive ANA increases with age and is also higher in females.[15]
- A positive ANA is found in a large percentage of the healthy population; 25–30% have a titer of 1:40, 10–15% a titer of 1:80, and 5% a titer of 1:160.[1]
- Some variability exists among different nationalities:
  - Brazil: 13% had titer 1:80.[13]
  - India: 12% had titer 1:40.[16]
  - Japan: 26% had titer 1:40.[17]
  - China: 14% had titer 1:100.[18]

Etiology

The differential for a positive ANA is very broad and includes the following[19]:

- Healthy individual
- Other autoimmune connective tissue disease (Table 43-1)
- Malignancy
- Chronic infection (e.g., TB, viral hepatitis, endocarditis)
- Acute infection (e.g., viral, some parasites)
- Drug-induced lupus, or simply caused by drug without signs of lupus
- Autoimmune hematologic disorders (e.g., idiopathic thrombocytopenia purpura, hemolytic anemia)
- Autoimmune GI disorders (e.g., autoimmune hepatitis, inflammatory bowel disease, primary biliary cholangitis)
- Autoimmune endocrine disorders (e.g., type I diabetes mellitus, Hashimoto thyroiditis, Graves disease)
- Autoimmune neurologic disorder (e.g., multiple sclerosis, myasthenia gravis)

Pathophysiology

Typically, autoantibodies tend to form years before the onset of clinical disease.[20] Patients with a high ANA titer may need to be followed for any developing signs of connective tissue disease, though many patients will never develop disease, and 25% of healthy patients will eventually revert to a negative titer.[13] Despite this, serial testing of ANA is **not** recommended.

Risk Factors

Increasing age,[15] female sex,[15] and having a first-degree relative with positive ANA[14] or an actual autoimmune disorder[21] are all risk factors for having a positive ANA.

DIAGNOSIS

Clinical Presentation

History

The most important step in evaluating the patient is to obtain a good history with emphasis on rheumatic symptoms. The American College of Rheumatology classification criteria

TABLE 43-2 1997 UPDATE OF THE 1982 AMERICAN COLLEGE OF RHEUMATOLOGY REVISED CRITERIA FOR CLASSIFICATION OF SYSTEMIC LUPUS ERYTHEMATOSUS

4 of the Following 11 Criteria Must be Met

Criterion	Description
Malar rash	Fixed erythema, flat or raised, over the malar eminences tending to spare the nasolabial folds
Discoid rash	Erythematosus raised patches with adherent keratotic scaling and follicular plugging. Atrophic scarring may occur.
Photosensitivity	Skin rash as a result of unusual reaction to sunlight
Oral or nasopharyngeal ulcers	Usually painless
Arthritis	Nonerosive, inflammatory in two or more peripheral joints
Serositis	Pleuritis *OR* pericarditis
Renal disorder	Persistent proteinuria >0.5 g/24 h or >3+ on spot *OR* cellular casts
Neurologic disorder	Seizures *OR* psychosis in absence of known cause
Hematologic	Hemolytic anemia, *OR* leukopenia (<4000/mm^3), *OR* lymphopenia (<1500/mm^3), *OR* thrombocytopenia (<100,000/mm^3)
Immunologic disorder	Antibodies to dsDNA or Smith (Sm) *OR* positive antiphospholipid antibodies (IgG or IgM anticardiolipin antibodies, lupus anticoagulant, or false-positive serologic test for syphilis for at least 6 mo)
Antinuclear antibody	Positive test

Data from Tan EM Cohen AS, Fries JF, et al. The 1982 revised criteria for the classification of systemic lupus erythematosus. *Arthritis Rheum* 1982;25(11):1271–7; Hochberg MC. Updating the American College of Rheumatology revised criteria for the classification of systemic lupus erythematosus. *Arthritis Rheum* 1997;40(9):1725.

(Table 43-2)[22,23] for the diagnosis of lupus can help guide clinical suspicion regarding pretest probability of a positive ANA, and these features should be sought when evaluating any patient with a positive ANA.

Physical Examination

The presence of rheumatologic signs may be varied and subtle in patients with a connective tissue disease, but a careful exam includes looking for the following:

- Head, ears, eyes, nose, and throat: uveitis, dry eyes or oropharynx, oral ulcers, or malar rash
- Chest: crackles or pleural rub
- Cardiovascular: pericardial rub
- Musculoskeletal: joint tenderness, effusion, or chronic destruction/deformity

- Skin: rash, palpable purpura, sclerotic skin changes, or Raynaud phenomenon
- Neurologic: proximal muscle weakness, psychosis without other known cause

Diagnostic Testing

- Again, the most important workup of a positive ANA is a thorough history and physical. Many times, the diagnosis of a false-positive ANA can be made on this basis alone.
- Other basic studies including CXR, urinalysis, complete blood count, and comprehensive metabolic panel are helpful to evaluate for organ involvement.
- Many tests are available for further workup of a positive ANA, but like the ANA itself, many are relatively nonspecific and the workup should be guided by clinical suspicion. Only test for ANA subserologies (below) with a positive ANA **AND** clinical suspicion of immune-mediated disease.[24]
- Factors of the ANA that would favor a **true positive**:
  - Higher ANA titers >1:160.[5]
  - Very high titer >1:640 should be given special attention, as the positive predictive value for autoimmune rheumatic disease at this titer is 25%.[4]
  - Certain patterns of the ANA, including nuclear homogenous, nuclear coarse speckled, and nuclear centromeric, are nearly 100% specific for autoimmune rheumatic diseases.[5]
- Factors that favor a **false-positive** ANA[5]:
  - Titer <1:160
  - Nuclear dense fine speckled pattern, which is only seen in healthy individuals.
- Rheumatology consultation may be considered if high-risk factors are present on clinical or laboratory evaluation. Interestingly, in a 2003 retrospective study, positive ANA was detected in 78% of patients who were eventually diagnosed with SLE, up to 9 years prior to the diagnosis being made.[20] This would suggest a pre-SLE state and would imply a need for follow-up for patients with positive ANA, especially those with high-risk factors, in order to monitor for the manifestation of other clinical hallmarks of connective tissue disease. This follow-up may be with the primary care physician or rheumatology.
- ANA subserologies can be ordered based on positive ANA AND clinical suspension, as discussed above. ANA subserologies include the following[6]:
  - **Extractable nuclear antigens (ENA) panel**: this test encompasses a panel of saline-soluble nuclear antigens usually including, but not limited to, Smith (Sm), Sjögren syndrome-A/Ro (SS-A) and Sjögren Syndrome-B/La (SS-B), and ribonucleoprotein (RNP) antigens. While so named because of the laboratory method originally used to discover these antigens, the term ENA has come to be used mainly to denote a panel of autoantibodies and may include autoantibodies that are neither extractable nor nuclear.
  - **Anticentromere antibodies**: directed against 70/13 kDa proteins making up the centromere complex of the chromosome and are associated with limited systemic sclerosis (aka CREST syndrome).
  - **Anti-dsDNA antibodies**: directed against double-stranded DNA, specific for SLE. One of the few autoantibodies that correlate with disease activity; can be used for monitoring.
  - **Antihistone antibodies**: commonly seen in patients with drug-induced lupus.
  - **Anti–Jo-1 antibodies**: directed against histidyl tRNA synthetase and associated with myositis.
  - **Antiphospholipid antibodies**: includes IgG, IgM, and IgA anticardiolipin antibodies, lupus anticoagulant antibody, anti-β2 glycoprotein I, and antiphosphatidylserine. Can be seen in antiphospholipid antibody syndrome alone or as part of SLE.
  - **Anti-RNP antibodies**: directed against U1 snRNP protein–RNA complex. Highly associated with mixed connective tissue disease (MCTD); also found in SLE.

- **Anti–Scl-70 antibodies**: directed against topoisomerase I; is associated with diffuse systemic sclerosis.
- **Anti–SS-A/Ro and anti–SS-B/La**: antibodies against a 52/60 and 47 kDa proteins, respectively. Associated with Sjögren syndrome and SLE.
- **Anti-Smith antibodies**: named after the patient in whom it was discovered, antibody system of multiple antibodies against a series of protein–RNA complexes called snRNPs. Highly specific for SLE.
- **Anticyclic citrullinated peptide (CCP)**: directed against a citrullinated form of the protein filaggrin; associated with rheumatoid arthritis. More specific than RF.
- **Rheumatoid factor (RF)**: an immune complex of IgM that binds to the F_c portion of IgG. RF is elevated in ~80% of patients with RA, but this test is nonspecific, also being positive in Sjögren syndrome, sarcoidosis, chronic infections, and other conditions where immune complexes are formed.
- **Erythrocyte sedimentation rate (ESR)**: the ESR is a very nonspecific indicator of inflammation and is often elevated in any inflammatory condition. Anemia, kidney disease (especially proteinuria), and aging can all elevate the ESR in the absence of inflammation.
- **C-reactive protein (CRP)**: CRP is an acute-phase reactant and a component of the innate immune system that rises rapidly with inflammation and infection and falls quickly as inflammation resolves. Unlike the ESR, the CRP is not influenced by anemia or abnormal erythrocytes.
- **Complement**: usually C3 and C4, often CH50 (total complement); part of the complement cascade; ordered to assess immune complex–mediated disease activity in SLE.

TREATMENT

Generally, treatment is directed toward the underlying disease and is etiology specific. No treatment is needed for ANA-positive patients without underlying autoimmune rheumatic disease.

REFERENCES

1. Solomon DH, Kavanaugh AJ, Schur PH. Evidence-based guidelines for the use of immunologic tests: antinuclear antibody testing. *Arthritis Rheum* 2002;47:434–44.
2. Slater CA, Davis RB, Shmerling RH. Antinuclear antibody testing: a study of clinical utility. *Arch Intern Med* 1996;156:1421–5.
3. Qaseem A, Alguire P, Dallas P, et al. Appropriate use of screening and diagnostic tests to foster high-value, cost-conscious care. *Ann Intern Med* 2012;156:147–9.
4. Abeles AM, Abeles M. The clinical utility of a positive antinuclear antibody test result. *Am J Med* 2013;26:342–8.
5. Emlen W, O'Neill L. Clinical significance of antinuclear antibodies: comparison of detection with immunofluorescence and enzyme-linked immunosorbent assays. *Arthritis Rheum* 1997;40:1612–8.
6. Chan EK, Damoiseaux J, Carballo OG, et al. Report of the first international consensus on standardized nomenclature of antinuclear antibody HEp-2 cell patterns 2014–2015. *Front Immunol* 2015;6:1–13.
7. Kavanaugh AF, Solomon DH. Guidelines for immunologic laboratory testing in the rheumatic diseases: anti-DNA antibody tests. *Arthritis Rheum* 2002;47:546–55.
8. Benito-Garcia E, Schur PH, Lahita R. Guidelines for immunologic laboratory testing in the rheumatic diseases: anti-Sm and anti-RNP antibody tests. *Arthritis Rheum* 2004;51:1030–44.
9. Shiboski SC, Shiboski CH, Criswell LA, et al. American College of Rheumatology classification criteria for Sjögren syndrome: a data-driven, expert consensus approach in the SICCA cohort. *Arthritis Care Res* 2012;64:475–87.
10. Reveille JD, Solomon DH. Evidence-based guidelines for the use of immunologic tests: anticentromere, Scl-70 and nucleolar antibodies. *Arthritis Rheum* 2003;49:399–412.

11. Zampieri S, Ghirardello A, Iaccarino L, et al. Anti-Jo-1 Antibodies. *Autoimmunity* 2005;38:73–8.
12. Agmon-Levin N, Damoiseaux J, Kallenberg C, et al. International recommendations for the assessment of autoantibodies to cellular antigens referred to as anti-nuclear antibodies. *Ann Rheum Dis* 2014;73:17–23.
13. Mariz, HA, Sato EI, Barbosa SH, et al. Pattern on the antinuclear antibody-HEp-2 test is a critical parameter for discriminating antinuclear antibody-positive healthy individuals and patients with autoimmune rheumatic diseases. *Arthritis Rheum* 2011;63:191–200.
14. Fitch-Rogalsky C, Steber W, Mahler M, et al. Clinical and serological features of patients referred through a rheumatology triage system because of positive antinuclear antibodies. *PLoS One* 2014;9:e93812.
15. Tan EM, Smolen JS, McDougal JS, et al. A critical evaluation of enzyme immunoassays for detection of antinuclear autoantibodies of defined specificities: I. Precision, sensitivity, and specificity. *Arthritis Rheum* 1999;42:455–64.
16. Minz RW, Kumar Y, Anand S, et al. Antinuclear antibody positive autoimmune disorders in North India: an appraisal. *Rheumatol Int* 2012;32:2883–8.
17. Hayashi N, Koshiba M, Nishimura K, et al. Prevalence of disease-specific antinuclear antibodies in general population: estimates from annual physical examinations of residents of a small town over a 5-year period. *Mod Rheumatol* 2008;18:153–60.
18. Guo YP, Wang CG, Liu X, et al. The prevalence of antinuclear antibodies in the general population of China: a cross-sectional study. *Curr Ther Res Clin Exp* 2014;76:116–9.
19. Kavanaugh AF, Tomar R, Reveille J. Guidelines for clinical use of the antinuclear antibody test and tests for specific autoantibodies to nuclear antigens. *Arch Pathol Lab Med* 2000;124:71–81.
20. Arbuckle MR, McClain MT, Rubertone MV, et al. Development of autoantibodies before the clinical onset of systemic lupus erythematosus. *N Engl J Med* 2003;349:1526–33.
21. Van der Linden MW, Westendorp RG, Zidane M, et al. Autoantibodies within families of patients with systemic lupus erythematosus are not directed against the same nuclear antigens. *J Rheumatol* 2001;28:284–7.
22. Tan EM Cohen AS, Fries JF, et al. The 1982 revised criteria for the classification of systemic lupus erythematosus. *Arthritis Rheum* 1982;25:1271–7.
23. Hochberg MC. Updating the American College of Rheumatology revised criteria for the classification of systemic lupus erythematosus. *Arthritis Rheum* 1997;40:1725.
24. Yazdany, J, Schmajuk G, Robbins M, et al. Choosing wisely: the American College of Rheumatology's top 5 list of things physicians and patients should question. *Arthritis Care Res* 2013;65:329–39.

Approach to Low Back Pain

44

Mosmi Surati

GENERAL PRINCIPLES

- Low back pain (LBP) is a common condition, occurring in 85% of people during their lifetime,[1] with over a quarter of the American population experiencing LBP within the last 3 months.[2]
- The medical costs are substantial, with >$85 billion in health expenditures annually.[3]
- Furthermore, LBP can have a major impact on self-assessed health status, work limitation, and social functioning, contributing to the number of temporarily and permanently disabled individuals in the United States.[1,3]
- Given the economic and social costs attributed to LBP, proficiency in its evaluation and management is critical. With rising costs of care and concerns about the quality of care, it is imperative that evidence-based guidelines are considered.
- The differential diagnosis for LBP is presented in Table 44-1.[4]
- The causes of LBP are varied and are influenced by both anatomic considerations as well as individual risk factors including age, occupation, exercise, smoking status, and genetics.[1]
- Mechanical causes of back pain account for the vast majority of cases—about 97%, with nonmechanical and visceral disease accounting for the balance.[4]
  - Mechanical back pain stems from an injury or alteration to an anatomic structure that causes work to be diverted to nearby structures.
  - Examples include lumbar strain, degenerative disease, disc herniation, spinal stenosis, and fracture.
- This contrasts with back pain caused by nonmechanical or systemic disorders, such as malignancy, infection, or inflammatory disease. Visceral disease is inflammation of pelvic, renal, or gastrointestinal structures that is referred to the back.
- Despite this classification, in ~85% of cases, a specific cause of LBP cannot be found.[4]
- Guidelines suggest that attempting to identify specific anatomic causes of acute LBP may not actually impact outcomes and instead, the focus should be on looking for serious pathology and identification of factors causing disability.[5]

DIAGNOSIS

Clinical Presentation

- The goal of a focused LBP history and physical should be to rule out serious spinal pathology, to try to identify specific causes of pain, to evaluate degree of neurologic involvement, and to assess the severity of symptoms and their influence on function.[6]
- The term **red flag** has been used in the literature to identify features that suggest critical spinal pathology that warrant urgent or emergent evaluation and/or treatment. There is disagreement among various guidelines as to which features characterize red flags and limited data to support the use of these red flags as indications for routine imaging, aside from history of cancer.[6–8] This is in part due to the low prevalence of serious causes of LBP in the primary care setting, that is, malignancy (0.7%), compression fracture (4%), spinal infection (0.01%), and cauda equina syndrome (0.04%).[9,10] However, given the

TABLE 44-1 DIFFERENTIAL DIAGNOSIS OF LOW BACK PAIN

Mechanical or Activity Related

Lumbosacral myofascial strain, strain, "spasm"

Degenerative changes of the vertebrae, discs, facet joints (spondylosis)

Herniated intervertebral disc[a]

Lumbar spinal stenosis[a]

Discogenic low back pain[b]

Facet joint syndrome[b]

Sacroiliac joint dysfunction without sacroiliitis/spondyloarthropathy[b]

Compression fractures

Osteoporotic compression fracture

Traumatic fractures

Other anatomic/congenital abnormalities

Spondylolisthesis

Kyphosis

Scoliosis

Referred Pain

Vascular

Abdominal aortic aneurysm

Aortic dissection

Genitourinary

Nephrolithiasis

Pyelonephritis

Pelvic inflammatory disease

Endometriosis

Prostatitis

Gastrointestinal

Cholecystitis

Pancreatitis

Peptic ulcer disease

Medical Conditions of the Spine

Rheumatologic

Spondyloarthropathies (e.g., ankylosing spondylitis, psoriatic arthritis, reactive arthritis, inflammatory bowel disease related)

Rheumatoid arthritis

Neoplastic

Primary tumors or metastatic disease (e.g., multiple myeloma, lymphoma, carcinoma)

TABLE 44-1	DIFFERENTIAL DIAGNOSIS OF LOW BACK PAIN (*Continued*)

Infectious
Discitis
Epidural abscess
Vertebral osteomyelitis
Metabolic
Paget disease

---

[a]Often associated with neurogenic leg pain.
[b]Validity of the diagnosis, method of precise diagnosis, and optimal unique management not universally accepted.
Adapted from Deyo RA, Weinstein JN. Low back pain. *N Engl J Med* 2001;26:153–59.

---

absolute number of patients presenting with LBP and the various settings in which patients present (including specialty clinics, urgent care, emergency room, and hospitals), clinicians commonly use these elements to influence the decision-making process.

History
- Symptoms and historical features suggestive of spinal **malignancy** include the following:
  - History of cancer[7]
  - Age > 50
  - Unexplained weight loss
  - Lack of improvement after 1 month of conservative management
  - Night pain
  - Pain at multiple sites
  - Urinary retention
- Symptoms and historical features suggestive of **infection** include the following:
  - Human immunodeficiency virus (HIV) or immunosuppression
  - Chronic use of steroids or other immunosuppression
  - History of IV drug abuse
  - Active or recent infection such as urinary tract infection, osteomyelitis/abscess, or endocarditis
  - Fever
  - History of spinal intervention
- Those that suggest **fracture** include the following:
  - Increasing age[8]
  - History of osteoporosis or risk factors (i.e., prolonged steroid use)
  - Trauma
- Symptoms compatible with **cauda equina syndrome** include the following:
  - Fecal incontinence
  - Urinary retention
  - Gait abnormality
  - Saddle anesthesia
  - Bilateral lower extremity sciatica, sensory changes, and/or weakness
- Individuals with acute back pain should also be evaluated for yellow flags or psychosocial barriers to recovery. These are stronger predictors of pain outcomes than either exam findings or intensity or duration of pain.[5,11] Assessment for maladaptive coping behaviors, psychiatric comorbidities, and baseline functional impairment can help predict

which patients are more likely to go on to develop chronic pain.[11–15] These yellow flags of acute back pain are important to inquire about:[16]
  ○ Belief that back pain is harmful or potentially severely disabling
  ○ Fear or avoidance behavior and reduced activity levels
  ○ Tendency to low mood and withdrawal from social interaction
  ○ Expectation that passive treatments rather than active participation will help
  ○ Early identification of these beliefs can identify which patients stand a greater chance for future disability and allow for targeted interventions such as counseling, antidepressant use, and early referral to specialists.[15]
- It is helpful to classify patients by the duration of their symptoms: acute, subacute, or chronic.
  ○ **Acute back pain** is generally classified as back pain lasting <4 weeks. The majority of cases are self-limited and improve within 2–4 weeks,[17] though recurrences are common. Once serious pathology is ruled out, the next step is to determine if the pain is radiating or nonradiating. Radiating pain is frequently the result of disc herniation but can also be due to foraminal stenosis, spondylolisthesis, and other causes. The presence of sciatica, defined as a sharp or burning pain radiating along the posterior or lateral aspect of the leg, often associated with numbness or tingling, suggests nerve irritation. It may be exacerbated by coughing, sneezing, or Valsalva. Sciatica is sensitive, but not specific, for lumbar disc herniation.[10] With spinal stenosis, patients describe pain in the legs worsened by standing and walking and relieved by leaning forward. Patients with radiating LBP tend to have a poorer outcomes and slower recoveries, compared with those with nonradiating symptoms.
  ○ **Patients with subacute back pain** (4–12 weeks) and **chronic back pain** (>12 weeks) are less likely to experience spontaneous improvement in symptoms. The focus on their assessment is to seek a diagnosis, ensure no treatable pathology exists, and improve function. Frequently, this will require a multidisciplinary approach with referral to physical therapists, physical medicine and rehabilitation specialists, spinal interventionalists, and surgeons.

Physical Examination
- The physical exam can aid in the diagnosis of LBP. There are many limitations of the physical exam, and reviews suggest varied sensitivities and specificities of exam findings.[18] However, due to the prevalence of abnormalities seen on imaging in both in asymptomatic and symptomatic individuals,[10,19–21] information gained from the exam can guide management. Though this is not meant to be a comprehensive list of findings and maneuvers, salient features are described.
- Physical exam features include the following:
  ○ **Inspection of gait, posture, and tenderness**. Trendelenburg gait suggests weakness of the gluteus medius and possible L5 involvement. Abnormal spine curvature can lead to loading stress on surrounding structures. Focal tenderness of the spinous process can suggest infection, malignancy, or fracture.
  ○ **Evaluation of mobility**. Increased pain with forward flexion suggests anterior column or discogenic source of pain. Increased pain with extension suggests a source in the posterior column as from the facets, foraminal stenosis, or spondylolysis.[22]
  ○ **Neurogenic evaluation** including reflexes, strength, and sensation (Table 44-2). Over 90% of symptomatic lumbar disc herniations occur at L4/5 and L5/S1. A focused exam includes evaluation of knee strength and reflexes (L4), great toe and foot dorsiflexion (L5), plantar flexion and ankle reflexes (S1), and distribution of sensory deficits.[5]
  ○ **Straight-leg and crossed straight-leg raising**. This is done by raising the ipsilateral leg, while transmitting tension to the nerve root, in the supine position. Pain should be elicited between 30 and 60 degrees of elevation. The crossed testing is done on the contralateral leg and elicits symptoms in the leg with sciatica.[10]

TABLE 44-2 NEUROLOGIC EXAMINATION FOR SCIATICA

Test	Comment
Knee reflex	Disc herniation usually L3–L4
Ankle reflex	Disc herniation usually L5–S1
Ankle dorsiflexion	Disc herniation usually L4–L5
Great toe dorsiflexion	Disc herniation either L4–L5 or L5–S1
Pinprick, medial foot	Suggests L4 compression
Pinprick, dorsal foot	Suggests L5 compression
Pinprick, lateral foot	Suggests S1 compression
Straight-leg raise	Positive if leg pain at <60 degrees (sensitivity 0.35–0.81, specificity 0.37–1.0)[a]
Crossed straight-leg raise	Positive if pain in contralateral leg (sensitivity 0.22–0.35, specificity 0.85–0.94)[a]

[a]From van der Windt DAWM, Simons E, Riphagen II, et al. Physical examination for lumbar radiculopathy due to disc herniation in patients with low-back pain. *Cochrane Database Syst Rev* 2010;(2):CD007431.

- **Other features**. Fever and tachycardia may be clues to infection or inflammatory arthropathy. A rectal exam is necessary to examine S2–S4 if there is concern for cord compression and can also help assess prostatic disease. An abdominal–pelvic exam can help assess for other causes of pain listed in Table 44-1.
- **Waddell signs**. Though these are not diagnostic for nonorganic disease, they can serve as "yellow flags." These include overreaction to examination, simulation of pain with sham maneuvers, nonreproducibility of pain with distraction, nonanatomic distribution of deficits, and tenderness to superficial touch in nonanatomic patterns.[23]

Diagnostic Testing

Among patients with LBP without worrisome features, it is reasonable to defer imaging for the first month, because the majority of patients will be significantly improved at the end of that time with or without intervention. Furthermore, meta-analysis of RCT data suggests that immediate, routine imaging does not improve clinical outcomes.[22]

Laboratories

The use of lab tests should be guided by the history and physical. The majority of patients will not need any lab tests specifically for the purpose of elucidating the cause of LBP. However, if the history and physical suggest the possibility of a serious diagnosis (i.e., malignancy, infection, rheumatologic disease, conditions that cause referred LBP), appropriate labs should be done. Some have advocated checking the erythrocyte sedimentation rate (ESR) among those at a higher risk for cancer in whom a malignant lesion is suspected.[24]

Imaging

- **Plain radiographs**: Routine use of lumbar imaging among those with nonspecific back pain is not recommended.
  - Many patients without back pain have degenerative changes and many patients with back pain will have no or nondiagnostic radiographic abnormalities.
  - Degenerative changes increase with age and are extremely common in the elderly. Therefore, when degenerative changes are present, it is very difficult to know if they are causative.[25]

- Plain films cannot detect disc herniation or nerve root impingement and may not clearly show evidence of infection or malignancy.
- Furthermore, lumbar radiography may be harmful due to exposure of reproductive organs to ionizing radiation, particularly in young, female patients.[9]
- **Plain lumbar radiographs are recommended for the initial evaluation of a vertebral fracture in at-risk patients.**[5]
- **Radiography can also be performed in those with persistent pain with lesser risk factors for cancer and in patients for whom ankylosing spondylitis is being considered.**[24]
- When obtaining plain films, anteroposterior and lateral views are generally sufficient except when evaluating certain conditions.[9]
* The advantage of **CT and MRI** over plain films is clearer delineation of bone and soft tissue abnormalities. Both modalities are capable of disclosing disc herniation, spinal stenosis, nerve root and spinal cord compression, malignancy, fractures, and infection.
  - CT or MRI is indicated when there is serious consideration of malignancy, infection, cauda equina syndrome, fracture undiagnosed by plain films, spinal cord compression, or severe radiculopathy.
  - These modalities should also be considered in patients with prolonged (>1 month) moderate to severe radicular symptoms who are reasonable surgical candidates and are open to surgical treatment.[5]
  - MRI is generally preferred in patients without contraindications since it provides better visualization of soft tissue, vertebral marrow, and the spinal canal and does not subject patients to ionizing radiation.
  - However, when bony anatomy is critical, CT is preferable.[9]

TREATMENT

This chapter primarily focuses on the evaluation and management of LBP in the primary care setting and provides guidance on indications for specialty referral. Special groups who were not considered in this review include pregnant women, athletes, and those with disabilities. Aside from cases with worrisome features, noninvasive interventions are typically first recommended in the treatment of acute LBP. Guidelines at present recommend:

Medications
* **Analgesics** such as acetaminophen and nonsteroidal anti-inflammatory drugs (NSAIDs) are modestly helpful. Risks of each class of medicine should be weighed against the benefits given a patient's risk factors. Opioids may be considered as a time-limited option for severe acute LBP. Failure to respond to a time-limited course of opioids should lead to consideration of alternative therapies and reassessment of its use.[26]
* **Systemic steroids** including both oral corticosteroids and intravenous methylprednisolone are not recommended for the treatment of LBP with or without sciatica.[5]
* **Muscle relaxants** have been shown to be superior to placebo for acute LBP. There is insufficient evidence to suggest that one muscle relaxant is better than another. Adverse effects associated with their use, including sedation, addiction, and hepatotoxicity, demand that caution is used when prescribing these drugs.[26,27]
* **Antidepressants**, particularly those that inhibit norepinephrine reuptake (tricyclic and serotonin–norepinephrine reuptake inhibitors), may be used to treat chronic LBP in patients without contraindication to their use. Depression is common among patients with LBP and it should also be assessed.[24]
* **Anticonvulsants** including gabapentin, carbamazepine, and pregabalin have limited efficacy in patients with radiculopathy. There is insufficient evidence to recommend their use in patients without radiculopathy.[24]

Other Nonpharmacologic Therapies

- **Patient education** regarding the nature and prognosis of the majority of cases of LBP. Providers should explain the high likelihood of improvement within the first month, counsel regarding the limitations of early and routine imaging, and review indications for reassessment.
- **Continuation of usual activities of daily living** should be stressed for most patients. Bed rest should be minimized as it may contribute to reduced functional recovery. Advice should be individualized regarding a patient's age and occupational status. Work restrictions and worker's compensation claims should refer to regulations in one's area of practice, and there is insufficient evidence to guide general recommendations.
- **Moderate, low-stress aerobic activity** is generally safe. Patients often worry that any increase of pain is a harbinger of significant, perhaps permanent worsening of LBP and, therefore, avoid such activities. Based on findings from a Cochrane review, a graded-activity exercise program may be helpful for those with chronic and subacute back pain, though the benefit is less clear in acute back pain.[28]
- **Physical therapy** has not been clearly shown to be beneficial in acute LBP, although therapy should be considered as a part of an interdisciplinary rehabilitation program in subacute and chronic pain.
- **Back school** consists of educational group sessions focusing on spinal anatomy, biomechanics, ergonomics, lifting techniques, posture, and activity suggestions. Evidence is varied regarding back schools, but it may be more useful when provided in an occupational setting for those with chronic and recurrent pain.[29]
- **Spinal manipulation** can be helpful in acute, subacute, and chronic back pain in those who do not improve with self-care options. Spinal manipulation may be as effective as other therapies commonly prescribed for LBP, though benefits are usually short term and its use should depend on patient preference and access.[30,31]
- **Local heat application** has been efficacious in acute LBP and is relatively low in cost, with minimal risk of side effects. Patients should be warned against sleeping with heating pads, owing to the potential for burns.
- **Cognitive-behavioral therapies** provide small to moderate benefits for chronic LBP such as reduction in work absenteeism, though no differences were seen as compared with other active therapies.[5,31,32]
- **Multidisciplinary biopsychosocial therapy** attempts to address various aspects of LBP and involves physicians, psychologists, physical/occupational therapists, and social workers. It requires the patient to take part in substantial active therapies (>100 hours) that incorporate the concept of functional restoration. Though expensive and not widely available, it has been shown to be effective for chronic LBP.[5,31,33]
- Due to variation in the quality of studies, data are inconclusive for the use of acupuncture, massage, and TENS units. These practices are generally safe and depend on the preference of the individual. There is insufficient evidence to recommend lumbar supports or use of cold packs.

Surgical/Interventional Management

- **Injection therapies** with epidural glucocorticoids can be considered in subacute and chronic cases of lumbosacral radiculopathy that have not improved with conservative management in patients who desire nonsurgical treatment. Steroid injections show modest, short-term (3 month) improvements in pain for those with radiculopathy due to a herniated disc, but differences were not significant at 1 year.[34] These benefits should be weighed against risk of serious adverse effects. Steroid injections are not indicated for the management of acute lumbosacral radiculopathy, spinal stenosis, or nonspecific LBP.
- **Surgical interventions**: Patients with severe and progressive weakness, cauda equina syndrome, or spinal infection warrant immediate surgical referral and intervention to preserve neurologic function.[24] Most other cases of LBP do not require urgent referral.

Surgery can be considered for those with disabling symptoms and impaired quality of life who have not responded to conservative management.
- **Spinal stenosis** may remain stable or gradually worsen over time, and therefore, patients with persistent or worsening symptoms may benefit from surgery.[4,35] As compared with nonsurgical care, patients undergoing decompressive laminectomy had improved pain scores and outcomes after several years of follow-up.[36–38] In cases with spondylolisthesis, fusion may also be performed.
- **Lumbar disc prolapse with radiculopathy** should be managed nonsurgically for at least 1 month in the absence of progressive neurologic decline given a natural history that shows spontaneous regression in a majority of cases.[4,39] Surgery may result in faster improvement, and durable improvement in some symptoms was seen in carefully selected patients.[40–42]
- **Nonspecific low back pain with degenerative disease** without radiculopathy can be managed with spinal fusion, though a shared decision-making process is recommended given inconsistent evidence of benefit. Alternative therapies such as interdisciplinary rehabilitation should be offered, and discussion of average benefits, harms, and appropriate patient selection is important.[43]

REFERENCES

1. Hartigan AG. Epidemiology of back pain. In: Haig AJ, Colwell M, eds. *Back Pain*. Philadelphia: American College of Physicians, 2005:15–28.
2. Schiller JS, Lucas JW, Ward BW, Peregoy JA. Summary health statistics for U.S. adults: National Health Interview Survey, 2010. *Vital Health Stat 10* 2012;(252):1–207.
3. Martin BI, Deyo RA, Mirza SK, et al. Expenditures and health status among adults with back and neck problems. *JAMA* 2008;299:656–64.
4. Deyo RA, Weinstein JN. Low back pain. *N Engl J Med* 2001;344:363–70.
5. Chou R, Qaseem A, Snow V, et al. Diagnosis and treatment of low back pain: a joint clinical practice guideline from the American College of Physicians and the American Pain Society. *Ann Intern Med* 2007;147:478–91.
6. Dagenais S, Tricco AC, Haldeman S. Synthesis of recommendations for the assessment and management of low back pain from recent clinical practice guidelines. *Spine J* 2010;10:514–29.
7. Henschke N, Maher CG, Ostelo RWJG, et al. Red flags to screen for malignancy in patients with low-back pain. *Cochrane Database Syst Rev* 2013;(2):CD008686.
8. Downie A, Williams CM, Henschke N, et al. Red flags to screen for malignancy and fracture in patients with low back pain: systematic review. *BMJ* 2013;347:1–9.
9. Jarvik JG, Deyo RA. Diagnostic evaluation of low back pain with emphasis on imaging. *Ann Intern Med* 2002;137:586–97.
10. Deyo RA, Rainville J, Kent DL. What can the history and physical examination tell us about low back pain? *JAMA* 1992;268:760–5.
11. Chou R, Shekelle P. Will this patient develop persistent disabling low back pain? *JAMA* 2010;303:1295–302.
12. Pincus T, Burton AK, Vogel S, Field AP. A systematic review of psychological factors as predictors of chronicity/disability in prospective cohorts of low back pain. *Spine* 2002;27:109–20.
13. Wertli MM, Eugster R, Held U, et al. Catastrophizing—a prognostic factor for outcome in patients with low back pain: a systematic review. *Spine J* 2014;14:2639–57.
14. Wertli MM, Rasmussen-Barr E, Weiser S, et al. The role of fear avoidance beliefs as a prognostic factor for outcome in patients with nonspecific low back pain: a systematic review. *Spine J* 2014;14:816–36.
15. Young IA. Yellow flags: predicting disability. In: Haig AJ, Colwell M, eds. *Back Pain*. Philadelphia: American College of Physicians, 2005:111–8.
16. Kendall NAS, Linton SJ, Main CJ. *Guide to assessing psychosocial yellow flags in acute low back pain: risk factors for long-term disability and work loss.* 2004 ed. Wellington, New Zealand: Accident Compensation Corporation and the New Zealand Guidelines Group.
17. Coste J, Delecoeuillerie G, Cohen de Lara A, et al. Clinical course and prognostic factors in acute low back pain: an inception cohort study in primary care practice. *BMJ* 1994;308:577–80.
18. van der Windt DAWM, Simons E, Riphagen II, et al. Physical examination for lumbar radiculopathy due to disc herniation in patients with low-back pain. *Cochrane Database Syst Rev* 2010;(2):CD007431.

19. Jensen MC, Brant-Zawadzki MN, Obuchowski N, et al. Magnetic resonance imaging of the lumbar spine in people without back pain. *N Engl J Med* 1994;331:69–73.
20. Boden SD, Davis DO, Dina TS, et al. Abnormal magnetic-resonance scans of the lumbar spine in asymptomatic subjects. *J Bone Joint Surg Am* 1990;72:403–8.
21. Brinjikji W, Diehn FE, Jarvik JG, et al. MRI findings of disc degeneration are more prevalent in adults with low back pain that in asymptomatic controls: a systematic review and meta-analysis. *AJNR Am J Neuroradiol* 2015;36:2394–9.
22. Chou R, Fu R, Carrino JA, Deyo RA. Imaging strategies for low-back pain: systematic review and meta-analysis. *Lancet* 2009;373:463–72.
23. Laidlaw A. Physical examination for acute back pain. In: Haig AJ, Colwell M, eds. *Back Pain*. Philadelphia: American College of Physicians, 2005:91–8.
24. Chou R. In the clinic. Low back pain. *Ann Intern Med* 2014;160:ITC6-1.
25. Chou R, Qaseem A, Owens D, et al. Diagnostic imaging for low back pain: advice for high-value health care from the American College of Physicians. *Ann Intern Med* 2011;154:181–9.
26. Chou R, Huffman LH. Medications for acute and chronic low back pain: a review of the evidence for an American Pain Society/American College of Physicians clinical practice guideline. *Ann Intern Med* 2007;147:505–14.
27. van Tulder MW, Touray T, Furlan AD, et al. Muscle relaxants for nonspecific low back pain: a systematic review within the framework of the Cochrane collaboration. *Spine* 2003;28:1978–92.
28. Hayden J, van Tulder MW, Malmivaara A, Koes BW. Exercise therapy for treatment of non-specific low back pain. *Cochrane Database Syst Rev* 2005;(3):CD000335.
29. Heymans MW, van Tulder MW, Esmail R, et al. Back schools for nonspecific low back pain: a systematic review within the framework of the Cochrane collaboration back review group. *Spine* 2005;30:2153–63.
30. Rubinstein SM, van Middelkoop M, Assendelft WJJ, et al. Spinal manipulative therapy for chronic low-back pain. *Cochrane Database Syst Rev* 2011;(2):CD008112.
31. Chou R, Huffman LH. Nonpharmacologic therapies for acute and chronic low back pain: a review of the evidence for an American Pain Society/American College of Physicians clinical practice guideline. *Ann Intern Med* 2007;147:492–504.
32. Henschke N, Ostelo RWJG, van Tulder MW, et al. Behavioural treatment for chronic low-back pain. *Cochrane Database Syst Rev* 2010;(7):CD002014.
33. Guzmán J, Esmail R, Karjalainen K, et al. Multidisciplinary bio-psycho-social rehabilitation for chronic low-back pain. *Cochrane Database Syst Rev* 2002;(1):CD000963.
34. Pinto RZ, Maher CG, Ferreira ML, et al. Epidural corticosteroid injections in the management of sciatica. *Ann Intern Med* 2012;157:865–77.
35. Issack PS, Cunningham ME, Pumberger M, et al. Degenerative lumbar spinal stenosis: evaluation and management. *J Am Acad Orthop Surg* 2012;20:527–35.
36. Weinstein JN, Tosteson TD, Lurie JD, et al. Surgical versus nonsurgical therapy for lumbar spinal stenosis. *N Engl J Med* 2008;358:794–810.
37. Atlas SJ, Keller RB, Robson D, et al. Surgical and nonsurgical management of lumbar spinal stenosis. *Spine* 2000;25:556–62.
38. Atlas SJ, Keller RB, Wu Y, et al. Long-term outcomes of surgical and nonsurgical management of lumbar spinal stenosis: 8 to 10 year results from the Maine lumbar spine study. *Spine* 2005;30(8):936–43.
39. Bozzao A, Gallucci M, Masciocchi C, et al. Lumbar disk herniation: MR imaging assessment of natural history in patients treated without surgery. *Radiology* 1992;185:135–41.
40. Weinstein JN, Lurie JD, Tosteson TD, et al. Surgical versus non-operative treatment for lumbar disc herniation: four-year results for the spine patient outcomes research trial. *Spine* 2008;33:2789–800.
41. Lurie JD, Tosteson TD, Tosteson ANA, et al. Surgical versus non-operative treatment for lumbar disc herniation: eight-year results for the spine patient outcomes research trial. *Spine* 2014;39:3–16.
42. Atlas SJ, Keller RB, Wu YA, et al. Long-term outcomes of surgical and nonsurgical management of sciatica secondary to a lumbar disc herniation: 10 year results from the Maine lumbar spine study. *Spine* 2005;30:927–35.
43. Chou R, Loeser JD, Owens DK, et al. Interventional therapies, surgery, and interdisciplinary rehabilitation for low back pain. *Spine* 2009;34:1066–77.

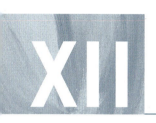

XII Allergy and Immunology

Anaphylaxis

Erin L. Reigh and Jennifer M. Monroy

GENERAL PRINCIPLES

Anaphylaxis is an immediate, immunoglobulin E (IgE)-mediated, life-threatening systemic allergic reaction caused by massive release of vasoactive mediators from mast cells and basophils. It can be fatal if not recognized and treated promptly with epinephrine, the only appropriate therapy for anaphylaxis.

Epidemiology

Lifetime prevalence of anaphylaxis is around 2%, and it causes up to 1000 deaths annually.[1,2] The vast majority (80–87%) of fatal cases did not receive epinephrine or it was delayed.[2] It remains underdiagnosed and undertreated, with 60–80% of cases in the emergency department (ED) never receiving epinephrine.[3]

Etiology

In adults, the **most common causes** of anaphylaxis are drugs (>50%), insect venom, and foods.[1,4,5] Drugs are the most common cause of fatal anaphylaxis (59%).[5,6] **Other common causes** include radiocontrast medium, latex, blood products, NSAIDs, anesthetic agents, and exercise.[4,6] Cause remains unknown in up to 60% of cases.[7]

Pathophysiology

Anaphylaxis is caused by the sudden, massive release of allergic mediators from mast cells and basophils, leading to a multisystem allergic response that can affect any part of the body.

- Preformed mediators such as histamine cause vasodilation, capillary leakage, and smooth muscle contraction. Onset is typically within minutes of exposure but may be delayed by 1–2 hours. Reactions that begin more rapidly tend to become more severe.[1,3,4]
- Synthesized mediators such as leukotrienes have a slower onset and may lead to recurrence of symptoms several hours later, the so-called biphasic reaction. Biphasic reactions occur in up to 25% of cases, typically within 10 hours, but can occur later.[1]
- **Fatalities** are most commonly due to asphyxia (45%) or cardiovascular collapse (41%).[2] In fatal cases, median time to cardiovascular collapse was 30 minutes for foods, 15 minutes for venom, and 5 minutes for drugs.[1,3,4]
- **Can be triggered by** IgE-mediated antigen recognition (allergic anaphylaxis) or by non-specific mast cell stimulation (nonallergic hypersensitivity reactions, formerly "pseudoallergic reactions"). The presentation and acute management are the same.

Risk Factors

- **Risk of severe reactions and death** are increased in patients on β-blockers, ACE inhibitors, and ARBs; those with underlying respiratory or cardiovascular disease; and old age.[2–5]
- **A history of anaphylaxis** increases risk of recurrence when reexposed.[1,2] Severity of subsequent reactions can vary due to route of exposure (oral is least immunogenic), time since last exposure (responses can wane over time), and amount of allergen.

DIAGNOSIS

Clinical Presentation

- Due to the systemic nature of the response, the clinical manifestations can be highly variable and affect any organ system.
  - **Skin:** hives, rash, flushing, pruritus, angioedema
  - **Respiratory tract:** nasal congestion, sneezing, cough, laryngeal edema, wheezing, dyspnea
  - **Gastrointestinal tract:** nausea, vomiting, diarrhea, abdominal pain
  - **Genitourinary tract:** uterine cramps, incontinence
  - **Nervous system:** dizziness, confusion, sense of impending doom
  - **Cardiovascular system:** hypotension, syncope, chest pain, tachycardia, bradycardia
- When possible, a history of food ingestion, drugs, insect bites, and other exposures should be taken.

Diagnostic Criteria

- The symptoms can be highly variable, so the key to diagnosing anaphylaxis is recognizing the system nature of the reaction. Diagnosis is largely clinical and depends on the presence of two major criteria[1]:
  - **Exposure to a *likely* allergen** prior to onset (e.g., foods, drugs, insects)
  - **Symptoms involving two or more organ systems**
- Common diagnostic errors include the following:
  - **Cutaneous involvement is *not* required to make a diagnosis of anaphylaxis**, though it occurs in 80–90% of patients.[1–3]
  - **Hypotension is *not* required to make a diagnosis of anaphylaxis.** Waiting to treat a patient until he or she develops hypotension with epinephrine can be fatal. While hypotension is not a requirement for diagnosis, a patient who develops hypotension after exposure to a ***known*** **allergen** should be treated for presumed anaphylaxis regardless of other symptoms.[1–3]

Differential Diagnosis

The differential diagnosis for anaphylaxis includes sepsis/distributive shock, myocardial infarction, acute respiratory distress, urticaria and angioedema, vasovagal reactions and syncope, panic attacks, mast cell disorders, carcinoid syndrome, scombroidosis, and postmenopausal flushing.[1,2]

Diagnostic Testing

Serum **tryptase** may be elevated if checked within 4 hours of the reaction.

TREATMENT

Assess **airway, breathing, and circulation**. Intubate if evidence of respiratory compromise.

Medications

- **Epinephrine is the only therapy** proven to prevent progression to respiratory or cardiovascular collapse.[1]
  - **Give immediately if there is any suspicion for anaphylaxis**, even if uncertain or reaction appears mild; reactions can progress rapidly and early epinephrine reduces the risk of death.[1,2,4]
  - There are **no absolute contraindications for the use of epinephrine** in anaphylaxis, including cardiovascular disease.[1,2,4]
  - **Initial therapy:** 0.2–0.5 mg of 1:1000 epinephrine IM q5–10min. PRN

- IM preferred over IV and SC due to better safety profile and efficacy; lateral thigh preferred over deltoid.[1–4]
- Up to 30% of patients need more than one dose.[1,3]
  - **Refractory cases:** continuous infusion of 1:100,000 epinephrine (starting dose 5–15 μg/min, titrate to effect). Bolus IV dosing is not recommended due to inferior efficacy and safety profile.[1,3]
- Consider **glucagon** in patients on β-blockers (1–5 mg bolus over 5 minutes, followed by infusion with starting dose 1–15 μg/min, titrated to response).[1–3]
- Patient should be admitted to the ICU for cardiac monitoring.
- Adjunctive therapies can be used in addition to, but should never replace, epinephrine. In particular, **antihistamines and glucocorticoids do not prevent progression of anaphylaxis** and should never be used as first-line therapy. Expert opinion lists the adjunctive therapies in order of importance[1]:
  - **Supine position** with legs elevated (to avoid death from empty heart syndrome)
  - **Oxygen** for prolonged reactions
  - **IV fluids** 5–10 mL/kg bolus over 5 minutes, then continuous and titrated to response
  - **Nebulized bronchodilators** for wheezing
  - **Vasopressors** (dopamine 2–20 μg/kg/min initial dose) if epinephrine maximized[1]
  - **Antihistamines** (diphenhydramine 25–50 mg IV) may improve cutaneous symptoms.[1,3]
  - **Glucocorticoids** (methylprednisolone 1–2 mg/kg) may reduce biphasic reactions.[1,3]

MONITORING/FOLLOW-UP

- **Close observation** is advised for 6–8 hours for patients who respond to therapy.
- **Refer to an allergist** for assistance in identifying the trigger and avoiding it.
- **Prescribe an epinephrine autoinjector** and instruct on its use.

REFERENCES

1. Lieberman P, Nicklas R, Oppenheimer J, et al. The diagnosis and management of anaphylaxis practice parameter: 2010 update. *J Allergy Clin Immunol* 2010;126:477–80.
2. Lee JK, Vadas P. Anaphylaxis: mechanisms and management. *Clin Exp Allergy* 2011;41:923–38.
3. Campbell RL, Li JC, Nicklas RA, et al. Emergency department diagnosis and treatment of anaphylaxis: a practice parameter. *Ann Allergy Asthma Immunol* 2014;113:599–608.
4. Kim H, Fischer D. Anaphylaxis. *Allergy Asthma Clin Immunol* 2011;7:S6.
5. Sicherer SH, Leung DM. Advances in allergic skin disease, anaphylaxis, and hypersensitivity reactions to foods, drugs, and insects in 2014. *J Allergy Clin Immunol* 2015;135:357–67.
6. Jerschow E, Lin RY, Scaperotti MM, et al. Fatal anaphylaxis in the United States, 1999–2010: temporal patterns and demographic associations. *J Allergy Clin Immunol* 2014;134:1318–28.
7. Webb LM, Lieberman P. Anaphylaxis: a review of 601 cases. *Ann Allergy Asthma Immunol* 2006;97:39–43.

Drug Reactions

Jennifer M. Monroy

GENERAL PRINCIPLES

- An **adverse drug reaction** (ADR) is an undesired or unintended response that occurs when a drug is given for the appropriate purpose.
- The etiology of a drug reaction can be immunologic, toxic, or idiosyncratic in nature.
- An allergic drug reaction is due to an immune response that is mediated by immunoglobulin E (IgE) or T cells.

Classifications

- **Type A** reactions are predictable, often dose dependent, and related to the pharmacokinetics of the drug.
- **Type B** reactions are unpredictable and are not related to the dose or the drug's pharmacokinetics. They account for 10–15% of all ADRs.
- Immune-mediated adverse reactions can be from a variety of mechanisms (see below). They usually occur upon reexposure to the offending drug.
- **Pseudoallergic reactions**, formerly called anaphylactoid reactions, are caused by IgE-independent degranulation of mast cells.

Epidemiology

- From 1966 to 1996, 15.1% of hospitalized US patients experienced an ADR with an incidence of 3.1–6.2% of hospital admissions due to ADRs.[1]
- Mortality incidence from ADRs is significant and ranges from 0.14% to 0.32%.[2]

Pathophysiology

Immunologic mechanisms of drug allergy can be stratified by the Gell and Coombs classification.

- **Type I reaction:** IgE-mediated and immediate onset. Presents as anaphylaxis, urticaria, angioedema, asthma, and rhinitis.
- **Type II reaction:** IgG antibody–mediated cytotoxic hypersensitivity; causes cell destruction via the complement system. Includes immune cytopenias such as hemolytic anemia due to antibodies formed against erythrocyte-bound penicillin.
- **Type III reaction:** IgG:antigen complex–mediated hypersensitivity; examples of agents implicated in causing serum sickness include antithymocyte globulin, rituximab, infliximab, and certain immunizations. Onset is delayed >1 week after drug exposure.
- **Type IV reaction:** delayed-type hypersensitivity that is mediated by sensitized T cells and classically represented by contact dermatitis and various exanthems.

Risk Factors

- Route of administration (cutaneous most immunogenic), size and structure of drug, dose, duration, and frequency of drug use.
- Patients who are atopic, who have a personal history of multiple drug allergies, a family history of drug allergy, genetic factors (HLA types), and certain predisposing disease

states (human immunodeficiency virus [HIV], infectious mononucleosis, cystic fibrosis) are at a higher risk of having a drug allergy.

Prevention
- HLA testing may be indicated in susceptible populations for prevention of a severe ADR for some drugs such as abacavir and carbamazepine.
- It is important to note that **hypersensitivity wanes with time**. A study of 55 patients with a history of an immediate-type reaction to penicillin and a positive skin test revealed that, after 5 years, only 40% of patients still had a positive skin test.[3]

DIAGNOSIS
Clinical Presentation
- A detailed history is essential in evaluating a possible drug reaction. Questions should be directed at establishing the following information:
  - Sign and symptoms: Where and what order did the symptoms begin, progress, and resolve?
  - Timing of the reaction: From the first dose of suspected drug to the peak of the reaction and resolution after discontinuing therapy.
  - Purpose of drug: Was it prescribed for the appropriate treatment, and can the signs and symptoms be explained by a concurrent illness?
  - Other medications the patient is receiving: This includes over-the-counter drugs and dietary supplements.
  - Prior exposure to the drug or another drug in the same or related class: If so, when was it given, and what was the outcome?
  - History of other allergic drug reactions: Did the patient ever see an allergist and receive skin testing? What was the reaction, and how long ago was the reaction?
- Skin and mucous membrane alterations are the most common manifestations of drug hypersensitivity:
- Urticaria, angioedema, wheezing, and anaphylaxis are all characteristics of IgE-mediated (**type 1**) reactions.
  - Symptoms do not typically occur on the first exposure to the medication unless the patient has been exposed to a structurally related medication. On reexposure, however, symptoms tend to manifest acutely (often <1 hour).
  - IgE-mediated reactions tend to worsen with repeated exposure to offending medication.
  - Pseudoallergic reactions (non–IgE mediated) can be clinically indistinguishable from IgE-mediated reactions because the final common pathway for their reaction is mast cell degranulation.
- **Maculopapular or morbilliform** skin eruptions are seen most often.
  - An eruption is usually symmetric, sparing palms and soles, and consists of erythematous macules and papules. Onset is usually 4–7 days into a course of therapy, often beginning on the lower extremities or over pressure points.
  - Ampicillin is implicated quite frequently in morbilliform rashes. Sulfonamides and nonsteroidal anti-inflammatory drugs (NSAIDs) can also cause these reactions.
- **Fixed drug eruptions** occur at the same body location with each exposure to a given drug.
  - Hands, feet, mouth, and genitals are the most common sites.
  - Typically, the lesion is round and well delineated. It starts as an area of edema and then becomes erythematous and darkens to a violaceous-colored area. The lesion is raised and nonpruritic.

- Begins 30 minutes to 8 hours after reexposure to the drug. After withdrawal of the drug, the lesion will resolve in 2–3 weeks leaving an area of desquamation and then hyperpigmentation.
- Drugs commonly implicated in fixed drug reactions include phenolphthalein, barbiturates, sulfonamides, tetracycline, and NSAIDs.
- **Erythema multiforme (EM), Stevens-Johnson syndrome (SJS), and toxic epidermal necrolysis (TEN)** are all serious drug reactions primarily involving the skin.
  - EM is characterized most typically by target lesions.
  - SJS and TEN manifest with varying degrees of sloughing of the skin and mucous membranes (<10% of the epidermis in SJS and >30% in TEN).
  - Mortality with SJS can be 10% in severe cases and with TEN up to 40%.
  - Drugs associated include sulfonamides, anticonvulsants, barbiturates, phenylbutazone, piroxicam, allopurinol, and aminopenicillins.
  - **Readministration or future skin testing with the offending drug is absolutely contraindicated as symptoms will recur.**
- **Serum sickness syndrome** is a type III hypersensitivity reaction with soluble immune complexes that activate the complement system.
  - It encompasses a broad spectrum of symptoms, including fever, malaise, rash (palpable purpura and urticaria), leukopenia, lymphadenopathy, arthralgias, myalgias, and arthritis.
  - It usually begins within 1–4 weeks of drug ingestion and resolves only when the offending agent or its metabolite is completely eliminated from the body.
- **Drug reaction with eosinophilia and systemic symptoms (DRESS)** or hypersensitivity syndrome is a serious ADR, often presenting with rash and fever.[4]
  - Systemic involvement can manifest as hepatitis, eosinophilia, pneumonitis, lymphadenopathy, and nephritis.
  - Symptoms tend to present 2–6 weeks after introduction of medication.
  - First described with antiepileptic (carbamazepine) agents but has also been reported to occur with allopurinol, NSAIDs, some antibiotics, and β-blockers.
- **Drug-induced hepatitis** presents with symptoms similar to those of viral hepatitis including fever, jaundice, nausea, dark urine, and clay-colored stools.
  - Begins 1–5 weeks after initiating drug. Liver injury occurs via hepatocellular and extracellular (cholestatic) mechanisms.
  - Numerous drugs have been implicated including isoniazid, tetracycline, halothane, methotrexate, acetaminophen, and amoxicillin–clavulanic acid.
- **Drug fever** may be the only evidence of hypersensitivity to a drug.
  - Fever often reaches high levels; associated findings may include eosinophilia, transaminitis, leukocytosis, rash, and an elevated erythrocyte sedimentation rate (ESR).
  - Typically, it develops around days 7–10 and disappears within 36–72 hours after the drug is stopped, although it can persist for days.
  - While any drug can theoretically cause a **drug fever**, certain classes, such as anticonvulsants, antipyretics, and antibiotics, are the most frequent culprits.
- **Acute interstitial nephritis** is rare and includes mild proteinuria, microhematuria, and eosinophiluria.
  - Symptoms start days to weeks after initiating the drug. Associated with fever, rash, and eosinophilia. Renal insufficiency resolves once offending drug is removed.
  - Can be seen with β-lactams, in particular methicillin, as well as rifampin, NSAIDs, sulfonamides, captopril, and allopurinol.
- There are multiple other types of drug eruptions, including acneiform, erythema nodosum, erythroderma, palpable purpura, photosensitivity (phototoxic and photoallergic), bullous (e.g., pemphigus and pemphigoid), lichenoid, lupus-like, alopecia, Sweet disease (erythematous plaques infiltrated by neutrophils, fever, and leukocytosis), and acute generalized exanthematous pustulosis.

Diagnostic Testing

Laboratories
- Tryptase is a mediator released by mast cells and can indicate an allergic reaction if elevated.
  - Serum tryptase should be obtained within 3 hours from start of symptoms.
  - It is more sensitive than serum or urine histamine levels.
- Decreases in total hemolytic complement (CH_{50}) or C3 and C4 levels can be seen in drug reactions involving complement activation.
- A complete blood count is useful to determine if eosinophilia is present.
- Total IgE level is not useful for drug allergy.
- Immunoassays such as radioallergosorbent test (RAST) testing can detect drug-specific IgE antibodies although these are considered investigational and primarily used in research.

Diagnostic Procedures
- Prick and intradermal skin tests help to measure an IgE response. A patient with a positive wheal-and-flare response identifies a drug that can cause a type 1 reaction.
  - High molecular weight drugs such as antisera, egg-containing vaccines, monoclonal antibodies, latex, and toxoids can be used directly as skin testing reagents.
  - Penicillin has established sensitivity and specificity for skin testing. The major determinant of penicillin (Pre-Pen) is approved to evaluate for penicillin allergy.
  - For skin testing, it is important for patients to abstain from using antihistamines and tricyclic antidepressants, which can interfere with the wheal-and-flare response.
  - There is a refractory period of 2–4 weeks after an episode of acute anaphylaxis where skin tests are invalid.
- Patch testing can be used to asses for a type IV contact hypersensitivity to topical agents. A series of antigens are placed on the skin under occlusive dressing and results read 48–72 hours later.
- Provocative test dosing provides a direct challenge to the patient to confirm that a suspected drug caused the clinical manifestations.
  - This approach has the risk of a potentially serious adverse reaction and must be performed by a person with experience in managing hypersensitivity reactions.
  - A graded challenge, or incremental test dosing, administers small doses that would not cause a serious reaction and increases the dose by safe increments over hours to weeks until therapeutic dose is achieved.
  - Desensitization differs from provocative testing as those with desensitization have established a true drug allergy. A patient undergoing provocative testing has a low probability of a true drug allergy but requires cautious administration of the drug to avoid a serious reaction.

TREATMENT

- **Discontinuation** of the suspected drug or drugs is the most important initial approach in managing an allergic drug reaction.
- Treatment of the reaction depends on the mechanism of drug allergy.
  - Urticarial reactions are treated with antihistamines and steroids.
  - Anaphylaxis is treated with epinephrine and antihistamines.
  - Severe reactions such as TEN can be treated with immunosuppressive drugs and intravenous immunoglobulin.
  - Serum sickness is treated with antihistamines and steroids. Rarely, plasmapheresis is used.
- Administer an alternative (not cross-reactive) drug. With sulfonamide allergy, the cross-reactivity between antibiotic and nonantibiotic sulfa-containing drugs is low.
- Administer a potentially cross-reactive drug under close medical supervision.
  - The cross-reactivity between β-lactam antibiotics is variable and largely determined by their side-chain structure attached to the β-lactam ring.

TABLE 46-1 PRETREATMENT PROTOCOL FOR PATIENTS WITH A HISTORY OF REACTIONS TO RADIOCONTRAST MEDIA

Time Before Procedure	Drug and Dose		
	Prednisone[a]	Cimetidine[b]	Diphenhydramine[c]
13 h	50 mg PO	300 mg PO or IV	—
7 h	50 mg PO	300 mg PO or IV	—
1 h[d]	50 mg PO	300 mg PO or IV	50 mg PO or IV

[a]Or methylprednisolone 40 mg IV.
[b]Or ranitidine 150 mg PO.
[c]Or chlorpheniramine 10–12 mg PO.
[d]Ephedrine 25 mg PO may also be given 1 h before a procedure.

- Prior to the 1980s, cephalosporins had a higher cross-reactivity to penicillin as they were contaminated with a small amount of penicillin.[5]
- Risk of a cross-reaction with a first-generation cephalosporins is 5.0% to 16.5%, second generation is 4%, and third or fourth generation is 1–3%.[6]
- Skin test cross-reactivity has been documented between carbapenems and penicillins. Patients undergoing a graded carbapenem challenge with a positive penicillin skin test and a negative carbapenem skin test did not have any hypersensitivity reactions.[5]
- The monobactam aztreonam rarely cross-reacts with penicillins. Ceftazidime does share an identical side chain to aztreonam and is highly cross-reactive.[7]
* Pretreatment protocols are available for some drugs to prevent or mitigate any reaction that might occur. Table 46-1 outlines such a protocol for reactions to radiocontrast media.
* **Drug desensitization** is performed when the patient has an identified IgE-mediated reaction and no alternative medication is available.
  - The exact mechanism by which desensitization prevents anaphylaxis is unclear.
  - Desensitization should be performed only under the supervision of a trained allergist in a location outfitted with resuscitative equipment for treating anaphylaxis.
  - The drug must be taken daily at a specified dose to maintain the desensitized state.
  - If a dose of drug is missed for >48-hour period following a desensitization procedure, the patient will often need to undergo a repeat desensitization.
  - Successful desensitization or graded challenge does not preclude the development of a non–IgE-mediated, delayed reaction (e.g., rash).

REFERENCES

1. Lazarou J, Pomeranz BH, Corey PN. Incidence of adverse drug reactions in hospitalized patients: a meta-analysis of prospective studies. *JAMA* 1998;279:1200–5.
2. Gomes ER, Demoly P. Epidemiology of hypersensitivity drug reactions. *Curr Opin Allergy Clin Immunol* 2005;5:309–16.
3. Bianca M, Torres MJ, Garcia JJ, et al. Natural evolution of skin test sensitivity in patients allergic to beta-lactam antibiotics. *J Allergy Clin Immunol* 1999;103:918–24.
4. Gogtay NJ, Bavdekar SB, Kshirsagar NA. Anticonvulsant hypersensitivity syndrome: a review. *Expert Opin Drug Saf* 2005;4:571.
5. Khan DA, Solensky R. Drug allergy. *J Allergy Clin Immunol* 2010;125:S126–37.
6. Greenberger PA. 8. Drug allergy. *J Allergy Clin Immunol* 2006;117:S464–70.
7. Frumin J, Gallagher JC. Allergic cross-sensitivity between penicillin, carbapenem, and monobactam antibiotics: what are the chances? *Ann Pharmacother* 2009;43:304–15.

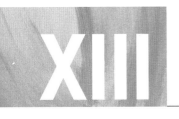

XIII Toxicology

Alcohol Withdrawal

Stephen Hasak and Geoffrey Cislo

GENERAL PRINCIPLES

Alcohol withdrawal syndrome is a common problem seen in the hospitalized patient, with 20% of patients in most medical settings having an alcohol use disorder.[1] Of these patients, about 50% will exhibit symptoms of alcohol withdrawal when they reduce or discontinue their alcohol consumption and about 5% of these will go on to have delirium tremens (DTs) or withdrawal seizures.[2]

DIAGNOSIS

Clinical Presentation

History

- **Autonomic hyperactivity** typically begins within 6 hours after alcohol cessation and subsides within 48 hours, although in severe cases it can last >7 days.[3] Signs and symptoms include tremulousness, tachycardia, hypertension, diaphoresis, low-grade fever, nausea, anxiety, and headache.[4]
- **Alcohol withdrawal seizures** occur in 3% of alcoholic patients.[5]
  - A history of previous alcohol withdrawal seizures increases risk, and up to 50% of patients who seize have other risk factors, such as a history of traumatic brain injury (36%), epilepsy (22%), or cerebrovascular accident (CVA) (8%).[5]
  - Most withdrawal seizures occur in the first 24 hours, and >90% occur in the first 48 hours.[5]
  - They are typically brief, generalized tonic–clonic seizures without status epilepticus, although partial seizures and status both can occur.[5]
  - Patients frequently do not show other signs of alcohol withdrawal before seizing, but alcohol withdrawal seizures predict a high risk of progression to DTs.[6]
- **Alcoholic hallucinosis** occurs in ~25% of people with alcohol withdrawal, typically beginning within 12–24 hours of abstinence and ending within 6 days.[6]
  - This is distinguished from DTs by the lack of generalized confusion.[6]
  - The hallucinations may be tactile (e.g., formication, the sensation of insects crawling on the skin), visual (e.g., seeing deceased relatives), auditory, or olfactory.[6]
- **DTs** usually begin at 48–96 hours and peak on the fourth to fifth day of alcohol cessation. It can persist for up to 2 weeks.[3]
  - In addition to hallucinations, patients have altered sensorium and prolonged autonomic hyperactivity with tachycardia, hypertension, diaphoresis, low-grade fever, and agitation.[4]
  - Mortality in untreated patients has been reported to be as high as 35%; but with adequate treatment, the mortality is very low (<3%).[7]
  - Death usually results from hyperthermia, cardiac arrhythmias, complication of withdrawal seizures, or concomitant medical disorders.[7,8]
  - Affective disturbances such as depression, anxiety, insomnia, and tremor often persist for weeks or months post withdrawal.[9]

- **Wernicke encephalopathy** is the result of chronic thiamine deficiency.
  - It can be precipitated by administration of glucose without thiamine.[10]
  - Left untreated, clinical cases have a mortality of 20%, with cognitive deficits in 75% of patients.[10]
  - Subclinical cases are surprisingly common, with about 2% of unselected autopsies in the United States having findings consistent with a history of Wernicke encephalopathy.[11]
  - Wernicke encephalopathy classically presents with the triad of **confusion, oculomotor dysfunction** (nystagmus, diplopia, rectus muscle weakness), and **ataxia** (typically of the lower extremities).[11]
  - The long-term sequela of Wernicke encephalopathy is Korsakoff psychosis, denoted by short-term memory loss, confabulation, and memory gaps.[12]

Physical Examination
Every patient should undergo a careful physical exam to identify other possible diagnoses. Patients frequently stop drinking owing to another medical problem that prevents alcohol intake. Common problems include gastrointestinal (GI) bleeding, infection, electrolyte or glucose imbalance, or liver failure. Signs of cirrhosis should be sought.

Diagnostic Testing

- Evaluation virtually always includes a complete metabolic panel, complete blood count (CBC), serum alcohol level, and urine toxicology screen.
- Other tests may be guided by symptoms and include prothrombin time/partial thromboplastin time (PT/PTT), urinalysis (UA), lumbar puncture, electrocardiogram, chest radiograph, magnesium, phosphorus, and computed tomography (CT) of the head.
- A bedside glucose should be performed in all patients with altered sensorium or seizures.
- Stool guaiac aids in identifying GI bleeding.
- Common abnormalities are hypokalemia, hypomagnesemia, hyponatremia, and elevated transaminases (aspartate aminotransferase > alanine aminotransferase [AST > ALT]). In a meta-analysis, initial labs revealing thrombocytopenia and/or hypokalemia were found to correlate with severe alcohol syndrome, which includes life-threatening complications of alcohol withdrawal such as withdrawal seizures and DTs.[13]
- An arterial blood gas usually reveals a respiratory alkalosis.
- Seizures should precipitate a brain imaging, such as noncontrast CT of the head or magnetic resonance imaging (MRI). Seizures may also warrant a neurology consultation in all alcoholic patients with new-onset seizure, patients with more than six seizures during withdrawal, partial seizure, status epilepticus, head trauma, new focal neurologic deficit, meningeal irritation, family history of seizures in relatives who do not abuse alcohol, or prolonged postictal state.[5,14] If an alcohol-dependent patient presents with a recurrent seizure unchanged from the pattern set by previous alcohol withdrawal seizures that have already been fully evaluated, repeat imaging is not necessary.

TREATMENT

- Empiric treatment for all alcohol-dependent patients should start with thiamine, 100 mg IV or IM.
- In patients with evidence of Wernicke encephalopathy, administration of 500 mg IV thiamine three times per day for 2–3 days followed by oral thiamine supplementation

guided by response to initial therapy is standard practice.[10,15] Oral administration at presentation is not adequate owing to poor GI uptake.[10,15]
- Administration of folate and a multivitamin to all alcohol-dependent patients is also standard practice.
- Fluid repletion must be individualized for each patient, as alcohol has variable effects on sodium and water balance depending on the chronicity of use, although most patients are volume depleted.
- Glucose should be administered to those with severe alcohol withdrawal, but never before thiamine, although a review reported little evidence that IV dextrose precipitates the syndrome.[16]
- Potassium and magnesium should be repleted if low, but empiric magnesium in alcohol-withdrawing patients has not been shown to alter seizure frequency, DTs, or other symptoms.[17]
- **Benzodiazepines** (BZDs) have been shown to be the drugs of choice in meta-analyses and literature reviews to reduce the severity of alcohol withdrawal, occurrence of delirium and seizures, and side effects of medication, as well as entry into rehabilitation following detoxification.[18,19] Symptom-based administration using the **Clinical Institute Withdrawal Assessment for Alcohol Scale** (CIWA-Ar) is effective and often results in decreased use of BZDs and earlier discharge compared with fixed dosing, or front-loading dosing, but requires careful and frequent monitoring.[4,20] A score of <10 is very mild withdrawal, 10–15 is mild withdrawal, 16–20 is modest withdrawal, and >20 is severe withdrawal (Fig. 47-1).[21] High doses are needed in the first 24 hours and can be tapered over 3–7 days in uncomplicated patients or 1–2 weeks in patients with DTs.[22]
  - For stable patients treated on a medical or surgical floor, the oral agents chlordiazepoxide and oxazepam are common choices. **Chlordiazepoxide** is used at 25–100 mg PO q6–8h but is contraindicated in hepatic insufficiency.[23] **Oxazepam**, 15–30 mg PO q6–8h, is preferred in patients with liver disease.[22]
  - Diazepam and lorazepam have the advantage of both IV and PO dosing, allowing for rapid initial therapy if there is concern for a seizure or the patient cannot take medications PO. **Diazepam** has a longer half-life and is a common choice in the emergency department (ED), with initial therapy of 5–10 mg IV q10min until the patient is calm.[24] **Lorazepam** is typically given at 2–4 mg IV q10min as needed and is a common choice for patients in DTs requiring a drip in the intensive care unit (ICU), sometimes requiring >24 mg/h.[24]
- In patients with refractory DTs, phenobarbital can be effective when given with BZDs.[14] There is also some evidence for the use of propofol or dexmedetomidine in refractory patients in the ICU.[7,25]
- β-Blockers, such as propranolol, and α-blockers, including dexmedetomidine and **clonidine**, should not be used as monotherapy but can be helpful in controlling autonomic symptoms.[4,25]
- The anticonvulsant **carbamazepine** is also an acceptable supplement of BZDs to reduce autonomic symptoms. It has been shown to be equal in efficacy to phenobarbital and oxazepam for patients with mild to moderate withdrawal symptoms but has not been evaluated for treating DTs.[4] Valproate may also reduce the symptoms of alcohol withdrawal.[4] On the other hand, phenytoin has not been shown to be effective in controlling withdrawal seizures.[26] Despite their proven benefit as adjunctive medications, anticonvulsants should not be used for monotherapy for alcohol withdrawal, including seizures.
- Neuroleptics cannot be used as solo therapy, but haloperidol is a useful adjunct to BZDs for alcoholic hallucinosis or DTs.[7] Haloperidol can lower the seizure threshold

and prolong the QTc interval, but it is safe at low doses (5 mg PO, IM, or IV q8h PRN) if the patient's electrolytes have been corrected and he or she is receiving BZDs.[7] Newer antipsychotics, like risperidone and olanzapine, may have a better safety profile but have not been evaluated thoroughly in the treatment of alcohol withdrawal.[14]

Clinical Institute Withdrawal Assessment of Alcohol Scale, Revised (CIWA-Ar)

Patient: _____ **Date:** _____ **Time:** _____ (24 hour clock, midnight = 00:00)

Pulse or heart rate, taken for one minute: _____ **Blood pressure:** _____

NAUSEA AND VOMITING – Ask "Do you feel sick to your stomach? Have you vomited?" Observation.
0 no nausea and no vomiting
1 mild nausea with no vomiting
2
3
4 intermittent nausea with dry heaves
5
6
7 constant nausea, frequent dry heaves and vomiting

TACTILE DISTURBANCES – Ask "Have you experienced any itching, pins and needles sensations, any burning, any numbness, or do you feel bugs crawling on or under you skin?"
0 none
1 very mild itching, pins and needles, burning or numbness
2 mild itching, pins and needles, burning or numbness
3 moderate itching, pins and needles, burning or numbness
4 moderately hallucinations
5 severe hallucinations
6 extremely severe hallucinations
7 continuous hallucinations

TREMOR – Arms extended and fingers spread apart.
0 no tremor
1 not visible, but can be felt fingertip to fingertip
2
3
4 moderate, with patient's arms extended
5
6
7 severe, even with arms not extended

AUDITORY DISTURBANCES – Ask "Are you more aware of sounds around you? Are they harsh? Do they frighten you? Are you hearing anything that is disturbing to you? Are you hearing things you know are not there?"
0 not present
1 very mild harshness or ability to frighten
2 mild harshness or ability to frighten
3 moderate harshness or ability to frighten
4 moderately severe hallucinations
5 severe hallucinations
6 extremely severe hallucinations
7 continuous hallucinations

PAROXYSMAL SWEATS – Observation.
0 no sweat visible
1 barely perceptible sweating, palms moist
2
3
4 beads of sweat obvious on forehead
5
6
7 drenching sweats

VISUAL DISTURBANCES – Ask "Does the light appear to be too bright? Is its color different? Does it hurt your eyes? Are you seeing anything that is disturbing to you? Are you seeing things you know are not there?"
0 not present
1 very mild sensitivity
2 mild sensitivity
3 moderate sensitivity
4 moderately hallucinations
5 severe hallucinations
6 extremely severe hallucinations
7 continuous hallucinations

FIGURE 47-1 Clinical Institute Withdrawal Assessment of Alcohol Scale, revised (CIWA-Ar). From Sullivan JT, Sykora K, Schneiderman J, et al. Assessment of alcohol withdrawal: the revised Clinical Institute Withdrawal Assessment for Alcohol Scale [CIWA-Ar]. *Br J Addict* 1989;84:1353–7.

ANXIETY – Ask "Do you feel nervous?" Observation. 0 no anxiety, at ease 1 mildly anxious 2 3 4 moderately anxious, or guarded, so anxiety is inferred 5 6 7 equivalent to acute panic states as seen in severe delirium or acute schizophrenic reactions	**HEADACHE, FULLNESS IN HEAD** – Ask "Does your head feel different? Does it feel like there is a band around your head? Do not rate dizziness or lightheadedness. 0 not present 1 very mild 2 mild 3 moderate 4 moderately severe 5 severe 6 very severe 7 extremely severe
AGITATION – Observation. 0 normal activity 1 somewhat more than normal activity 2 3 4 moderately fidgety and restless 5 6 7 paces back and forth or constantly thrashes about	**ORIENTATION AND CLOUDING OF SENSORIUM** – Ask "What day is this? Where are you? Who am I?" 0 oriented and can do serial additions 1 cannot do serial additions or is uncertain about date 2 disoriented to date by no more than 2 calendar days 3 disoriented to date by more than 2 calendar days 4 disoriented to place/or person

Total **CIWA-Ar** Score _____

Rater's Initials _____

Maximum Possible Score 6, 7

The **CIWA-Ar** is not copyrighted and may be preproduced freely. This assessment for monitoring withdrawal symptoms requires approximately 5 minutes to administer. The maximum score is 67 (see instrument). Patients scoring less than 10 do not usually need additional medication for withdrawal. Scale—0–9: absent or minimal withdrawal; 10–19: mild to moderate withdrawal; >20: severe withdrawal.

FIGURE 47-1 (*Continued*)

SPECIAL CONSIDERATIONS

Hospitalization is a good opportunity to arrange referral for long-term treatment of alcohol dependence.

- The American Psychiatric Association (APA) treatment guidelines suggest screening for comorbid psychiatric conditions and trying to engage the patient in long-term outpatient relapse prevention.[27]
- Best practice for early postdetoxification involves 28-day residential care, intensive outpatient therapy with frequent visits, or day hospital care.[22]
- **Alcoholics Anonymous** (AA) and other 12-step self-help programs are effective for many people.[22] If a patient shows an interest in change, such a meeting should be identified for his or her attendance after discharge.
- A brief **motivational interview** has been shown to be effective in decreasing alcohol abuse among ED patients but has not proved successful in improving long-term outcomes in hospitalized patients.[28] More in-depth counseling sessions by nurses on the medicine floor have been shown to improve long-term outcomes, however.[28]
- Various types of behavioral therapies including **cognitive behavioral therapy** and marital therapy have shown benefit in long-term outcomes.[29]

- Medications available for the treatment of alcohol dependency are **naltrexone**, **acamprosate**, and **disulfiram**. A large, randomized trial published in 2006 looked at optimal therapy for alcoholism by comparing different combinations of medical management with naltrexone, acamprosate, or placebo with or without behavioral therapy.[30] Medical management consisted of a nine-session intervention focused on medication compliance and encouragement of abstinence. The percentage of days abstinent was best with medical management and naltrexone alone (81%) followed by medical management, placebo, and behavioral therapy (79%).[30] Medical management and placebo without behavioral therapy (75%) were superior to behavioral therapy without medical management or pills (66%).[30] Acamprosate showed no benefit over placebo.[30] Other medication that can been used with varying levels of success and evidence include baclofen, ondansetron, sertraline, and topiramate.[31]

REFERENCES

1. Schuckit MA. Alcohol-use disorders. *Lancet* 2009;373:492–501.
2. American Psychiatric Association. *Diagnostic and Statistical Manual of Mental Disorders*. 5th ed. Washington: American Psychiatric Publishing, 2013.
3. Bayard M, McIntyre J, Hill KR, Woodside J. Alcohol withdrawal syndrome. *Am Fam Physician* 2004;69:1443–50.
4. Kosten TR, O'Connor PG. Management of drug and alcohol withdrawal. *N Engl J Med* 2003;348:1786–95.
5. Rathlev NK, Ulrich AS, Delanty N, D'Onofrio G. Alcohol related seizures. *J Emerg Med* 2006;31:157–63.
6. Tovar R. Diagnosis and treatment of alcohol withdrawal. *J Clin Outcomes Manage* 2011;18:361–70.
7. Schuckit MA. Recognition and management of withdrawal delirium (delirium tremens). *N Engl J Med* 2014;371:2109–13.
8. Khan A, Levy P, Dehorn S, et al. Predictors of mortality in patients with delirium tremens. *Acad Emerg Med* 2008;15:788–90.
9. Duka T, Gentry J, Malcolm R, et al. Consequences of multiple withdrawals from alcohol. *Alcohol Clin Exp Res* 2004;28:515–9.
10. Day E, Bentham PW, Callaghan R, et al. Thiamine for prevention and treatment of Wernicke-Korsakoff syndrome in people who abuse alcohol. *Cochrane Database Syst Rev* 2013;(7):CD004033.
11. Torvik A. Wernicke's encephalopathy—prevalence and clinical spectrum. *Alcohol Alcohol Suppl* 1991;1:381–384.
12. Thomson AD, Marshall EJ. The natural history and pathophysiology of Wernicke's encephalopathy and Korsakoff's psychosis. *Alcohol Alcohol* 2006;41:151–158.
13. Goodson CM, Clark BJ, Douglas IS. Predictors of severe alcohol withdrawal syndrome: a systematic review and meta-analysis. *Alcohol Clin Exp Res* 2014;38:2664–77.
14. Kattimani S, Bharadwaj B. Clinical management of alcohol withdrawal: a systematic review. *Ind Psychiatry J* 2013;2:100–8.
15. Thomson AD, Guerrini I, Marshall EJ. Wernicke's encephalopathy: role of thiamine. *Pract Gastroenterol* 2009;23:21–30.
16. Schabelman E, Kuo D. Glucose before thiamine for Wernicke encephalopathy: a literature review. *J Emerg Med* 2012;42:488–94.
17. Sarai M, Tejani AM, Chan AW, et al. Magnesium for alcohol withdrawal. *Cochrane Database Syst Rev* 2013;(6):CD008358.
18. Mayo-Smith MF. Pharmacological management of alcohol withdrawal: a meta-analysis and evidence-based practice guideline: American Society of Addiction Medicine Working Group on Pharmacological Management of Alcohol Withdrawal. *JAMA* 1997;278:144–51.
19. Lejoyeux M, Solomon J, Ades J. Benzodiazepine treatment for alcohol-dependent patients. *Alcohol Alcohol* 1998;33:563–75.
20. Cassidy EM, O'Sullivan I, Bradshaw P, et al. Symptom-triggered benzodiazepine therapy for alcohol withdrawal syndrome in the emergency department: a comparison with the standard fixed dose benzodiazepine regimen. *Emerg Med J* 2012;29:802–4.

21. Sullivan JT, Sykora K, Schneiderman J, et al. Assessment of alcohol withdrawal: the revised Clinical Institute Withdrawal Assessment for Alcohol scale (CIWA-Ar). *Br J Addict* 1989;84:1353.
22. Connor JP, Haber PS, Hall WD. Alcohol use disorders. *Lancet* 2015;15:S0140–6736.
23. Saitz R, Mayo-Smith MF, Roberts MS, et al. Individualized treatment for alcohol withdrawal. A randomized double-blind controlled trial. *JAMA* 1994;272:519–23.
24. Saitz R, O'Malley SS. Pharmacotherapies for alcohol abuse. Withdrawal and treatment. *Med Clin North Am* 1997;81:881–97.
25. Albertson TE, Chenoweth J, Ford J, et al. Is it prime time for alpha2-adrenocepter agonists in the treatment of withdrawal syndromes? *J Med Toxicol* 2014;10:369–81.
26. Chance JF. Emergency department treatment of alcohol withdrawal seizures with phenytoin. *Ann Emerg Med* 1991;20:520–2.
27. Kleber H, Weiss R, Anton R, et al. *Practice Guidelines for the Treatment of Patients with Substance Use Disorders*. 2nd ed. Arlington, VA: American Psychiatric Association, 2006.
28. Saitz R, Palfai TP, Cheng DM, et al. Brief intervention for medical inpatients with unhealthy alcohol use: a randomized, controlled trial. *Ann Intern Med* 2007;146:167–76.
29. Magill M, Kiluk BD, McCrady BS, et al. Active ingredients of treatment and client mechanisms of changes in behavioral treatments for alcohol use disorders: progress 10 years later. *Alcohol Clin Exp Res* 2015;39:1852–62.
30. Anton RF, O'Malley SS, Ciraulo DA, et al. Combined pharmacotherapies and behavioral interventions for alcohol dependence: the COMBINE study: a randomized controlled trial. *JAMA* 2006;295:2003–17.
31. Thompson A, Owens L, Pushpakon SP, et al. Pharmacotherapies for alcohol dependence: a stratified approach. *Pharmacol Ther* 2015;153:10–24.

General Toxicology and Opioid Intoxication and Withdrawal

48

David B. Liss and Anna Arroyo-Plasencia

GENERAL PRINCIPLES

- In 2011, there were over two million human exposures logged into the National Poison Data System.[1]
- Analgesic exposure was the substance class with the highest exposure frequency, with over 11% of the calls, while sedatives/hypnotics/antipsychotics were the fourth most common substance class with over 6% of the calls.[1]
- Furthermore, there were over 48,000 poisoning deaths in the United States in 2013 alone.[2]
- This chapter discusses the approach to the undifferentiated poisoned patient, aspirin and acetaminophen overdoses, general toxidromes, and finally opioid intoxication and withdrawal.

APPROACH TO THE UNDIFFERENTIATED POISONED PATIENT

When presented with an undifferentiated overdose patient, certain physical exam and laboratory findings can give clues to the specific exposure. In addition to a complete history, each patient presenting following an unknown overdose should receive the following evaluation.

- The complete physical exam should pay special attention for signs for specific toxidromes.
- An ECG should evaluate for cardiac effects of potential ingestants.
- An acetaminophen concentration and aspartate transaminase (AST) to evaluate for acetaminophen toxicity
- Obtaining a serum salicylate concentration should be considered. A serum salicylate concentration must be obtained in any patient demonstrating signs of or reporting an aspirin overdose.
  - It has been suggested that a serum salicylate concentration may not be required for fully conscious asymptomatic patients who deny taking aspirin.
  - However, the inappropriate attribution of the vague signs and symptoms of salicylate toxicity to other diagnoses could result in significant consequences.
- A urine drug screen should be obtained.

ASPIRIN OVERDOSE

- As with the undifferentiated poisoned patient, patients presenting after an aspirin overdose should undergo a full history and physical.
- A reported history of ingesting 150 mg/kg of body weight or 6.5 g of aspirin (whichever is less) is concerning for potential systemic toxicity.
- Abdominal pain, nausea, emesis, tinnitus, and lethargy are clinical characteristics of patients presenting with an aspirin overdose.

- Following ingestion, aspirin is rapidly hydrolyzed to salicylate, and a serum salicylate concentration will guide treatment.
- A basic metabolic panel and anion gap, lactate concentration, arterial or venous blood gas determination, and serum or urine ketones may lend clues to an unrecognized aspirin overdose.
- Classically, salicylate poisoning is associated with a primary respiratory alkalosis and a primary metabolic acidosis resulting in net alkalemia.
- Salicylate concentrations need to be interpreted in the context of the reported units.
  - In the United States, serum salicylate concentrations are commonly reported in mg/dL.
  - Serum salicylate concentrations may also be reported in mg/L and µg/mL.
  - This become particularly problematic for patients transferred from an institution using a different reporting system from the receiving facility as the difference in result could be falsely interpreted as improvement or incorrectly interpreted as requiring aggressive therapy.
- Salicylate concentrations need to be repeated every 2–4 hours with more frequent monitoring for cases of significant salicylate toxicity. Monitoring can stop once the salicylate concentration is clearly down trending and <30 mg/dL based on a minimum of two levels with one being done a minimum of 8 hours after the time of ingestion. Pharmacokinetics are altered in overdose, and consultation with a medical toxicologist or the local poison control center (1-800-222-1222) should be obtained in any patient with altered metal status attributable to aspirin and any detectible salicylate concentration or with an increasing serum salicylate concentration at or above 30 mg/dL.
- There is no antidote for aspirin; treatment for aspirin overdose is supportive and based on levels.
  - Following an acute aspirin overdose, sodium bicarbonate therapy dosed as 150 mEq NaHCO$_3$ in one liter of D5W with 40 mEq KCl added to each liter should be started when the salicylate concentration is at or above 30 mg/dL.
  - Sodium bicarbonate administration is influenced by the acid–base status of the patient but is generally initiated at a rate of 1.5–2 times maintenance to alkalinize the urine and aid in renal salicylate excretion, which is highly dependent on urine pH.[3] The goal urinary pH is 7.5–8. Alkalemia is essential to preventing salicylate penetration into the central nervous system. Caution should be used when administering sodium bicarbonate therapy in patients with congestive heart failure or any medical condition where they may experience difficulty with the volume of infusion, and the rate should be adjusted accordingly.
- Renal consultation for hemodialysis should be considered once the salicylate concentration reaches 80 mg/dL as this will allow setup of hemodialysis before the serum concentration reaches >90 mg/dL, an indication for dialysis in an acute overdose.
  - Caution should be used in cases of respiratory failure where sedation and mechanical ventilation can impair minute ventilation and become rapidly fatal if PCO$_2$ is allowed to rise with a fall in pH. Consultation with a medical toxicologist or the local poison center can help guide treatment in cases of respiratory failure.

ACETAMINOPHEN OVERDOSE

- After obtaining a complete history and physical, patients presenting following an acetaminophen overdose should undergo laboratory evaluation including an acetaminophen concentration and an AST.
- Patients reporting an acetaminophen ingestion of 150 mg/kg or greater are at risk for hepatic toxicity. However, overdose histories are not always accurate. An acetaminophen concentration is essential for evaluating potential toxicity risk.

TABLE 48-1 ACETYLCYSTEINE IN ACETAMINOPHEN OVERDOSE

Time Since Ingestion	Level At or Above Which Acetylcysteine Should Be Started
4 h	150 µg/mL
8 h	75 µg/mL
12 h	37.5 µg/mL
16 h	18.75 µg/mL
20 h	9.375 µg/mL

Data from Rumack BH. Acetaminophen hepatotoxicity: the first 35 years. *Clin Toxicol (Phila)* 2002;40:3–20.

- An acetaminophen concentration should be obtained at least 4 hours after the reported start time of their ingestion and as soon as possible if more than 4 hours have past since their ingestion. Acetaminophen concentrations from patient's presenting within 24 hours of their acute ingestion can be interpreted using the Rumack-Matthew Nomogram[4] if their AST is normal.
  - Acetylcysteine is the antidote used for patients at risk for possible or probable acetaminophen toxicity and should be started for anyone with a concentration of 150 µg/mL or higher at 4 hours following their ingestion. Table 48-1[5] lists acetaminophen concentrations and the time following ingestion where acetylcysteine should be started, and Table 48-2[6] lists acetylcysteine dosing for patients presenting within 24 hours of their ingestion.
  - Acetylcysteine can be discontinued after the 21-hour infusion protocol if laboratory data sent following 20 hours of continuous acetylcysteine therapy demonstrates an undetectable acetaminophen concentration, an INR < 2, an AST that has not increased, and the patient is otherwise clinically stable and at their baseline.
  - A medical toxicologist or the local poison center should be contacted for any patient presenting 24 hours or more following their ingestion with a detectible acetaminophen level or an elevated AST.
  - A medical toxicologist or the local poison center should also be contacted for any patient with an elevated AST following an acetaminophen overdose regardless of their time of presentation.

TABLE 48-2 ACETYLCYSTEINE DOSING FOR PATIENTS WEIGHING >40 kg

Loading dose	150 mg/kg in 200 mL of diluent infused over 60 min
Dose 2	50 mg/kg in 500 mL of diluent infused over 4 h at a rate of 12.5 mg/kg/h
Dose 3	100 mg/kg in 1000 mL of diluent administered over 16 h at a rate of 6.25 mg/kg/h

From Acetadote (acetylcysteine) injection. In: *Highlights of Prescribing Information.* Nashville, TN: Cumberland Pharmaceuticals Inc, 2006. Available from http://www.accessdata.fda.gov/drugsatfda_docs/label/2006/021539s004lbl.pdf (last accessed: 3/14/2016).

TOXIDROMES

- Toxidromes are a pattern of physical exam findings that can suggest a specific class of xenobiotic exposure; once recognized, this can help guide patient treatment. Consultation with a medical toxicologist or the poison center may be necessary.
- Below are characteristics of selected toxidromes.

Anticholinergic (Antimuscarinic) Toxidrome

- Anticholinergics medications include antihistamines, scopolamine, atropine, and tricyclic antidepressants to name a few. This class of medications is found in prescription and many over-the-counter medications. There are also plants that produce anticholinergic effects. Thus, a careful medication and exposure history is important.
- Signs and symptoms of the anticholinergic toxidrome include: mydriasis, tachycardia, anhidrosis, hypoactive bowel sounds altered sensorium (hallucinations, psychosis, and delirium), flushing, and urinary retention.
- Treatment of patients presenting with signs of an anticholinergic toxidrome is mostly supportive, including IV fluids and benzodiazepines as needed for agitation.
- In selected cases of severe antimuscarinic toxicity consider administering physostigmine. A medical toxicologist or the local poison center should be contacted for advice on physostigmine administration.

Cholinergic Toxidrome

- Cholinergic agents include organophosphates and carbamates. These agents include medical and nonmedical applications. Medications include acetylcholinesterase inhibitors such as neostigmine and central acetylcholinesterase inhibitors such as donepezil. Nonmedical applications include pesticides.
- Signs and symptoms of the cholinergic toxidrome include diarrhea, urination, miosis, bronchorrhea and bronchospasm, emesis, lacrimation, and salivation.
- Treatment is supportive.
  - Severe intoxication may require atropine administration at 0.5–1 mg IV with increasing doses if needed.
  - Seizures should be treated with IV benzodiazepines.
  - If there is concern for organophosphate poisoning, a medical toxicologist or the local poison center should be consulted and pralidoxime administration should be considered. Pralidoxime can be dosed at 1–2 g IV once followed by bolus dosing or a continuous infusion if symptoms remain or recur.

Sympathomimetic Toxidrome

- Sympathomimetic agents include medications (e.g., ephedrine containing medications) as well as illicit substances, including cocaine, and amphetamines.
- Signs and symptoms of the sympathomimetic syndrome include tachycardia, hypertension, hyperthermia, diaphoresis, mydriasis, and agitation.
- Treatment is supportive and includes IV fluids, benzodiazepines IM, IV, or PO, and cooling if the patient has significantly hyperthermia.

Sedative-Hypnotic Toxidrome

- Sedative-hypnotic agents are generally prescribed for treating sleep disorders. Medications include benzodiazepines (e.g., temazepam) and nonbenzodiazepines (e.g., zolpidem).
- Signs and symptoms of the sedative-hypnotic syndrome include somnolence, coma, slurred speech, ataxia, and respiratory depression.

- Treatment is supportive.
  - Isolated benzodiazepine exposure is relatively safe even with substantial ingestion; however, coingestions may cause significant abnormalities.
  - It is not recommended to give the reversal agent flumazenil in a patient with unknown tolerance, with chronic benzodiazepine use, or with a mixed overdose.

OPIOID INTOXICATION

- There is an epidemic of opioid related overdose deaths currently in the United States. There has been a 200% increase in the number of opioid-related overdose deaths since 2000.[7] Opioid-related overdose can occur from the usage of opioids in any form.
- Signs and symptoms of opioid intoxication include sedation and coma, euphoria, bradycardia and orthostatic hypotension, respiratory depression/hypopnea/apnea, miosis, hypoactive bowel sounds, cyanosis, and possibly seizure (tramadol,[8] meperidine[9]).
- Laboratory evaluation can include basic serum electrolytes and glucose. Opioid-intoxicated patients may be under the influence of other substances; frequently, a urine drug screen is sent on patients presenting with altered mental status. Results can suggest potential exposure but are not indicative of a level of intoxication.
- ECG is indicated in any patient intoxicated with is methadone that can prolong the QTc and when coingestants with cardiac toxicity are suspected.
- Treatment of opioid-intoxicated patients is primarily supportive.
  - Depending on the severity of the intoxication, intubation may be necessary.
  - Naloxone should be given to rapidly reverse the effects of opioid intoxication in any patient demonstrating significant respiratory depression.[10]
    - Caution should be used when administering naloxone to opioid-dependent patients as this can precipitate acute withdrawal.
    - In cases of opioid dependence, low dose naloxone should be administered with dose titration as needed to reverse respiratory depression and prevent intubation.
  - Naloxone is available in 0.4 mg/mL and 1 mg/mL concentrations and should be diluted in normal saline to a concentration of 0.04 mg/mL.
  - For symptomatic respiratory depression, administer an initial dose of 0.04 mg and monitor for every 2 minutes until respiratory depression improves (up to 10 mg of naloxone).[11]
  - Naloxone's onset of action is ~2 minutes after intravenous administration. The duration of action of naloxone is shorter than that of most opioid analgesics; be prepared to repeat the dose or begin a continuous naloxone infusion (two-thirds of the effective dose administered converted into an hourly rate).
  - If there is no clinical improvement after 10 mg of naloxone, an alternative diagnosis is likely.
  - Some opioids are thought to be more resistant to naloxone (e.g., buprenorphine, codeine, fentanyl) and may require higher initial doses (10 mg) for full response.
  - Alternative routes of administration include intramuscular, subcutaneous, intranasal, and endotracheal routes. These offer different bioavailability and onset of action when compared to intravenous naloxone.[12]
  - Gastric decontamination with activated charcoal is not indicated for opioid ingestion alone, given the risk of aspiration and the efficacy of naloxone therapy and supportive care.

OPIOID WITHDRAWAL

- Opioid withdrawal may be seen in any patient on chronic opioid therapy following its abrupt discontinuation.
- Signs and symptoms of withdrawal may begin as early as 4–6 hours after the last dose of a short-acting opioid and up to 24–48 hours after cessation of a long-acting opioid such as methadone.[13]

- Opioid withdrawal is extremely unpleasant but generally not life-threatening in otherwise healthy adults.[13]
- Typical signs and symptoms of opioid withdrawal are shown in Table 48-3.
- Treatment of opioid withdrawal is focused on symptomatic and supportive care.
  - **The Clinical Opioid Withdrawal Scale** (COWS) and the **Clinical Institute Narcotic Assessment** (CINA) withdrawal instrument were validated as for monitoring patients for signs of opioid withdrawal.[14]
  - Methadone has been used to treat the objective signs of opioid withdrawal[15]; however, caution needs to be used when prescribing methadone for opioid withdrawal as opioid toxicity is possible.
    - Consultation with an addiction medicine specialist should be considered before prescribing methadone for opioid withdrawal in nonpregnant patients.
    - Consultation with pain management and obstetrics should be obtained in any pregnant patient with signs of opioid withdrawal as withdrawal can be detrimental to the fetus and fetal viability needs to be documented.
    - Methadone can be used in pregnancy to treat opioid withdrawal as its benefits outweigh its potential for fetal risk, despite being pregnancy category C.[16]
    - Physician's need to remember that they are not permitted to prescribe methadone for opioid maintenance treatment, unless specially licensed.[17] However, physicians can administer methadone for the temporary treatment of acute opioid withdrawal in patients hospitalized for a separate medical condition.[17]
    - The initial dose of methadone is 20–30 mg daily with an additional 5–10 mg given after 2–4 hours if the patient is symptomatic. The dose is titrated to a goal of preventing symptoms for 24 hours.[18]
    - Obstetrics and pain management can help guide methadone dosing and titration in pregnancy.
  - Clonidine can be used to treat symptoms of opioid withdrawal. Given at an initial dose of 0.1–0.2 mg orally, clonidine can be increased to a maximum of 1 mg/d as needed until symptoms resolve. The patient can then be maintained at up to 1.2 mg/d divided into three doses and tapered gradually over 7–10 days after opioid cessation to prevent clonidine withdrawal. Clonidine should be held and the dose adjusted for hypotension and bradycardia.[19]
  - Benzodiazepines can also be added to clonidine therapy, especially when opioid therapy cannot be used (e.g., lorazepam 1–2 mg PO or IV q4h PRN).
  - Additional symptom-specific therapies include
    - Ondansetron 4–8 mg PO or IV q6h or prochlorperazine 5–10 mg PO or IV q6h, both PRN for nausea.
    - Loperamide 4 mg PO then 2 mg PO PRN diarrhea up to 16 mg/d as needed for diarrhea.
- Refer any patient with a substance use disorder to drug rehabilitation and Narcotics Anonymous programs.

TABLE 48-3 SIGNS AND SYMPTOMS OF OPIOID WITHDRAWAL

Flu-like symptoms, myalgias	Diaphoresis, hot and cold flashes	Pruritus	Frequent yawning	Hypertension (Alternatively, hypotension may be present if volume depletion has resulted from vomiting and diarrhea)
Rhinorrhea, lacrimation	Insomnia, anxiety, irritability	Mydriasis	Hyperactive bowel sounds	
Nausea, vomiting, and diarrhea	Intense drug craving	Piloerection	Tachycardia	

REFERENCES

1. Bronstein AC, Spyker DA, Cantilena LR Jr, et al. 2011 Annual report of the American Association of Poison Control Centers' National Poison Data System (NPDS): 29th annual report. *Clin Toxicol (Phila)* 2012;50:911–1164.
2. Xu J, Murphy SL, Kochanek KD, Bastian BA. Deaths: final data for 2013. *Natl Vital Statistics Report* 2016;64:1–118.
3. Prescott LF, Balali-Mood M, Critchley JA, et al. Diuresis or urinary alkalinisation for salicylate poisoning? *Br Med J* 1982;285:1383–6.
4. Rumack BH, Matthew H. Acetaminophen poisoning and toxicity. *Pediatrics* 1975;55:871–6.
5. Rumack BH. Acetaminophen hepatotoxicity: the first 35 years. *Clin Toxicol (Phila)* 2002;40:3–20.
6. Acetadote (acetylcysteine) injection. In: *Highlights of Prescribing Information*. Nashville, TN: Cumberland Pharmaceuticals Inc., 2006. Available at: http://www.accessdata.fda.gov/drugsatfda_docs/label/2006/021539s004lbl.pdf (last accessed: 3/14/2016).
7. Rudd R, Aleshire N, Zibbell JE, Gladden M. Increases in drug and opioid overdose deaths—United States, 2000–2014. *MMWR* 2016;64:1378–82.
8. Ultram (tramadol hydrochloride) tablets. In: *Prescribing Information*. Gurabo, Puerto Rico: Janssen Ortho, LLC, 2008. Available at: http://www.accessdata.fda.gov/drugsatfda_docs/label/2009/020281s032s033lbl.pdf (last accessed: 3/14/2016).
9. Demerol (meperidine hydrochloride, USP). In: *Prescribing Information*. Bridgewater, NJ: Sanofi-Aventis U.S. LLC, 2014. Available at http://products.sanofi.ca/en/demerol.pdf (last accessed: 3/14/2016).
10. Kim HK, Nelson LS. Reducing the harm of opioid overdose with the safe use of naloxone: a pharmacologic review. *Expert Opin Drug Saf* 2015;14:1137–46.
11. Boyer EW. Management of opioid analgesic overdose. *N Engl J Med* 2012;367:146–55.
12. Dowling J, Isbister GK, Kirkpatrick CM, et al. Population pharmacokinetics of intravenous, intramuscular, and intranasal naloxone in human volunteers. *Ther Drug Monit* 2008;30:490–6.
13. Farrell M. Opiate withdrawal. *Addiction* 1994;89:1471–5.
14. Tompkins DA, Bigelow GE, Harrison JA, et al. Concurrent validation of the Clinical Opiate Withdrawal Scale (COWS) and single-item indices against the Clinical Institute Narcotic Assessment (CINA) opioid withdrawal instrument. *Drug Alcohol Depend* 2009;105:154–9.
15. Amato L, Davoli M, Minozzi S, et al. Methadone at tapered doses for the management of opioid withdrawal. *Cochrane Database Syst Rev* 2005:CD003409.
16. Methadose (methadone hydrochloride) tablet. In: *Prescribing Information*. Hazelwood, MO: Mallinckrodt, Inc., 2014. Available at: http://www.accessdata.fda.gov/drugsatfda_docs/label/2008/017116s021lbl.pdf (last accessed: 3/14/2016).
17. Center for Substance Abuse Treatment. *Medication-Assisted Treatment for Opioid Addiction in Opioid Treatment Programs. Treatment Improvement Protocol (TIP) Series 43. DHHS Publication No. (SMA) 05-4048*. Rockville, MD: Substance Abuse and Mental Health Services Administration, 2005.
18. Nicholls L, Bragaw L, Ruetsch C. Opioid dependence treatment and guidelines. *J Manag Care Pharm* 2010;16:S14–21.
19. Gowing L, Farrell MF, Ali R, White JM. Alpha2-adrenergic agonists for the management of opioid withdrawal. *Cochrane Database Syst Rev* 2014;(3):CD002024.

Index

Note: Page numbers followed by f refer to figures; page numbers followed by t refer to tables.

A

α_1-antitrypsin deficiency, 147
α_2-agonists, 9
Abdominal compartment syndrome, 160
Abdominal exam, 125
Abdominal pain
  diagnosis
    clinical presentation, 139–144
    diagnostic testing, 144
    differential diagnosis of, 141t–142t
    history, 139–143
    imaging, 144
    laboratories, 144
    physical examination, 143–144
  etiology, 139
  general principles, 139
  treatment, 145
ABGs. *See* Arterial blood gases (ABGs)
Ablation, 80
Abnormal liver enzymes
  diagnosis
    clinical presentation, 147–148
    diagnostic testing, 148–151
    history, 147–148
    physical examination, 148
    predominantly hepatocellular pattern, 148–150
    predominately cholestatic pattern, 150–151
  etiology, 146–147
  general principles, 146
Acamprosate, 372
ACE inhibitors. *See* Angiotensin-converting enzyme (ACE) inhibitors
Acetaminophen overdose, 375–376, 376t
Acetylcysteine, 376t
Acoustic neuroma, 250, 251
ACS. *See* Acute coronary syndromes (ACS)
Acute adrenal crisis, 331
Acute asthma exacerbations, 110–112
Acute back pain, 349
Acute coronary syndromes (ACS)
  diagnosis
    diagnostic procedures, 43
    diagnostic testing, 42–43
    differential diagnosis, 42
    ECG, 43
    history, 40–41, 41t
    laboratories, 42
    physical exam, 41–42
  pathophysiology, 40
  STEMI, treatment
    medications, 51
    reperfusion, 51–52
  UA/NSTEMI, treatment
    anticoagulation therapy, 47–48
    anti-ischemic therapy, 43–45
    antiplatelet therapy, 46–47
    early invasive approach, 49
    ischemia-guided approach, 49
    TIMI or GRACE risk scores, 49, 50t, 51
Acute glomerulonephritis, 156
Acute heart failure
  clinical presentation, 73
  diagnosis, 73
  general principles
    etiology, 72
    pathophysiology, 72
    special considerations, 74
    treatment, 73–74
Acute hemodialysis, 74
Acute infective endocarditis, 224
Acute interstitial nephritis, 156, 362
Acute kidney injury (AKI), 20
  diagnosis
    clinical presentation, 156–158
    diagnostic procedures, 158
    diagnostic testing, 158, 159f
    history, 157
    imaging, 158
    laboratories, 158
    physical examination, 157–158
  general principles, 155–156
    classification, 155
    definition, 155
    etiology, 155–156
  perioperative care of, 20
  special considerations, 160
  treatment, 159
Acute Kidney Injury Network (AKIN), 155
Acute myocardial infarction, 315
Acute onset of hyponatremia, 170
Acute tubular necrosis (ATN), 156
Acute viral hepatitis, 15

Index

ADA. *See* American Diabetes Association (ADA)
Addiction, 304
Adjuvant pain therapies, 300
ADR. *See* Adverse drug reaction (ADR)
Adrenal incidentaloma
  diagnosis
    clinical presentation, 333–334
    diagnostic procedures, 334
    diagnostic testing, 334
    imaging, 334
    laboratories, 334
  general principles, 333
  treatment, 334, 336
Adrenal insufficiency (AI)
  causes of, 330t
  diagnosis
    clinical presentation, 329–330
    diagnostic testing, 330–331
    history, 329
    imaging evaluation, 331
    laboratories, 330–331
    physical exam, 329–330
  general principles, 329
  treatment, 331
Adrenal tumors, imaging characteristics of, 334, 335t
Adverse drug reaction (ADR)
  diagnosis
    clinical presentation, 361–362
    diagnostic procedures, 363
    diagnostic testing, 363
    history, 361
    laboratories, 363
    physical examination, 361–362
  general principles
    classifications, 360
    epidemiology, 360
    pathophysiology, 360
    prevention, 361
    risk factors, 360–361
  treatment, 363–364
AEDs. *See* Antiepileptic drugs (AEDs)
AF. *See* Atrial fibrillation (AF)
Age
  low back pain, 348
  preoperative pulmonary evaluation, 10
  solitary pulmonary nodule, 115
Agranulocytosis, 323
AHA. *See* American Heart Association (AHA)
AI. *See* Adrenal insufficiency (AI)
Airway inflammation, 105, 107
AKI. *See* Acute kidney injury (AKI)
AKIN. *See* Acute Kidney Injury Network (AKIN)
Alanine aminotransferase (ALT), 146
Alcohol withdrawal seizures, 367
Alcohol withdrawal syndrome
  diagnosis
    clinical presentation, 367–368
    diagnostic testing, 368
    history, 367–368
    physical examination, 368
  general principles, 367
  medications, 368–370
  special considerations, 371–372
  treatment, 368–370
Alcoholic hallucinosis, 367
Alcoholic hepatitis, 15
Alcoholics Anonymous (AA), 371
Aldosterone receptor antagonists, 67t, 68
Alimentary feedings, inpatient diabetes management, 317
Alkaline phosphatase, 146
Allergy testing, 110
ALT. *See* Alanine aminotransferase (ALT)
Altered mental status
  causes of, 243t
  diagnosis
    clinical presentation, 242–244
    diagnosis, 242–245
    diagnostic testing, 245
    history, 242–243
    imaging, 245
    laboratories, 245
    physical exam, 234–244
  general principles, 241–242
  historical features of, 244t
  treatment, 245–246
Alternate cover test, 251
Ambulatory ECG (Holter) monitoring, 61
American Association of Clinical Endocrinologists (AACE), 313
American College of Chest Physicians (ACCP) guidelines, 88, 117
American College of Rheumatology classification, 341–342, 342t
American College of Surgeons (ACS), 7
American Diabetes Association (ADA), 313
American Gastroenterological Association, 123
American Heart Association (AHA), 230
American Psychiatric Association (APA), 371
American Thoracic Society (ATS), 187
American Urologic Association (AUA), 182
Amiodarone, 79, 80t
ANA. *See* Antinuclear antibodies (ANA)
Analgesics, 351
  nonopioid, 300, 303
  opioid, 301
Anaphylaxis
  diagnosis
    clinical presentation, 358

diagnostic criteria, 358
diagnostic testing, 358
differential diagnosis, 358
general principles
epidemiology, 357
etiology, 357
pathophysiology, 357
risk factors, 357
medications, 358–359
monitoring/follow-up, 359
treatment, 358–359
Anemia, 157
diagnosis
clinical presentation, 267
diagnostic procedures, 269
diagnostic testing, 268–269
history, 267
laboratories, 268–269
physical exam, 267
general principles, 265–267
postoperative anemia, special considerations in, 269
treatment
chronic renal failure, 270
folate deficiency, 270
iron deficiency anemia, 270
vitamin B_{12} deficiency, 270
Angina
historical features associated with, 35t
typical, 41
Angiodysplasia, 136
Angiography, 137, 255
Angiotensin II receptor blockers (ARBs)
acute coronary syndromes, 45
heart failure, 67t, 68
hypertension, 10
Angiotensin-converting enzyme (ACE) inhibitors
acute coronary syndromes, 45
heart failure, 66, 68
hypertension, 10
Antibiotic prophylaxis, 230
Antibiotics
bacteremia, 216
COPD, acute exacerbations of, 103
endocarditis, 231
preoperative pulmonary evaluation, 12
Anti-CD-20 agent, 276
Anticentromere antibodies, 343
Anticholinergic agents, 127–128
Anticholinergic (antimuscarinic) toxidrome, 377
Anticoagulation, 47, 256, 287
determining risk
major bleeding, 86–87
thrombosis, 87

disease-specific perioperative anticoagulation management
atrial fibrillation, 88
prosthetic heart valves, 89
venous thromboembolism, 87–88, 88t
general principles, 86
pharmacokinetics and dosing, 288t
treatment, 89–91, 90t
Anticoagulation therapy, 47–48
Anticonvulsants, 351
Anticyclic citrullinated peptide (CCP), 344
Antidepressants, 300, 351
Anti-dsDNA antibodies, 343
Antiepileptic drugs (AEDs), 300
Antifungal therapy, 309
Antihistamines, 127, 359
Antihistone antibodies, 343
Anti-ischemic therapy, 43–45
Anti–Jo-1 antibodies, 343
Antimitochondrial antibodies (AMA), 151
Antinuclear antibodies (ANA), 150, 275
diagnosis
clinical presentation, 341–343
diagnostic testing, 343–344
history, 341–342
physical examination, 342–343
general principles
classification, 339–341
definition, 339
epidemiology, 341
etiology, 341
pathophysiology, 341
risk factors, 339
treatment, 344
Antiphospholipid antibodies, 343
Antiplatelet therapy, 46–47
Antipseudomonal β-lactam agent, 307
Anti-RNP antibodies, 343
Anti–Scl-70 antibodies, 344
Anti-Smith antibodies, 344
Antispasmodic agents, 301
Anti-SS-A/Ro, 344
Anti-SS-B/La, 344
Antivirals, 309
Aortic dissection, 33, 34, 38
Aortic stenosis (AS), 4
Aortic valve replacements (AVR), 89
APA. *See* American Psychiatric Association (APA)
Apixaban, 84
Apparent mineralocorticoid excess, 167, 167t
Aprepitant, 128
ARBs. *See* Angiotensin II receptor blockers (ARBs)
ARISCAT Risk Index, 12
Arrhythmias, 60–62

Index

Arterial blood gases (ABGs), 11, 110
Arthritis, 148
Ascites, 15
Aseptic meningitis, etiologic differential diagnosis, 233, 234t
Aspartate aminotransferase (AST), 146
Aspirin (ASA), 9, 46, 255, 256, 374–375
Asthma, 10
  diagnosis
    clinical presentation, 107–108
    diagnostic procedures, 108, 110
    diagnostic testing, 108–110
    differential diagnosis, 108
    history, 107–108
    imaging, 110
    physical examination, 108
  general principles
    classification, 105–106, 106t
    definition, 105
    pathophysiology, 106–107
  treatment
    of acute exacerbations, 110–112
    chronic asthma, 112, 113t
Asymptomatic aortic stenosis, 4
Asymptomatic bacteriuria, 194
Ataxia, 248, 250, 368
Atenolol, 45
ATN. *See* Acute tubular necrosis (ATN)
Atrial fibrillation (AF)
  anticoagulation and surgery, 88
  diagnosis
    diagnostic procedures, 78
    diagnostic testing, 77–78
    electrocardiography, 77
    history, 77
    imaging, 77
    laboratories, 77
    physical exam, 77
  general principles, 76
    classification, 76
    etiology, 76
    risk factors, 76–77
  treatment, 78
    rate control, 78–79
    sinus rhythm, restoration and maintenance of, 79–80
    thromboembolic risk reduction, 81–84
Atrial flutter, 80
Atypical antipsychotics, 246
AUA. *See* American Urologic Association (AUA)
Audiometry, 251
Autoimmune hepatitis, 148
Autologous blood donation, 14
Autonomic hyperactivity, 367
AVR. *See* Aortic valve replacements (AVR)
Azithromycin, 103

B

β_2-adrenergic agents, 165
Back school, 352
Bacteremia, 213
  diagnosis
    clinical presentation, 214–215
    diagnostic testing, 215
    history, 214–215
    laboratories, 215
    physical examination, 215
  epidemiology, 213–214
  general principles, 213–214
  risk factors, 214
  treatment, 216–218, 216t–217t
Bacterial meningitis, 233
Balloon-occluded retrograde transvenous obliteration (BRTO), 136
β-blockers, 324, 369
  acute coronary syndromes, 44
  atrial fibrillation, 78
  heart failure, management of, 66
  perioperative hypertension, 10
  preoperative cardiac evaluation, 8–9
Behavioral therapy, 62, 63
Benign paroxysmal positional vertigo (BPPV), 249
Benzodiazepines (BZDs), 128, 246, 369, 379
Bethanechol, 128
Bilateral edema, 27
Biliary disorders, 146
Bisphosphonates, 301
Bivalirudin, 48
Biventricular pacing, 71
Bleeding diathesis, 20
Bleeding time (BT), 275
Blood cultures, 226, 307
Blood stream infection (BSI), 213, 216t–217t
Blood transfusions, 162
BNP. *See* B-type natriuretic peptide (BNP)
BODE index scores, 104
Bone infections, 200
Bone marrow biopsy, 275
Bone pain, 298
BPPV. *See* Benign paroxysmal positional vertigo (BPPV)
Brandt-Daroff habituation exercises, 251
Bronchial challenge testing, 108
Bronchodilators, 103
Bronchoscopic biopsy, 119
BRTO. *See* Balloon-occluded retrograde transvenous obliteration (BRTO)
Brudzinski sign, 235
BSI. *See* Blood stream infection (BSI)
β-thalassemia trait, 269
B-type natriuretic peptide (BNP)

acute heart failure and CPE, 73
chronic heart failure and cardiomyopathy, 65
Bumetanide, 69
BZDs. *See* Benzodiazepines (BZDs)

C
CAD. *See* Coronary artery disease (CAD)
Calcium channel blockers (CCB), 45, 69, 78
Calcium gluconate, 165
Caloric testing, 250
CAM. *See* Confusion Assessment Method (CAM)
Cancer history, 235
Candida bloodstream infection, 218
Cannabinoids, 128
CAP. *See* Community-acquired pneumonia (CAP)
Capsule endoscopy, 137
Carbamazepine, 369
Cardiac cause, 56, 58
Cardiac enzymes, 65, 73
Cardiac resynchronization therapy (CRT), 71
Cardiac transplantation, 71–72
Cardiogenic pulmonary edema (CPE), 72
  clinical presentation, 73
  diagnosis, 73
  general principles
    etiology, 72
    pathophysiology, 72
  special considerations, 74
  treatment, 73–74
Cardiomyopathy
  diagnosis
    history, 65
    physical exam, 65
  diagnostic testing
    electrocardiography, 65
    imaging, 66
    laboratories, 65
  general principles
    classification, 64
    epidemiology, 64
    general principles, 64
    pathophysiology, 64
  treatment
    lifestyle/risk modification, 72
    medications, 66–71, 67t
    nonpharmacologic therapies, 71
    surgical management, 71–72
Carotid angioplasty, 256
Carotid angioplasty and stenting (CAS), 255
Carotid bruit
  diagnosis
    clinical presentation, 253–254
    diagnostic procedures, 255
    diagnostic testing, 254–255
    imaging, 254–255
    physical examination, 254
  general principles, 253
  history, 253–254
  treatment, 255–256
Carotid Dopplers, 61
Carotid endarterectomy (CEA), 255, 256
Carotid sinus hypersensitivity
  diagnostic procedures, 61
  diagnostic testing, 59
  etiology, 56
  history, 58
  treatment, 63
Carotid sinus massage, 61
Carvedilol, 66
CAS. *See* Carotid angioplasty and stenting (CAS)
Catheter-associated urinary tract infections (CAUTI), 194
Catheter-directed therapies, 290
Catheter-related bloodstream infection (CRBSI), 221
Cation-exchange resins, 165
Cauda equina syndrome, 348
CAUTI. *See* Catheter-associated urinary tract infections (CAUTI)
CBC. *See* Complete blood count (CBC)
CCB. *See* Calcium channel blockers (CCB)
CEA. *See* Carotid endarterectomy (CEA)
Cefazolin, 202, 203
Cefepime, 203
Ceftriaxone, 202, 203
Cellulitis
  diagnosis
    clinical presentation, 196–197
    diagnostic testing, 197
    history, 196–197
    imaging, 197
    laboratories, 197
    physical exam, 197
  etiology, 196
  general principles, 196
  treatment, 197–199
Central pontine myelinolysis, 174
Central vertigo
  causes of, 250t
  history and exam features, 249t
Cerebral angiography, 251
Cerebral infarction, 250
Chemoreceptor trigger zone (CTZ), 123
Chemotherapy-induced peripheral neuropathy (CIPN), 297
Chest discomfort, 25, 33, 42
Chest pain
  diagnosis

Chest pain (*Continued*)
    disease-specific confirmatory testing, 36–38
    electrocardiography, 35, 37t
    history, 33–34
    imaging, 36
    laboratories, 35
    physical exam, 35, 36t
  differential diagnosis, 34t
  general principles, 33
  historical features associated with angina, 35t
  treatment, 38
Chest radiograph, 36, 66, 228
Chest X-ray (CXR), 77
Chlordiazepoxide, 369
Chlorpromazine, 127
Chlorthalidone, 69
Cholestasis, 323
Cholestatic disorders, 146
Cholinergic toxidrome, 377
Chronic asthma, 110
Chronic back pain, 349
Chronic bronchitis, 99
Chronic heart failure
  diagnosis
    history, 65
    physical exam, 65
  diagnostic testing
    electrocardiography, 65
    imaging, 66
    laboratories, 65
  general principles
    classification, 64
    epidemiology, 64
    general principles, 64
    pathophysiology, 64
  treatment
    lifestyle/risk modification, 72
    medications, 66–71, 67t
    nonpharmacologic therapies, 71
    surgical management, 71–72
Chronic hepatitis, 15
Chronic hyponatremia, 171
Chronic kidney disease (CKD), 20
  general principles, 19
  stigmata of, 148
  treatment, 19–20
Chronic obstructive pulmonary disease (COPD), 10
  diagnosis
    clinical presentation, 100–101
    diagnostic procedures, 102
    diagnostic testing, 101–102
    differential diagnosis, 101
    history, 100–101
    imaging, 102
    laboratories, 101–102
    physical examination, 101
  general principles
    classification, 99, 100t
    definition, 99
    etiology, 99
    pathophysiology, 99
    risk factors, 100
  outcome/prognosis, 104
  treatment
    acute exacerbations, 103–104
    stable, 102–103
Chronic renal failure, anemia of, 265, 270
CINA. *See* Clinical Institute Narcotic Assessment (CINA)
CIPN. *See* Chemotherapy-induced peripheral neuropathy (CIPN)
Ciprofloxacin, 203
CKD. *See* Chronic kidney disease (CKD)
Clindamycin, 203
Clinical Institute Narcotic Assessment (CINA), 379
Clinical Institute Withdrawal Assessment for Alcohol Scale (CIWA-Ar), 369, 370f–371f
Clinical Opioid Withdrawal Scale (COWS), 379
Clinical Trial of Metabolic Modulation in Acute Myocardial Infarction Treatment Evaluation—Estudios Cardiologicos Latinoamerica (CREATE-ECLA), 315
Clonidine, 10, 369, 379
Clopidogrel, 46, 256
Coagulase-negative staphylococcal infective endocarditis, 230
Coagulase-negative staphylococci (CoNS), 213
Coagulase-negative *Staphylococcus*, 216
Coagulation abnormalities, 275, 277t
Coagulation inhibitors, 282
Coagulopathy, 15
Cognitive-behavioral therapies, 352, 371
Colonoscopy, 137
Community-acquired pneumonia (CAP), 187, 190
Complement, 344
Complete blood count (CBC), 126, 226, 235
Complicated cystitis, 192, 193
Comprehensive metabolic panel (CMP), 126
Computed tomographic angiography (CTA), 137, 254
Computed tomography (CT), 202, 210, 215
Computed tomography pulmonary angiography (CTPA), 286
Confusion, 148, 242, 368

Confusion Assessment Method (CAM), 241
Congestive hepatopathy, 148
CoNS. *See* Coagulase-negative staphylococci (CoNS)
Constipation, 303
Contamination, 213
Continuous external cardiac monitoring, 61–62
Continuous insulin infusion, 17
Contrast venography, 286
Contrast-induced nephropathy, 160
COPD. *See* Chronic obstructive pulmonary disease (COPD)
Coronary artery disease (CAD), 40
Coronary revascularization, 71
Corticosteroids, 128, 300
  diagnosis
    history, 18
    laboratories, 18–19
    physical examination, 18
  general principles, 18
  pathophysiology, 18
  treatment, 19
Cosyntropin stimulation test, 18, 330
Cough-variant asthma, 105
COWS. *See* Clinical Opioid Withdrawal Scale (COWS)
CPE. *See* Cardiogenic pulmonary edema (CPE)
CRBSI. *See* Catheter-related bloodstream infection (CRBSI)
C-reactive protein (CRP), 344
CREATE-ECLA. *See* Clinical Trial of Metabolic Modulation in Acute Myocardial Infarction Treatment Evaluation-Estudios Cardiologicos Latinoamerica (CREATE-ECLA)
Creatine kinase-MB (CK-MB), 42, 42t, 43
Critical illness, 331
CRT. *See* Cardiac resynchronization therapy (CRT)
Cryoprecipitate, 20, 281
CT. *See* Computed tomography (CT)
CTZ. *See* Chemoreceptor trigger zone (CTZ)
CXR. *See* Chest X-ray (CXR)
Cyclooxygenase (COX) inhibitor, 46
Cycloxygenase-2 (COX-2) inhibitor, 135, 300
Cystitis, 192, 193

D
Dabigatran, 83–84
DCC. *See* Direct current cardioversion (DCC)
Deamino-8-d-arginine vasopressin (DDAVP), 177, 178
Deep venous thrombosis (DVT), 283
  clinical presentation, 284
  imaging modalities, 286
  pathophysiology, 283
  therapy duration, 290
  treatment, 287
  wells criteria for, 284, 285t
Degenerative disease, 353
Delirium, 241–242, 242t
Delirium tremens (DTs), 367
Demeclocycline, 175
Dementia, characteristics of, 242t
DES. *See* Drug-eluting stents (DES)
Desmopressin, 20
Dexamethasone, 128, 237
Dexamethasone suppression tests, 334
Diabetes, 162, 200
  inpatient management
    critically ill patients, 313
    general principles, 313
    glucocorticoid-induced diabetes mellitus, management of, 316
    inpatients on alimentary feedings, management of, 317
    noncritically ill patients, 314–315
    outpatient management, transition to, 317
    patients with acute myocardial infarction, 315
    perioperative period, management of diabetes in, 315–316
  management of
    classification, 16
    diagnosis, 16
    general principles, 15–16
    laboratory studies, 16
    treatment, 16–17
Diabetes and Insulin-Glucose Infusion in Acute Myocardial Infarction (DIGAMI 1), 315
Diagnostic and Statistical Manual of Mental Disorders, fifth edition (DSM-5), 241
Dialysis, 20
Diastolic dysfunction, 64
Diazepam, 369
Dietary, 162
Diet-controlled type 2 diabetes, 17
Differential time to positivity (DTP), 220
DIGAMI 1. *See* Diabetes and Insulin-Glucose Infusion in Acute Myocardial Infarction (DIGAMI 1)
Digitalis glycosides, 69
Digoxin, 79
Dimenhydrinate, 127
Diphenhydramine, 127
Dipyridamole, 256
Direct current cardioversion (DCC), 79
Direct hyperbilirubinemia, 146

Direct thrombin inhibitors (DTIs), 48
Disseminated intravascular coagulation (DIC), 282
Disulfiram, 372
Diuretic therapy, 15, 69
Diverticulosis, 136
Dix-Hallpike, 250
Dizziness, 248
Dobutamine, 70
Dolasetron, 127
Dopamine, 70
Dopamine receptor antagonists, 127
Doxycycline, 203
DRESS. *See* Drug reaction with eosinophilia and systemic symptoms (DRESS)
Dronabinol, 128
Droperidol, 127
Drug desensitization, 364
Drug fever, 362
Drug reaction with eosinophilia and systemic symptoms (DRESS), 362
Drug-eluting stents (DES), 8
Drug-induced hepatitis, 362
Drug-induced thrombocytopenia, 276
DTIs. *See* Direct thrombin inhibitors (DTIs)
DTP. *See* Differential time to positivity (DTP)
DTs. *See* Delirium tremens (DTs)
Duplex ultrasonography, 254
Duplex ultrasound, 286
DVT. *See* Deep venous thrombosis (DVT)
Dyspnea
  diagnostic testing
    diagnostic procedures, 97
    electrocardiography, 97
    imaging, 97
    laboratories, 96–97
  differential diagnosis, 96t
  general principles, 95
    diagnosis, 95–96
    etiology, 95
    history, 95–96
    physical examination, 96
  treatment, 97

E
Early Cushing syndrome, 333
Early prosthetic valve infective endocarditis, 225
ECF. *See* Extracellular fluid (ECF)
Echocardiography, 5, 36, 60, 61, 286
ED. *See* Emergency department (ED)
Edema
  diagnosis
    differential diagnosis, 27
    history, 25–26
    imaging, 27–28
    laboratories, 27
    physical examination, 26–27
  general principles, 25
  treatment, 28–29
    medications, 28–29
    nonpharmacologic therapies, 29
Edoxaban, 84
EEG. *See* Electroencephalography (EEG)
EIB. *See* Exercise-induced bronchoconstriction (EIB)
Electrocardiogram, 227
Electroencephalography (EEG), 61
Electrolyte abnormalities, 15, 19–20
Electrooculography, 251
Electrophysiologic (EP) testing, 60, 62
ELISA. *See* Enzyme-linked immunosorbent assay (ELISA)
Emergency department (ED), 33
Emphysema, 99
Empiric antibiotics, 216
Empiric CA-MRSA coverage, 198
Empiric therapy, 228
ENA panel. *See* Extractable nuclear antigens (ENA) panel
Encephalopathy, 15
Endocarditis
  diagnosis
    clinical presentation, 225–226
    diagnosis, 225–228
    diagnostic testing, 226–228
    electrocardiography, 227
    history, 225
    imaging, 228
    laboratories, 226–227
    physical examination, 225–226
  etiology, 224–225
  general principles, 224–225
  special considerations, 230–231
  treatment, 228–230
Endocarditis prophylaxis, 4
Endoscopic sclerotherapy (EST), 136
Endoscopic variceal ligation (EVL), 136
Endoscopy
  capsule, 137
  with push enteroscopy, 137
End-stage renal disease (ESRD)
  general principles, 19
  treatment, 19–20
Enterococcal bloodstream infection, 217–218
Enzyme-linked immunosorbent assay (ELISA), 339
Epidural spinal cord compression, 298
Epinephrine, 358
Epley maneuver, 251
EPR3. *See* Expert Panel Report 3 (EPR3)
Erythema multiforme (EM), 362

Erythrocyte sedimentation rate (ESR), 344
Erythromycin, 128
Esmolol, 45
Esophageal disease, 38
ESR. *See* Erythrocyte sedimentation rate (ESR)
ESRD. *See* End-stage renal disease (ESRD)
EST. *See* Endoscopic sclerotherapy (EST)
Ethacrynic acid, 69
Euthyroid sick syndrome
   diagnosis, 327
   general principles, 327
   treatment, 327
Euvolemic hyponatremia, 171–172
EVL. *See* Endoscopic variceal ligation (EVL)
Exercise
   cardiac evaluation, 5
   heart failure, management of, 72
Exercise stress test, 5
Exercise-induced bronchoconstriction (EIB), 105
Exit site infection, 220
Expert Panel Report 3 (EPR3), 105
Extracellular fluid (ECF), 173
Extractable nuclear antigens (ENA) panel, 343

F
Factor Xa inhibitors, 48
Family history, 148
Fe deficiency anemia, 268–269
Ferritin, 268, 275
Fever
   causes of, 206t–207t
   diagnosis
      clinical presentation, 209
      diagnostic testing, 209–211
      physical examination, 209
      physical examination findings in, 210
   general principles, 205–209
   pathophysiology, 208–209
   treatment, 211–212
Fever of unknown origin (FUO)
   common causes of, 206–207
   general principles, 205
FFP. *See* Fresh frozen plasma (FFP)
Fibrin degradation products/d-dimer, 275
Fixed drug eruptions, 361
Fluorodeoxyglucose positron emission tomography (^{18}F-FDG PET), 117, 119, 202
FOCUS trial, 13
Folate deficiency, 270, 275
Fondaparinux, 48
Fosaprepitant, 128
Fracture, 348
Free water deficit, 177
Free water restriction, 174

Fresh frozen plasma (FFP), 281
Fungemia, 214
FUO. *See* Fever of unknown origin (FUO)
Furosemide, 69, 73

G
Gas gangrene infections, 196
Gastric variceal obturation (GVO), 136
Gastrointestinal (GI) bleeding
   diagnosis
      causes of, 131t
      clinical presentation, 130–131
      diagnostic procedures, 133
      diagnostic testing, 133
      differential diagnosis, 131–132
      history, 130–131
      imaging, 133
      laboratories, 133
      physical examination, 131
   general principles, 130
   treatment, 133
      of lower bleeding, 136–138
      of upper bleeding, 134–136
Gastroparesis, 124
G-CSF. *See* Granulocyte colony-stimulating factor (G-CSF)
GDMT. *See* Guideline-directed medical therapy (GDMT)
Generalized edema, 27
Ghrelin, 129
GI bleeding. *See* Gastrointestinal (GI) bleeding
GINA. *See* Global Initiative for Asthma (GINA)
Global Initiative for Asthma (GINA), 112
Glomeruli, 156
Glucagon, 359
Glucocorticoid-induced diabetes mellitus, management of, 316
Glucocorticoids, 276, 359
Glucose infusions, 17
Glycoprotein IIb/IIIa inhibitors, 47
GM-CSF. *See* Granulocyte-macrophage colony-stimulating factor (GM-CSF)
GNB. *See* Gram-negative bacilli (GNB)
Gram-negative bacilli (GNB), 214
Gram-positive organisms, 214
Granisetron, 127
Granulocyte colony-stimulating factor (G-CSF), 309
Granulocyte–macrophage colony-stimulating factor (GM-CSF), 309
Graves disease (GD), 319
Guideline-directed medical therapy (GDMT), 8
GVO. *See* Gastric variceal obturation (GVO)

H

Haloperidol, 127, 246, 369–370
HAP. *See* Hospital-acquired pneumonia (HAP)
HCAP. *See* Health care–associated pneumonia (HCAP)
Head Impulse test, 250, 251
Headache, 298
Head-up tilt-table testing, 61
Health care–associated pneumonia (HCAP), 187
Hearing loss, 248–250
Heart failure
  acute heart failure and cardiogenic pulmonary edema
    clinical presentation, 73
    diagnosis, 73
    etiology, 72
    pathophysiology, 72
    special considerations, 74
    treatment, 73–74
  chronic heart failure and cardiomyopathy
    classification, 64
    diagnosis, 65
    diagnostic testing, 65
    electrocardiography, 65
    epidemiology, 64
    general principles, 64
    history, 65
    imaging, 66
    laboratories, 65
    pathophysiology, 64
    physical exam, 65
    treatment, 66–72, 67t
Helicobacter pylori, 135
Hematocrit (Hct), 275
Hematuria
  diagnosis
    diagnostic procedures, 184
    diagnostic testing, 182–184
    differential diagnosis of, 181t
    history, 180, 182
    imaging, 184
    laboratories, 183–184
    physical exam, 182
  etiology, 180
  general principles, 180
  monitoring/follow-up, 184
  treatment, 184
Hemochromatosis, 147
Hemodialysis, 19, 165
Hemoglobin (Hgb), 275
Hemoglobin A1c, 16
Hemoglobin electrophoresis, 269
Hemolytic anemias, 266t, 269
Heparin, 20, 47
Heparin-free dialysis, 20
Heparin-induced thrombocytopenia (HIT), 272
  four Ts of, 274t
  treatment, 276
Heparin–PF4 antibody, 275
Hepatic disorders, 146
Hepatitis C virus (HCV), 275
Hepatocellular injury, 146
High-bioavailability oral agents, 203
High-intensity statin therapy, 256
H.I.N.T.S exam, 250
HIV. *See* Human immunodeficiency virus (HIV)
Hospital-acquired pneumonia (HAP), 187, 190
Hospital-ventilator pneumonia, 190
Host inflammatory response, continuum of, 211t
Human immunodeficiency virus (HIV), 275
Hydralazine, 68
Hydrochlorothiazide, 69
Hydrocortisone, 324
Hydroxyzine, 127
Hypercoagulable workup, 290
Hyperglycemia Intensive Insulin Infusion in Infarction (Hi-5), 315
Hyperkalemia, 19–20
  causes of, 163t
  diagnosis
    clinical presentation, 162–164
    diagnostic testing, 164–165
    electrocardiography, 164–165
    history, 162–164
    laboratories, 164
    physical examination, 167–168
  etiology, 162
  general principles, 162
  treatment, 165–166
Hypernatremia
  definition, 176
  diagnosis
    diagnostic testing, 177
    laboratories, 177
    physical exam, 177
  general principles, 175
  history, 176
  pathophysiology, 176
  treatment, 177–178
Hypersensitivity syndrome, 362
Hypertension, 4
Hyperthyroidism
  clinical presentation
    history, 319
    physical examination, 320–321
  diagnostic testing, 321–322
    imaging, 322
    laboratories, 321–322

etiology, 319, 320
general principles, 319
special considerations, 323–324
treatment
  medications, 322–323
  nonpharmacologic therapies, 323
  surgical management, 323
Hypertonic hyponatremia, 173
Hypertriglyceridemia, 174
Hypervolemic hypernatremia, 176
Hypokalemia
  causes of, 166t
  diagnosis
    clinical presentation, 167–168
    diagnosis, 167–168
    diagnostic testing, 168
    electrocardiography, 168
    history, 167
    laboratories, 168
  etiology, 166
  general principles, 166
  primary/apparent excess aldosterone, 167
  treatment, 168
Hyponatremia, 15
  definition, 170
  diagnosis
    diagnostic testing, 171, 172
    laboratories, 171
    physical examination, 171
  general principles, 170
  history, 170–171
  hypertonic hyponatremia, 173
  hypotonic hyponatremia, 171–173
  pseudohyponatremia/isotonic hyponatremia, 173–174
  treatment, 174–175
Hypotension, 358
Hypothyroidism, 324
  causes of, 325
  diagnosis
    diagnostic testing, 326
    history, 324–325
    physical examination, 325
  etiology, 324
  general principles, 324
  special considerations, 326–327
  treatment, 326
Hypotonic hyponatremia, 171–173
Hypovolemic hypernatremia, 176
Hypovolemic hyponatremia, 172–173

I

IABP. See Intra-aortic balloon pump (IABP)
ICD. See Implantable cardioverter-defibrillator (ICD)
IDSA. See Infectious Disease Society of America (IDSA)
IDU. See Intravenous drug use (IDU)
Imbalance, 248
Immunoassays, 363
Immunoglobulin E (IgE), 107
Immunosuppression, 235
Implantable cardioverter–defibrillator (ICD), 71
Implantable loop recorders, 62
Impulsion, 248
In vitro allergy testing, 110
Indirect hyperbilirubinemia, 146
Indium-111, 202
Infectious Disease Society of America (IDSA), 187, 235
Inferior vena cava (IVC) filters, 290
Inflammatory cells, 107
Inflammatory mediators, 107
Influenza, 103
Injection therapies, 352
Inotropic agents, 70, 70t, 74
Inpatient diabetes management
  critically ill patients, 313
  general principles, 313
  glucocorticoid-induced diabetes mellitus, management of, 316
  inpatients on alimentary feedings, management of, 317
  noncritically ill patients
    NPO, management of patients, 314–315
    patients tolerating PO, management of, 314
  outpatient management, transition to, 317
  patients with acute myocardial infarction, 315
  perioperative period, management of diabetes in, 315–316
Insulin, 165, 314
  type 1 diabetes, 16
  type 2 diabetes, 17
Interstitium, 156
Intra-aortic balloon pump (IABP), 71
Intraoperative renal hypoperfusion, 160
Intravascular catheter infections
  definition, 220
  diagnosis
    clinical presentation, 221
    diagnostic testing, 221–222
  epidemiology, 220–221
  etiology, 221
  general principles, 220–221
  special considerations, 223
  treatment, 222
Intravenous drug use (IDU), 224
Intravenous magnesium sulfate, 111

Intrinsic azotemia, 156
Ipratropium bromide, 111
Iron deficiency anemia, 268–270
Irritant-induced asthma., 106
Ischemic colitis, 136
Ischemic heart failure, 64
Ischemic hepatitis, 148
Isotonic hyponatremia, 173–174
IV fluids, 359
IV immunoglobulin, 276
IV potassium, 168

J
Janeway lesions, 225

K
Kayser-Fleischer rings, 148
Kernig sign, 235
Ketogenesis, 315
Kingella kingae, 201

L
Lactate dehydrogenase (LDH), 275
Lactulose, 15
Late prosthetic valve IE, 225
Latex agglutination testing, 237
LBBB. *See* Left bundle-branch block (LBBB)
LBP. *See* Low back pain (LBP)
LDH. *See* Lactate dehydrogenase (LDH)
Left bundle-branch block (LBBB), 43
Levofloxacin, 203
Levothyroxine, 326
Listeria monocytogenes, 233
Lithium, 175
Liver disease
  classification, 14
  diagnosis, 14
  general principles, 14
  laboratories, 14
  treatment, 15
Liver transplantion, 136
LMWH. *See* Low molecular weight heparin (LMWH)
Local heat application, 352
Local/topical agents, 300–301
Long-acting sulfonylureas, 17
Long-term maintenance therapy, 331
Loop diuretics, 20, 165
  acute heart failure and CPE, 73
  chronic heart failure and cardiomyopathy, 69
Lorazepam, 246, 369
Low back pain (LBP)
  diagnosis
    clinical presentation, 346, 348–350
    diagnostic testing, 350–351
    imaging, 350–351
    laboratories, 350
    physical exam, 349–350
  differential diagnosis of, 347t–348t
  general principles, 346
  treatment
    medications, 351–352
    nonpharmacologic therapies, 352
    surgical/interventional management, 352–353
Low molecular weight heparin (LMWH), 47, 89, 289
Low reticulocyte count, 268
Lumbar disc prolapse, with radiculopathy, 353
Lumbar puncture, 245

M
MACE. *See* Major adverse cardiac events (MACE)
Macrocytic anemia, 265, 267, 268
Maculopapularmorbilliform skin eruptions, 361
Magnetic resonance angiography (MRA), 251, 254–255, 286
Magnetic resonance cholangiopancreatography (MRCP), 151
Magnetic resonance imaging (MRI), 202, 251
Major adverse cardiac events (MACE), 6
Major bleeding, 86–87
Major stress, 331
Malignancy, 249, 348
Massive pulmonary emboli, 283
Maximal bronchodilator therapy, 12
McConnell sign, 286
MCH. *See* Mean corpuscular hemoglobin (MCH)
Mean corpuscular hemoglobin (MCH), 268
Mechanical ventilation, 104
Meckel diverticulum, 137
Meclizine, 127
Medication-induced hepatotoxicity, causes of, 149t
Melatonin agonists, 246
MELD score. *See* Model for End-stage Liver Disease (MELD) score
Ménière disease, 251
Meningitis
  diagnosis
    clinical presentation, 235
    diagnostic testing, 235–237
    history, 235
    physical examination, 235
  epidemiology, 233
  etiology, 233, 234
  general principles, 233, 234

nonpharmacologic therapies, 237
treatment, 237, 238
Meningococcus, 329
Mesenteric angiography, 137
Metabolic acidosis, 20, 95
Metformin, 17
Methadone, 379
Methicillin-resistant *S. aureus* (MRSA), 202
Methicillin-sensitive *S. aureus* (MSSA), 202
Methimazole, 323
Methylxanthines, 104
Metoclopramide, 127
Metolazone, 69
Metoprolol, 45
Metronidazole, 203
Microcytic anemia, 265, 266t
Microscopic hematuria, 180, 182, 183f
Migrainous vertigo, 249
Milrinone, 71
Mineralocorticoid supplementation, 19
Mini Mental State Examination (MMSE), 244
Minocycline, 203
Minor stress, 331
Mitral stenosis, 4
MMSE. *See* Mini Mental State Examination (MMSE)
Model for End-stage Liver Disease (MELD) score, 14
Moderate exacerbation, 110
Moderate stress, 331
Modified Duke criteria, 226
Morning aldosterone-to-renin ratio, 334
Morphine sulfate, 44, 74
MRA. *See* Magnetic resonance angiography (MRA)
MRCP. *See* Magnetic resonance cholangiopancreatography (MRCP)
MRI. *See* Magnetic resonance imaging (MRI)
MRSA. *See* Methicillin-resistant *S. aureus* (MRSA)
MSSA. *See* Methicillin-sensitive *S. aureus* (MSSA)
Multidisciplinary biopsychosocial therapy, 352
Muscle relaxants, 301, 351
Musculoskeletal/somatic pain, 298
Myocardial infarction (MI), 3, 33, 42, 146
type I, 40
type II, 40
Myoglobin, 42, 42t
Myxedema coma, 327

N
Nabilone, 128
NAEPP. *See* National Asthma Education and Prevention Program (NAEPP)
Nafcillin, 202
Naltrexone, 372
Nasogastric lavage (NGL), 133
National Asthma Education and Prevention Program (NAEPP), 105
National Surgical Quality Improvement Program (NSQIP), 7
Native valve endocarditis, 214
Nausea
diagnosis
clinical presentation, 123–125
diagnostic procedures, 126
diagnostic testing, 126–127
differential diagnosis, 125, 125t
history, 124
imaging, 126
laboratories, 126
physical examination, 124–125
general principles, 123
medications, 127–129
pathophysiology, 123
treatment, 127
Nebulized bronchodilators, 359
Neisseria meningitidis, 233
Neurocardiogenic/vasovagal syncope
diagnostic procedures, 61
diagnostic testing, 59–60
etiology, 56
history, 57
treatment, 62
Neurokinin-1 receptor antagonists, 128
Neuroleptic agents, 246
Neurologic findings, 226
Neurologic imaging, 60, 126
Neurologic system, 164
Neuropathic pain, 298
Neutral protamine Hagedorn (NPH) insulin, 314
Neutropenic fever
causes, 306
clinical presentation
history, 306
physical exam, 306
diagnostic testing
laboratories, 307
physical exam, 306
general principles, 306
imaging evaluation, 307
medications, 307–309
special considerations, 309
treatment, 307–309
New York Heart Association (NYHA), 10
NGL. *See* Nasogastric lavage (NGL)
Nitrates
acute heart failure and CPE, 74
chronic heart failure and cardiomyopathy, 68
Nitroglycerin (NTG), 44, 71, 74

Nitroprusside, 74
NIV. *See* Noninvasive ventilation (NIV)
Nonalcoholic steatohepatitis, 148
Nondihydropyridines, 78
Nonhepatic causes, 146
Noninvasive positive pressure ventilation (NPPV) devices, 12
Noninvasive ventilation (NIV), 104
Nonischemic heart failure, 64
Nonmassive pulmonary emboli, 283
Nonopioid analgesics, 300
Nonpharmacologic methods, 80
Nonpitting edema, 26
Nonpurulent cellulitis, 198
Nonselective β-blocker, 136
Nonsteroidal anti-inflammatory drugs (NSAIDs), 300
Non-ST-segment elevation myocardial infarction (NSTEMI), 40
  diagnosis
    diagnostic procedures, 43
    diagnostic testing, 42–43
    differential diagnosis, 42
    ECG, 43
    history, 40–41, 41t
    laboratories, 42
    physical exam, 41–42
  pathophysiology, 40
  treatment
    anticoagulation therapy, 47–48
    anti-ischemic therapy, 43–45
    antiplatelet therapy, 46–47
    early invasive approach, 49
    ischemia-guided approach, 49
    TIMI or GRACE risk scores, 49, 50t, 51
Norepinephrine, 70
Normocytic anemias, 265
Normoglycemia in Intensive Care Evaluation—Survival Using Glucose Algorithm Regulation (NICE-SUGAR) trial, 313
Nosocomial endocarditis, 225
Nosocomial GNB, 214
Novel oral anticoagulants (NOACs), 287
  anticoagulation and surgery, 89, 91
  atrial fibrillation, 83
NPH insulin. *See* Neutral protamine Hagedorn (NPH) insulin
NPPV devices. *See* Noninvasive positive pressure ventilation (NPPV) devices
NSAIDs. *See* Nonsteroidal anti-inflammatory drugs (NSAIDs)
NSQIP. *See* National Surgical Quality Improvement Program (NSQIP)
NSTEMI. *See* Non-ST-segment elevation myocardial infarction (NSTEMI)

NTG. *See* Nitroglycerin (NTG)
NYHA. *See* New York Heart Association (NYHA)
Nystagmus, 250

O
OAC. *See* Oral anticoagulation (OAC)
Obesity, 10
Obstructive sleep apnea, 10
Obstructive uropathy, 164
Occupational asthma, 105–106
Octreotide, 136
Oculomotor dysfunction, 368
OIH. *See* Opioid-induced hyperalgesia (OIH)
Ondansetron, 127
Opioid analgesics, 301–304
Opioid intoxication, 378
Opioid withdrawal, 378–379, 379t
Opioid-induced hyperalgesia (OIH), 304
Opioids, 299
Oral anticoagulation (OAC), 86, 89
Oral therapy, type 2 diabetes managed with, 17
Oral urea, 175
ORSA. *See* Oxacillin-resistant *S. aureus* (ORSA)
Orthostasis, 58
Orthostatic hypotension
  abdominal pain, physical examination, 143
  etiology, 57
  treatment, 63
Osler nodes, 225
OSSA. *See* Oxacillin-sensitive *S. aureus* (OSSA)
Osteomyelitis
  clinical presentation, 201
    history, 201
    physical examination, 201
  diagnostic testing
    imaging, 202
    laboratories, 201–202
  etiology, 200–201
  general principles, 200–201
  medications, 202–203
  surgical management, 203
  treatment, 202–203
Oxacillin-resistant *S. aureus* (ORSA), 229–230
Oxacillin-sensitive *S. aureus* (OSSA), 229
Oxazepam, 369
Oxygen, 3, 359

P
$P2Y_{12}$ inhibitors, 46

Pacemaker therapy, 62, 63
Pain
  assessment, 297–298
  general principles, 297
  interventional therapies, 304–305
  medications, 300–304
  nonopioid medications, 300–301
  nonpharmacologic therapies, 304
  opioid analgesics, 301–304
  organ involvement and perceived locat ion of, 140t
  special considerations, 305
  treatment, 298–305
Palonosetron, 127
Palpation, 143
Paracentesis, 15
Paraproteinemia, 174
Parietal (somatic) pain, 139–140, 142t
PBC. *See* Primary biliary cirrhosis (PBC)
PCI. *See* Percutaneous coronary intervention (PCI)
PCMs. *See* Physical counterpressure maneuvers (PCMs)
Penicillin G, 203
Percussion, 143
Percutaneous coronary intervention (PCI), 51–52
Pericardial effusion, 37–38
Pericarditis, 34, 37–38
Perilymphatic fistula, 250
Perinephric abscesses, 194
Perioperative cardiac complications, 19
Perioperative care, 3
  acute renal failure, 20
  cardiac evaluation
    12-Lead ECG, 4
    diagnosis, 3–8
    diagnostic testing, 5
    epidemiology, 3
    exercise stress testing with imaging, 5
    exercise testing, 5
    follow-up, 9
    history, 3–4
    imaging, 5
    pathophysiology, 3
    pharmacologic stress testing, 5
    physical examination, 4
    revascularization, 8
    risk stratification, 5–8
    treatment, 8–9
  chronic kidney disease, 20
    general principles, 19
    treatment, 19–20
  corticosteroids, management of
    general principles, 18
    history, 18
    laboratories, 18–19
    pathophysiology, 18
    physical examination, 18
    treatment, 19
  diabetes, management of
    classification, 16
    diagnosis, 16
    general principles, 15–16
    laboratory studies, 16
    treatment, 16–17
  end-stage renal disease
    general principles, 19
    treatment, 19–20
  hypertension
    general principles, 10
    treatment, 10
  liver disease, surgery in patient with
    classification, 14
    diagnosis, 14
    general principles, 14
    laboratories, 14
    treatment, 15
  pulmonary evaluation
    diagnosis, 11
    diagnostic procedures, 12
    diagnostic testing, 11–12
    epidemiology, 10
    estimating risk, 12
    etiology, 10
    history, 11
    imaging, 11–12
    laboratories, 11
    modifiable patient-related risk factors, 12
    modifiable procedure-related risk factors, 12
    patient risk factors, 10–11
    physical examination, 11
    postoperative interventions, 12–13
    procedure-related risk factors, 11
    treatment, 12–13
  transfusion issues in surgery
    diagnosis, 13
    general principles, 13
    treatment, 13–14
Peripheral smear, 268
Peripheral vertigo
  causes of, 249t
  history and exam features, 249t
Peritoneal inflammation, 143
Persistent bloodstream infection, 218
Petechiae, 225
PFTs. *See* Pulmonary function tests (PFTs)
Pharmacologic agents, 79–80, 80t
Pharmacologic stress testing, 5
Pharmacologic therapy, 62
Pheochromocytoma, 334

Phlebitis, 220
Phosphodiesterase 4 inhibitor, 103
Phosphodiesterase inhibitors, 71
Physical counterpressure maneuvers (PCMs), 62
Physical therapy, 352
Pit recovery time (PRT), 26
Pitting edema, 26
Pituitary function tests, 331
Plain films, 202
Plain radiographs, 350
Plasmapheresis, 276
Platelet dysfunction, 20
Platelet transfusions, 276
Pneumococcal vaccines, 103
Pneumococcus, 329
Pneumonia
  clinical presentation, 188
  diagnosis
    diagnostic studies, 189
    differential diagnosis, 188–189
    history, 188
    pathophysiology, 187–188
    physical examination, 188
  epidemiology, 187
  general principles, 187–188
  treatment, 189–191
Pneumothorax, 33, 34
Pocket infection, 220
Portosystemic encephalopathy, 148
Postoperative fever, 208
Postrenal azotemia, 155
Posttransfusion purpura (PTP), 273, 276
Potassium, 369
  24-hour urine collection for, 168
  replacement, 168
Potassium chloride, 168
Potassium deficit, 168
PPD. *See* Purified protein derivative (PPD)
PPI. *See* Proton pump inhibitor (PPI)
Prasugrel, 46
Pregnancy, 150, 194–195
Preoperative erythropoietin, 14
Prerenal azotemia, 155
Presyncope, 56
Primary adrenal insufficiency, 18
Primary biliary cirrhosis (PBC), 148
Primary bloodstream infection, 213
Primary hyperaldosteronism, 167, 334
Primary sclerosing cholangitis, 148
Prochlorperazine, 127
Prokinetic drugs, 128
Promethazine, 127
Prophylactic antibiotics, 136
Propranolol, 324
Propylthiouracil (PTU), 323

Prosthetic heart valves, 89
Prothrombin complex concentrate, 278
Prothrombin time/partial thromboplastin time (PT/PTT), 279
  diagnosis
    clinical presentation, 279
    diagnostic testing, 279–280
    differential diagnosis of, 280t
    history, 279
    laboratories, 279–280
    physical examination, 279
  etiology, 279
  general principles, 279
  treatment, 280–282
Proton pump inhibitor (PPI), 135, 136
PRT. *See* Pit recovery time (PRT)
Prucalopride, 128
Pruritus, 304
Pseudoallergic reactions, 360
Pseudobacteremia, 213
Pseudohyponatremia, 173–174
Pseudomonas species, 329
Pseudosyncope, 57
Psychiatric causes, of syncope, 57, 59
Psychiatric evaluation, 61
PTP. *See* Posttransfusion purpura (PTP)
Pulmonary angiography, 61, 286
Pulmonary embolism (PE), 33, 38, 57, 58, 283
  clinical presentation, 284
  imaging modalities, 286
  pathophysiology, 283
  treatment, 287, 289
  wells criteria for, 284, 285t
Pulmonary function tests (PFTs), 12, 108
Pulmonary hypertension, 10
Pulmonary rehabilitation, 103
Pulmonary vein isolation, 80
Purified protein derivative (PPD), 209
Pyelonephritis, 192–194

R
Radiation therapies, 304
Radiculopathy, 298
  lumbar disc prolapse with, 353
  nonspecific low back pain with degenerative disease without, 353
Radioactive iodine, 323
Radioactive iodine (RAI), 322
Radioallergosorbent test (RAST), 363
Radiofrequency ablation, 80
Radionuclide imaging, 137, 210
Radionuclide therapies, 304
RADS. *See* Reactive airways dysfunction syndrome (RADS)
RAI. *See* Radioactive iodine (RAI)

Ramosetron, 127
Ramsay Hunt syndrome, 250, 251
RAST. *See* Radioallergosorbent test (RAST)
RCRI. *See* Revised Cardiac Risk Index (RCRI)
Reactive airways dysfunction syndrome (RADS), 106
Rebound tenderness, 143
Recombinant factor VIIa, 278
Recurrent urinary tract infection, 195
Red blood cell indices, 268
Red blood cell transfusions, 20
Red flag, 346
Referred pain, 142
Renal abscesses, 194
Renal function, 15, 16
Renal osteodystrophy, 157
Renal perfusion, 159
Respiratory depression, 303
Reticulocyte count, 268
Revised Cardiac Risk Index (RCRI), 7
Rheumatoid factor (RF), 344
Rifampin, 202
Right heart catheterization, 74
Rituximab, 276
Rivaroxaban, 84
Romifulast, 103
Roth spots, 225
Ruptured abdominal aortic aneurysm, 143

S
Sacubitril/valsartan, 69
Salicylate concentrations, 375
SBT. *See* Short Blessed Test (SBT)
Sciatica, 349, 350t
Scopolamine, 128
SCS. *See* Subclinical Cushing syndrome (SCS)
Secondary adrenal insufficiency, 18
Secondary bloodstream infection, 213
Secondary hyperaldosteronism, 167
Sedation, 304
Sedative-hypnotic toxidrome, 377–378
Sedatives, 15
Seizure, 57
Selective serotonin reuptake inhibitors (SSRIs), 300
Serotonin antagonists, 127
Serotonin-release assay, 275
Serum albumin, 11
Serum sickness syndrome, 362
Severe exacerbation, 111
Short Blessed Test (SBT), 244, 244t
Short-acting sulfonylureas, 17
SIADH. *See* Syndrome of inappropriate antidiuretic hormone (SIADH)

Sickle cell anemia, 14, 164
Sinus rhythm, restoration and maintenance of, 79–80
Situational syncope, 56
SJS. *See* Stevens-Johnson syndrome (SJS)
Skin rash, 148
Sliding scale insulin (SSI), 314
Small bowel enteroclysis, 137
Smoking cessation, 10
 acute exacerbations of COPD, treatment of, 104
 risk factors, COPD, 100
 stable COPD, treatment of, 103
Sodium bicarbonate, 165
Sodium nitroprusside, 71
Sodium polystyrene sulfonate (SPS) resins, 20
Solitary pulmonary nodule (SPN)
 diagnosis
  clinical presentation, 115–116
  diagnostic testing, 116–118
  differential diagnosis, 116t
  history, 115
  imaging, 116–118
  physical examination, 116
 etiology, 115
 general principles, 115
 recommendations, follow-up CT imaging, 119t
 surgical management, 119
 treatment, 118–119
Somatostatin, 136
Spinal manipulation, 352
Spinal stenosis, 353
Splenomegaly, 216
Splinter hemorrhages, 225
SPN. *See* Solitary pulmonary nodule (SPN)
SPS resins. *See* Sodium polystyrene sulfonate (SPS) resins
SSI. *See* Sliding scale insulin (SSI)
SSRIs. *See* Selective serotonin reuptake inhibitors (SSRIs)
Staphylococci, 203
Staphylococcus aureus, 196, 216
Statins, 9, 45
STEMI. *See* ST-segment elevation myocardial infarction (STEMI)
Stenting, 256
Steroids, 12
Stevens-Johnson syndrome (SJS), 362
Streptococci, 203
Streptococcus pneumoniae, 233
Streptococcus species, 196
Stress hyperglycemia, 16
Stress testing, 60, 61
Stroke, 57

ST-segment elevation myocardial infarction (STEMI), 37, 40
  diagnosis
    diagnostic procedures, 43
    diagnostic testing, 42–43
    differential diagnosis, 42
    ECG, 43
    history, 40–41, 41t
    laboratories, 42
    physical exam, 41–42
  pathophysiology, 40
  treatment
    medications, 51
    reperfusion, 51–52
Subacute back pain, 349
Subacute infective endocarditis, 214
Subclinical Cushing syndrome (SCS), 334
Subclinical hyperthyroidism, 324
Subclinical hypothyroidism, 324, 327
Subcutaneous fondaparinux, 289
Submassive pulmonary emboli, 283
Substance P, 128
Subtotal thyroidectomy, 323
Sundowning, 242
Superior semicircular canal dehiscence, 250
Supine position, 359
Supplemental oxygen therapy
  acute exacerbations of COPD, treatment, 103
  stable COPD, treatment of, 102
Surgical consultation, 218
Surgical embolectomy, 289–290
Suspected myocardial ischemia, 36
Sympathomimetic toxidrome, 377
Symptomatic aortic stenosis, 4
Syncope, 56
  diagnosis
    diagnostic procedures, 61–62
    history, 57–58
    imaging, 60–61
    physical exam, 58–60
  etiology, 56–57, 57t
  general principles, 56
  treatment, 62–63
Syndrome of inappropriate antidiuretic hormone (SIADH), 171–174
Systemic corticosteroids, 103, 111, 190, 351
Systolic dysfunction, 64

T
Tagged white blood cell scans, 202
TCAs. *See* Tricyclic antidepressants (TCAs)
Technetium-99, 202
TEE. *See* Transesophageal echocardiography (TEE)
TEN. *See* Toxic epidermal necrolysis (TEN)
Tertiary adrenal insufficiency, 18

Tertiary insufficiency, 329
Test of Skew deviation, 250
Tetrahydrocannabinol (THC), 128
Thalassemia, 269
THC. *See* Tetrahydrocannabinol (THC)
Therapeutic index, 69
Thiazide, 69
Thrombocytopenia, 15
  diagnosis
    clinical presentation, 272–275
    diagnostic procedures, 275
    diagnostic testing, 275
    history, 272–273
    laboratories, 275
    medications commonly associated with, 274t
    physical examination, 275
  etiologies of, 273t, 277
  general principles, 272
  management, 277t
  treatment, 276
Thrombolysis, 52, 52t, 289
Thrombopoetin recepter agonists, 276
Thrombosis, 87
Thrombotic thrombocytopenic purpura (TTP), 274, 276
Thyroid disease
  euthyroid sick syndrome
    diagnosis, 327
    general principles, 327
    treatment, 327
  hyperthyroidism, 319–324
    clinical presentation, 319–321
    diagnostic testing, 321–322
    etiology, 319, 320
    general principles, 319
    special considerations, 323–324
    treatment, 322–323
  hypothyroidism, 324
    causes of, 325
    diagnosis, 324–326
    etiology, 324
    general principles, 324
    special considerations, 326–327
    treatment, 326
Thyroid storm, 319, 324
Thyroid-stimulating hormones (TSH), 321
TIA. *See* Transient ischemic attack (TIA)
TIBC. *See* Total iron-binding capacity (TIBC)
Ticagrelor, 46
Tilt-table testing, 60, 61
Tinnitus, 248, 249
TIPS. *See* Transjugular intrahepatic portosystemic shunt (TIPS)
Tissue plasminogen activator, 289
Tolerance, 304

Torsemide, 69
Total iron-binding capacity (TIBC), 150
Toxic epidermal necrolysis (TEN), 362
Toxicology
  acetaminophen overdose, 375–376, 376t
  aspirin overdose, 374–375
  general principles, 374
  toxidromes
    anticholinergic (antimuscarinic) toxidrome, 377
    cholinergic toxidrome, 377
    sedative-hypnotic toxidrome, 377–378
    sympathomimetic toxidrome, 377
  undifferentiated poisoned patient, 374
Toxidromes
  anticholinergic (antimuscarinic) toxidrome, 377
  cholinergic toxidrome, 377
  sedative-hypnotic toxidrome, 377–378
  sympathomimetic toxidrome, 377
Transdermal fentanyl patches, 301
Transesophageal echocardiography (TEE), 38, 78, 215, 228
Transfusion
  diagnosis, 13
  general principles, 13
  treatment, 13–14
Transient bacteremia, 213
Transient ischemic attack (TIA), 57, 58, 250
Transjugular intrahepatic portosystemic shunt (TIPS), 15, 136
Transthoracic echocardiogram (TTE), 77, 228
Transthoracic needle aspiration (TTNA), 118
Tricyclic antidepressants (TCAs), 300
Trimethoprim–sulfamethoxazole (TMP–SMX), 203
Triple-phase bone scans, 202
Tropisetron, 127
Troponin I, 42
Troponin measurements, 9
Tryptase, 358, 363
TSH. *See* Thyroid-stimulating hormones (TSH)
TTE. *See* Transthoracic echocardiogram (TTE)
TTNA. *See* Transthoracic needle aspiration (TTNA)
TTP. *See* Thrombotic thrombocytopenic purpura (TTP)
Tubules, 156
Tullio phenomenon, 250
Tumarkin attacks, 249
Tunnel infection, 220
Type 1 diabetes, 16–17
Type 2 diabetes, 16, 17

U
UA. *See* Unstable angina (UA)
UFH. *See* Unfractionated heparin (UFH)
ULN. *See* Upper limit of normal (ULN)
Ultrafiltration, 29, 74
Uncomplicated cystitis, 192, 193
Unfractionated heparin (UFH), 47, 89, 289
Unstable angina (UA), 40
  diagnosis
    diagnostic procedures, 43
    diagnostic testing, 42–43
    differential diagnosis, 42
    ECG, 43
    history, 40–41, 41t
    laboratories, 42
    physical exam, 41–42
  pathophysiology, 40
  treatment
    anticoagulation therapy, 47–48
    anti-ischemic therapy, 43–45
    antiplatelet therapy, 46–47
    early invasive approach, 49
    ischemia-guided approach, 49
    TIMI or GRACE risk scores, 49, 50t, 51
Unsteady gait, 248
Upper limit of normal (ULN), 148
Urinalysis, 158, 226, 245, 307
Urinary tract infections (UTIs)
  diagnosis
    diagnostic testing, 193
    history, 192
    imaging, 193
    laboratories, 193
    physical examination, 193
  general principles, 192
  recurrent, 195
  risk factors, 192
  special considerations, 194–195
  treatment, 193–194
Urine culture, 307
UTIs. *See* Urinary tract infections (UTIs)

V
V_2-receptor antagonists, 175
VADs. *See* Ventricular assist devices (VADs)
Valsartan, 69
Vancomycin, 202, 308
Vancomycin-resistant enterococcus, 217
VAP. *See* Ventilator-associated pneumonia (VAP)
Variceal hemorrhage, 135
Vasculature, 156
Vasodilator therapy, 68–69
Vasopressors, 359

Vasovagal syncope
  diagnostic procedures, 61
  diagnostic testing, 59–60
  etiology, 56
  history, 57
  treatment, 62
Venoocclusive disease, 148
Venous thromboembolism (VTE)
  anticoagulation and surgery, 87–88, 88t
  clinical presentation, 284
  diagnosis
    diagnostic criteria, 284
    diagnostic testing, 284, 286
    electrocardiography, 286
    imaging, 286
    laboratories, 284
    physical examination, 284
  general principles, 283–284
  guidelines for, 291t
  history, 284
  interventional management, 289–290
  medications, 287–289
  pathophysiology, 283
  risk factors, 284
  special considerations, 290
  treatment, 287–290
Ventilation–perfusion (V/Q) scaning, 61, 286
Ventilator-associated pneumonia (VAP), 187
Ventricular assist devices (VADs), 71
Ventricular function, 66
Vertebrobasilar insufficiency, 250
Vertigo
  diagnosis
    clinical presentation, 248–251
    diagnostic testing, 251
    history, 248–250
    physical exam, 250–251
  epidemiology, 248
  exam features, 249t
  general principles, 248
  treatment, 251
Vestibular neuritis, 249, 251
Viral hepatitis, 148
Visceral pain, 140, 141, 142t, 298
Vitamin B_{12} deficiency, 270, 275
Vitamin K, 281
Volume status, 15, 157, 171, 176
Vomiting
  diagnosis
    clinical presentation, 123–125
    diagnostic procedures, 126
    diagnostic testing, 126–127
    differential diagnosis, 125, 125t
    history, 124
    imaging, 126
    laboratories, 126
    physical examination, 124–125
  general principles, 123
  medications, 127–129
  pathophysiology, 123
  treatment, 127
VTE. *See* Venous thromboembolism (VTE)

W

Waddell signs, 350
Warfarin, 81, 83, 287
Wernicke encephalopathy, 368
Wilson disease, 147, 148
Wong-Baker FACES Pain Rating Scale, 298
Work-aggravated asthma, 106